The New Politics of Old Age Policy

The New Politics of Old Age Policy

SECOND EDITION

Edited by Robert B. Hudson

The Johns Hopkins University Press

Baltimore

© 2005, 2010 The Johns Hopkins University Press
All rights reserved. Published 2010
Printed in the United States of America on acid-free paper
9 8 7 6 5 4 3 2 1

The Johns Hopkins University Press
2715 North Charles Street
Baltimore, Maryland 21218-4363
www.press.jhu.edu

Library of Congress Cataloging-in-Publication Data

The new politics of old age policy / edited by Robert B. Hudson. — 2nd ed.
    p. ;   cm.
Includes bibliographical references and index.
ISBN-13: 978-0-8018-9491-6 (hardcover : alk. paper)
ISBN-10: 0-8018-9491-3 (hardcover : alk. paper)
ISBN-13: 978-0-8018-9492-3 (pbk. : alk. paper)
ISBN-10: 0-8018-9492-1 (pbk. : alk. paper)
  1. Older people—Government policy—United States. 2. Older people—Services for—
United States. 3. Old age pensions—United States. 4. Medicaid. 5. Social security—United
States. 6. Old age—United States. I. Hudson, Robert B., 1944–
  [DNLM: 1. Public Policy—United States. 2. Aged—United States. 3. Medicaid.
4. Pensions—United States. 5. Social Security—United States. HQ 1064.U5 N532 2010]
  HV1461.N76 2010
  362.6'5610973—dc22   2009035554

A catalog record for this book is available from the British Library.

*Special discounts are available for bulk purchases of this book. For more information,
please contact Special Sales at 410-516-6936 or specialsales@press.jhu.edu.*

The Johns Hopkins University Press uses environmentally friendly book materials,
including recycled text paper that is composed of at least 30 percent post-consumer waste,
whenever possible. All of our book papers are acid-free, and our jackets and covers are
printed on paper with recycled content.

Contents

III. Public Policies on Aging

Contributors

Christina M. Andrews, M.S.W., Doctoral Student, School of Social Service Administration, University of Chicago, Chicago, Illinois

Jeffrey A. Burr, Ph.D., Professor of Gerontology, Associate Dean, McCormick Graduate School of Policy Studies, University of Massachusetts–Boston, Boston, Massachusetts

Andrea Louise Campbell, Ph.D., Associate Professor, Department of Political Science, Massachusetts Institute of Technology, Cambridge, Massachusetts

Caroline Cicero, M.P.L., Doctoral Candidate, Davis School of Gerontology, University of Southern California, Los Angeles, California

Kerstin Gerst, Ph.D., Postdoctoral Fellow, Sealy Center on Aging, University of Texas Medical Branch, Galveston, Texas

Judith G. Gonyea, Ph.D., Professor and Chair, Department of Social Research, Boston University School of Social Work, Boston, Massachusetts

Colleen M. Grogan, Ph.D., Associate Professor, School of Social Service Administration, University of Chicago, Chicago, Illinois

Madonna Harrington Meyer, Ph.D., Laura J. and Douglas Meredith Professor, Sociology, Senior Research Associate, Center for Policy Research, Syracuse University, Syracuse, New York

Christopher Howard, Ph.D., Pamela C. Harriman Professor of Government and Public Policy, The College of William and Mary, Williamsburg, Virginia

Robert B. Hudson, Ph.D., Professor and Chair, Department of Social Welfare Policy, Boston University School of Social Work, Boston, Massachusetts

Ryan King, S.B., Energy Resource Engineer, Renewable Energy Systems Americas, Denver, Colorado

Sandra R. Levitsky, Ph.D., Assistant Professor, Department of Sociology, University of Michigan, Ann Arbor, Michigan

Frederick R. Lynch, Ph.D., Associate Professor of Government, Claremont McKenna College, Upland, California

Laurie A. McCann, J.D., Senior Attorney–Litigation, AARP Foundation Litigation, Washington, D.C.

Kimberly J. Morgan, Ph.D., Associate Professor of Political Science and International Affairs, The George Washington University, Washington, D.C.

Jan E. Mutchler, Ph.D., Department Chairman, Gerontology Institute, University of Massachusetts–Boston, Boston, Massachusetts

John Myles, Ph.D., Canada Research Chair and Professor in the Department of Sociology and in the School of Public Policy and Governance, University of Toronto, Toronto, Ontario

Christy M. Nishita, Ph.D., Assistant Professor, Center on Disability Studies, University of Hawaii, Honolulu, Hawaii

Jon Pynoos, Ph.D., UPS Foundation Professor, Gerontology, Policy, and Planning, Davis School of Gerontology, University of Southern California, Los Angeles, California

Richard A. Settersten, Jr., Ph.D., Professor of Human Development and Family Sciences, Oregon State University, Corvallis, Oregon

Molly E. Trauten, M.G.S., Doctoral Student, Oregon State University, Corvallis, Oregon

Cathy Ventrell-Monsees, J.D., Attorney, Chevy Chase, Maryland

Janet M. Wilmoth, Ph.D., Professor of Sociology and Director, Gerontology Center, Syracuse University, Syracuse, New York

Preface

The politics and policy of aging continue to hold a central place on the American social policy agenda. Pressures associated with the inexorable growth in public sector spending on behalf of older Americans will soon be further exacerbated by the entrance of the baby boom generation into the formal ranks of the old. Yet longstanding problems facing many older persons, notably women and persons of color, remain unabated and underaddressed. As a result, in no arena of domestic policy is there a greater sense of an expanding scope of conflict than that surrounding the needs, interests, and demands of older Americans.

This edition of *The New Politics of Old Age Policy* seeks to bring clarity to this welter of cross-cutting issues and concerns. The first of the volume's three sections presents theoretical perspectives to help guide readers in understanding the challenges faced by aging policy today. The second section addresses the standing of persons understood as both *aged* and *aging*, the former calling attention to different groups within the older population and the latter underscoring the importance of employing a longitudinal view of aging across the life course as a means of accounting for those differences. The book's third section then turns to specific aging-related policies, providing readers with thorough accounts of trends, provisions, politics, and prospects in each of these policy areas.

In Part I, my introductory chapter presents a historical overview of developments in aging policy and a brief analysis of the current political situation associated with those policies. I pay particular attention to the enactment of the Medicare Part D prescription drug program and to the rejection of George W. Bush's plan to partially privatize Social Security. And, while one might well suspect a more progressive stance around aging (and other) policy topics from the Obama administration, I also note that the president has made clear an intention to "bring entitlement spending under control."

Madonna Harrington Meyer uses the lens of risk and inequality in laying out an overview of the major aging-based programs currently in place. She emphasizes how shifting risks from government and employers toward individuals and families in recent years have placed major and inequitable burdens on many vulnerable older Americans. In the following chapter, Janet Wilmoth employs the construct of structural lag to account for what she sees as the frequent poorness-of-fit between what many older people require and the policies in place to address their needs. Put differently, her analysis finds many of our policies to be dated and in need of major reworking to reflect the current realities of many aging populations. John Myles sets forth a thorough and nuanced assessment of how different generations may fare under current policies, and he offers a set of logical responses that might better promote both inter- and intragenerational equity.

Frederick Lynch presents a rigorous examination of arguments around senior power and, in particular, addresses the question of how singular, cohesive, and concentrated the presence of older people in American politics is. Because of the economic and fiscal pressures growing on aging-based programs, few political questions are more important than How powerful are the elderly? My chapter concluding this section reviews the major theoretical approaches scholars have developed in accounting for aging-related welfare state developments in the United States. There can be no question about the enormity of such programs, but multiple explanations are available for why that is the case.

Part II addresses the issues and concerns facing different populations of older Americans. Richard Settersten and Molly Trauten use a life-course perspective in assessing the contributions and needs of adults making the transition between middle age and old age. Drawing on a variety of policy materials, they contend that, while many policies affect the life course, they are not life-course policies, that is, ones that appreciate transitions individuals make throughout life, such as the critical one from work toward retirement. Jeffrey Burr, Jan Mutchler, and Kerstin Gerst center their attention on older populations of color, noting in particular how society's largely homogenized understanding of "the elderly" masks the often-extraordinary vulnerabilities facing these older populations. The authors pay particular attention, as well, to the policy challenges faced by older immigrant groups.

The final two chapters in this section focus on the oldest old and those who serve as caregivers for them. In her assessment of what is often the plight of these long-lived individuals, Judith Gonyea reviews a wealth of troubling data on their income, health, and social status, finding vulnerability along each of these often-reinforcing dimensions. She also makes clear that long-term care policy in the United States leaves a great deal to be desired. In a fascinating chapter exploring the absence of any meaningful political presence among the caregivers of those frail elders, Sandra Levitsky addresses that long-term care policy question. Using field data gathered in California, Levitsky employs social movement and other literatures to help explain the failure of caregivers to lend political voice to the burdens they bear and, in turn, bring long-term care policies into the mainstream.

The book's third and final section addresses the nation's major aging-related policies. Andrea Campbell and Ryan King provide a riveting analysis of recent developments in Social Security policy, paying particular attention to President Bush's failed attempt to partially privatize the program. They conclude that in particular it was the enormous transition costs that doomed the proposal, the irony being that the president's Social Security proposal was hoisted on the petard of his massive tax cuts, ones that helped transform the stunning budget surpluses of the later Clinton years into large and growing deficits. The following chapter by Kimberly Morgan addresses Medicare, placing overall emphasis on the pressures generated by a politically deserving population meeting exigencies to contain costs. She also disentangles the extraordinary politics that led to the passage of the Medicare Part D prescription drug program. That the biggest expansion in Medicare since its enactment took place under a conservative Republican president certainly deserves an explanation, and Morgan provides one that finds a mix of liberals and conservatives coming together momentarily in a legislative episode that proves once and for all that "politics makes strange bedfellows."

Colleen Grogan and Christina Andrews explore the place of elderly people in the context of the means-tested Medicaid program. As noted by Gonyea, Medicaid is the principal public source of support for elders in need of long-term care. Yet its stringent eligibility requirements make it the bane of many older people (and their families) who find themselves excluded from coverage. The authors show how, over time, various constructions of elderly people have led to their being understood differently in efforts to either expand or contract the program. In the subsequent chapter, I review the development and challenges faced by the so-called aging network that has developed largely under the aegis of the Older Americans Act. A confederation of agencies that once served largely to recognize the standing of older Americans has, over the course of 45 years, morphed into a major component of the nation's community-based long-term care delivery system. Jon Pynoos, Caroline Cicero, and Christy Nishita provide the third leg of these three chapters addressing health, social, and housing policy for vulnerable elders. These authors highlight efforts to move the senior housing template beyond nursing homes and assisted living to incorporate aging in place, a new direction that requires innovations in housing design and transportation as well as in social and health care.

The final two chapters in this section address policies that are too often ignored in discussions of aging policy. Christopher Howard, noting that the government can improve individual well-being through both transfers and taxes, turns his attention to the latter. While it is well known that transfers such as Social Security and Medicare benefit older persons, Howard emphasizes how many of the government's tax expenditures benefit them through various exemptions, deferrals, deductions, and allowances. While several interests enjoy these kinds of tax breaks, Howard shows how and why older Americans are very much one such interest. The final chapter by Laurie McCann and Cathy Ventrell-Monsees, addressing legislation on age discrimination, hones in on an arena where the policy outcomes for seniors are deemed to be much less favorable. The authors find the Age Discrimination in Employment Act located in a separate-but-unequal legal world when compared with laws addressing racial and gender discrimination. They go on to review the reasoning found in various court decisions that yields what they see as an unwarranted second-class standing for age discrimination grievances.

The New Politics of Old Age Policy provides theoretical perspectives on aging-related issues, material addressing the structured inequality among older populations in the United States, and accounts of how our principal policies work and why that is the case. While building on the book's earlier edition, the current volume contains ten chapters by new authors, updated or expanded ones by four previous contributors, and three prepared by the editor. In a phrase used frequently in social science publishing, this edition represents both change and continuity.

I. Perspectives on Aging Policy

1. Contemporary Challenges to Aging Policy

Robert B. Hudson, Ph.D.

Provisions benefiting older people have long been a hallmark of social policy in the United States. Given their life circumstances, it is perhaps not surprising that the aged receive a far greater volume of public benefits than do younger populations. Nonetheless, social policy in the United States is distinctive because it allocates a higher proportion of social welfare expenditures to old people than do other industrial nations, it employs age as an eligibility criterion more than is the case elsewhere, and, in using chronological age, the United States puts greater emphasis on the needs of the old than those of the young.

Old Age as a Policy Variable

There are compelling reasons, both historical and current, to recognize advanced age as a major variable in social policy. The most obvious is that age has long stood as a formidable proxy for demonstrable need and, in turn, for the receipt of support from society at large. Indeed, old age has long been understood—in addition to illness, disability, and unemployment—to be one of the "bad things" (Rubinow, 1934) that can happen to people in industrial society.

In the United States, greater attention has been given to old age as a bad thing than to other risks or contingencies associated with modern life. Outliving one's income was long considered the most dire prospect facing older persons. That prospect was far from remote, given that, as recently as 70 years ago, at least one-half of all older people are estimated to have been poor and that some three-quarters of elders' incomes in that period are estimated to have come from their adult children (Upp, 1982). Few would have argued with Franklin Roosevelt's contention, made while governor of New York, that "poverty in old age should not be regarded either as a disgrace or necessarily as a result of a lack of thrift or energy . . . it is a mere by-product of modern industrial life" (Rimlinger, 1971, p. 212). Or, as noted by Carole Haber (1983), beginning from an early time in U.S. history, the aged were consciously omitted from "the redeemable" (i.e., those who should be expected to earn their own support).

Historically, chronological age has served as a central proxy for need, as an important marker of an inability to work, and as an essentially inevitable predictor of illness and disability. Separately and in combination, these traits have given the old a uniquely legitimate claim to policy benefits in the U.S. context. If one cannot work due to age (or employers choose not to employ older people for real or alleged work-related limitations), provision should be made for income transfers in old age. If older people are understandably more ill than younger ones and if the private insurance market will not serve them, provision should be made for publicly sponsored health insurance. And, in those cases where advanced age creates especially desperate situations, means-tested supplements to existing income and health provisions may come into play. A "positive political construction" of the aged (Schneider and Ingram, 1993) has long held sway in the United States, and this construction goes a long way toward explaining the historic generosity public policy has shown toward older Americans.

An important contextual factor contributing to the old's positive political standing has been the nation's more ambivalent attitudes toward other population groups and social problems. In such prominent social policy arenas as public welfare, national health care, unemployment relief, mental health care provision, family support, or child care, the U.S. policy effort has been relatively limited and restrictive. The widely analyzed reasons for this distinctive U.S. profile extend to historical patterns of immigration (Hartz, 1955), a consensual political culture (Huntington, 1966), national devotion to individualism (Rimlinger, 1971), divided governmental institutions (Skocpol, 1985), and "the failure of socialism" (Esping-Andersen, 1990). Whatever the reasons (and justifications), the comparative level of benefits and the basis for benefit receipt in the United States have historically been more generous in the case of age-based policies than in the other social policy arenas.

Until the late 1970s, a comparatively benign economic and political environment, coupled with the aged's widely accepted deservingness, allowed for and fostered the growth of age-based public policy in the

United States. In more recent years, of course, that environment has changed fundamentally as the scope of conflict around aging policy has broadened and sharpened. The singular legitimacy long enjoyed by the aged—albeit largely based on a negative stereotype—has more recently morphed into an imposing institutional standing generated by a monumental policy presence and a new-found political identity (Hudson, 1999; Campbell, 2003). Yet this development itself has generated fiscal, generational, and ideological concerns which, in turn, have created the highly charged political atmosphere in which aging-based policy finds itself today.

The Development of Age-Based Policies

In both absolute and relative terms, the development of policies on aging in the United States has been impressive. The country's first national social policy took the form of Civil War pensions for Northern soldiers. Unprecedented in scale, these pensions were subject to large-scale fraud and abuse throughout the late nineteenth century, to the point where their policy legacy largely died with the passing of the veterans themselves (Skocpol, 1991). In the twentieth century, the dire needs of many of the elderly and widowed were first recognized in modest, state-level mothers' pensions and, in the 1930s, these needs were given federal recognition through Old Age Assistance, the Title I public assistance program for the destitute aged under the original Social Security Act.

The broader economic issue facing the aged centered on the transition from work to retirement and was addressed in the act's Old Age Insurance (OAI) title, the cornerstone for today's Social Security program. Roosevelt and his braintrust were able to overcome opposition to OAI by designing an insurance program that would reward only those who had contributed to Social Security during their working years and who would receive benefits based on those earnings only at the advanced age of 65, an age beyond which work was not to be expected. In 1939, benefits were made available to the survivors of deceased workers (the program expanding to Old Age and Survivors Insurance, or OASI), which was a matter of some controversy at the time because, unlike benefits for the deceased, the survivor benefit was independent of work history. In the 1950s, Disability Insurance— originally covering only individuals over the age of 50—was enacted, providing an important transitional benefit to older disabled individuals whose inability to work often turned older workers into younger retirees.

The high-water mark of aging-based public policy came in the decade from the mid-1960s to the mid-1970s. While much social legislation associated with Lyndon Johnson's Great Society was enacted during that period, policy for older Americans continued to stand out. Most notable was the passage of Medicare, a program that represented—in addition to economic need and an inability to work—the illness element of the elderly's deservingness triad. In Marmor's (1970, 17) well-known words, the elderly were "one of the few population groupings about whom one could not say the members should take care of their financial-medical problems by earning or saving more money."

The Medicaid program, also enacted in 1965, addressed both need and illness among the old by paying for the long-term care health costs of low-income frail elders. Medicaid primarily supported nursing home care in its early years, filling an important gap by recognizing the chronic care needs of many poor elders who were expressly omitted from Medicare coverage. Growing recognition of the needs of the elderly population led to additional enactments during this ten-year period. The Older Americans Act (OAA), a non-means-tested program that served in part as symbolic recognition of the growing policy place of the old in Washington, was also enacted in 1965. The OAA grew dramatically throughout the 1960s and 1970s, and it became the focal point of the *aging network*, an array of public and private sector planning and service agencies that now blanket the nation (Hudson, 1994).

Major civil rights legislation for the old was enacted in 1967 through the Age Discrimination in Employment Act (ADEA). The ADEA initially outlawed workplace bias against workers aged 40–65; in 1978, the upper age was raised to 70, and in 1986, the upper age was eliminated altogether, resulting in the effective elimination of mandatory retirement for the vast majority of older workers. The ADEA is also important for giving legislative acknowledgment to the contemporary reality that not all older individuals wish to cease working and that not all older individuals are beyond employment. In the years since, whether the old can, should, or—in light of the recession beginning in 2008—must work has become a matter of prominent policy debate, raising important questions about age-based employment and retirement policy.

The need for private pension protection for retired workers was recognized through the passage of the Employee Retirement Income Security Act (ERISA) in 1974. Under ERISA, workers in traditional or defined-benefit retirement plans were vested after five years' service, and the federal Pension Benefit Guarantee Corporation was established to insure employer pension plans in the case of bankruptcy or forfeiture. Finally, the National Institute on Aging (NIA) was created within the National Institutes of Health in 1974. Creation of the NIA represented a victory for researchers in geriatrics, who argued that the health needs and the particular health profiles of older people were not adequately recognized in disease-specific institutes directed to heart disease, cancer, and other illnesses.

Emerging Pressures on Age-Based Policy

By the late 1970s, known and anticipated age-based expenditures and program growth began garnering focused attention: Estes (1979) spoke of the "aging enterprise"; Hudson (1978) of "the graying of the federal budget"; and Samuelson (1978) of "shouldering the growing burden." Short-term economic pressures, emergent concerns about the aging of the United States, and a new conservative presence in Washington led to a halt in the enactment of additional age-based programs after a long expansionary period.

Nonetheless, expenditures under existing programs were continuing to grow "automatically" (Weaver, 1988), "unsustainably" (Concord Coalition, 2003), or even "understandably" (Ball, 2000). In the case of Social Security, retirement benefits had been increased by more than 60 percent between 1967 and 1972, and future benefits were now tied to cost-of-living increases. These liberalizations, and growing numbers of beneficiaries, resulted in expenditures from the OASI trust fund expanding from $33 billion in 1971 to $105 billion in 1980, and to $353 billion by 2000. Medicare costs began spiraling shortly after the program's enactment, with doctors' historical cry against the government promoting "socialized medicine" being replaced by their recognition that they were beneficiaries of a massive new health care funding stream. Indeed, critics suggested that Medicare had succeeded in socializing the costs of health care to the elderly while privatizing the benefits to physicians and other health care providers. Due to higher payments to providers, growing numbers of beneficiaries, and new technological developments, Medicare expenditures for the old rose from $8 billion in 1971 to $29 billion in 1980, and to $189 billion by 2000 (Congressional Budget Office, 2002).

Finally, nursing home and other long-term care costs were rising as well, even as concerns about the quality of long-term care for elderly or disabled people escalated (Walker, Bradley, and Wetle, 1998). Medicaid long-term care expenses, which totaled $24 billion in 1984, had risen to $44 billion by 1992, with long-term care accounting for 39 percent of all Medicaid expenditures (Coughlin, Ku, and Holahan, 1994).

Program developments in the 1980s and 1990s centered on concerns about these rising expenditures. Social Security legislation enacted in 1983—based on a commission headed by Alan Greenspan—incorporated both cuts in benefits (notably, a gradual rise in the normal retirement age to 67) and increases in payroll taxes. Also in the early 1980s, expenditure growth in the Medicare program led to the institution of a prospective payment system limiting how much Medicare would reimburse providers for particular medical procedures. Additional measures to curb Medicare spending, directed at physicians and at escalating home health care costs, were later imposed. In the late 1980s, the Medicare Catastrophic Coverage Act was enacted, a seemingly expansionary piece of legislation incorporating new hospital and drug benefits. However, the Reagan administration, invoking concern about the aging of the American population and data about new-found well-being among the old, insisted that these new benefits be paid through income tax surcharges on older people themselves rather than by current workers through the payroll tax system. The outcry by older voters in response to this provision was so heated that Congress was forced to repeal the law two years after its passage (Himelfarb, 1995).

The 1990s saw a major effort by Republicans in Congress to cut Medicare and Medicaid benefits—the stalemate leading to a government shutdown for several days—but legislation passed in 1997 imposed cuts that were less sweeping (Smith, 2002). During the late 1990s, several proposals to partially privatize Social Security were put forth, two of them being contained in the official report of the Social

Security Advisory Council. Proponents of privatization pointed to the need to rein in what they saw as unsustainable growth in program costs that would accompany retirements of baby boomers. Critics of these proposals, however, saw a different agenda at work, namely, to curtail the responsibility of the federal government to honor its obligations to these future old age cohorts. Finally, in what now seems a *fin de siècle* fiscal mirage, the booming economy and stock market of the late 1990s led the Clinton administration and other officials to predict that the entire federal budget debt could be retired by 2015, a development that would have dramatically eased long-term pressures on Social Security.

The dawning of the new century brought new challenges and new policies, with notions of surpluses and solvency coming to an abrupt halt. The bursting of the stock market dot-com bubble in 2000; homeland security concerns in the wake of the September 11, 2001, attacks; and expenses associated with the war in Iraq dramatically affected the receipts and expenditures of the federal government. In addition, President George W. Bush returned a conservative domestic policy agenda to center stage, one that had its origins in the Reagan years and in the efforts of right-wing think tanks such as the Heritage Foundation and the Cato Institute.

Aging policy became caught up in this highly charged political environment during the Bush years. The two major chapters in its development centered on the Medicare Part D prescription drug program, which became law, and the president's attempt to partially privatize the Social Security program, which did not. The effect of this growing politicization in aging-related policy was clearly seen in the debate leading to passage of the Part D program, the most significant expansion of Medicare since its inception. Eager to make inroads into the older voting constituency, Republicans had been promoting drug legislation and made it a major issue in the 2000 and 2002 elections. Because of Republican sponsorship and particular aspects of the plan, Democrats found themselves in the awkward position of opposing this major addition to the program. But there were tensions on both sides of the aisle: conservative Republicans were opposed to such a massive entitlement expansion, regardless of the political benefits, and Democrats found reason to oppose the legislation because of the central role private managed-care firms would play in program implementation (Pear, 2003). To further complicate matters, aging-based interest groups were divided on the issue, with AARP famously supporting the legislation while most other groups opposed it. The legislation passed in 2003 and has greatly expanded drug coverage for elders. However, as both sets of critics warned, it has proven to be expensive and has encouraged the expansion of Medicare Advantage plans to attract a growing proportion of Medicare beneficiaries into the quasi-private market.

The most contentious episode yet seen in aging politics took place in 2004–5 as President George W. Bush made partial privatization of Social Security the initial cornerstone of his second-term agenda. While an actual bill was never introduced, the president's proposal would have diverted a portion of workers' Social Security payroll tax payments into mandatory private retirement accounts akin to 401(k) defined-contribution plans. The president argued that this approach offered greater choice and control for plan participants. Republican operatives also believed that a cohort succession was building around Social Security, with a rising generation of baby boomers seen as more comfortable with equities and other private investment vehicles (Weisberg, 2005). They were viewed as more of a take-charge generation than the "silent generation" that had preceded them, and certainly more than the yet-earlier Depression generation, who had grown up leery of the stock market in light of their disastrous exposure to it.

Arrayed on the other side of the debate were those arguing that the Bush plan was more about undermining the current system than providing meaningful alternatives to an emerging generation of elders. Liberal think tanks such as the Center on Budget and Policy Priorities and columnists such as Paul Krugman and Robert Kuttner emphasized how weakening Social Security's universal and mildly redistributive aspects would threaten both lower-income seniors and erode the cornerstone of U.S. social insurance policy. After months of heated debate, it was clear by the end of 2005 that the president's ideas had failed in the court of public opinion and within much of the policy-elite community in Washington. The proposals were withdrawn without enabling legislation having ever been introduced in Congress.

Aging Policy Today

These shifts in the political and economic climate, coupled with the remarkable success of public policy in improving the overall well-being of the old, have generated policy debates that would have been hard to imagine thirty years ago. Have policy accomplishments (and expenditures) on behalf of the old gone beyond being a notable policy success to a form of policy excess? Do growing disparities in well-being among the aged call for a more-targeted and less-universal approach to age-based benefits? Are longstanding policy assumptions around the reciprocity of relations between the generations now dated and unfair to emerging generations? And, most fundamentally, what should the balance of responsibility be between individuals and their families, the private sector, and government in meeting a volume of needs that can only grow in the future. The tide of the past decade toward privatization appears to have receded, but the need to find resources from each of these three major sectors can only grow.

Federal Expenditures

The upward momentum in federal spending on behalf of older people seen earlier has not abated in more recent years and is certainly not expected to in the years ahead. By 2000, expenditures under the Old Age and Survivors Insurance program had risen to $351 billion, and by 2008 they had reached $507 billion, an increase of 44 percent. Medicare expenditures that had reached $215 billion by 2000 had more than doubled, to $455 billion, by 2006, an increase of 112 percent, illustrating why, as noted below, Medicare has become the chief social insurance budgetary worry in Washington. More remarkable yet, the Office of Management and Budget estimates that by 2014 Medicare expenditures will surpass those for OASI, $736 billion versus $694 billion (U.S. Office of Management and Budget, 2009). For their part, Medicaid long-term care expenditures have continued to rise as well, totaling $46 billion in 1994, $68 billion in 2000, and $99 billion in 2006. Importantly, the proportion of those funds directed toward home and community-based services rather than institutionally based ones nearly doubled, from 20 percent in 1996 to 39 percent in 2006 (Burwell, Sredl, and Eiken, 2007).

Structured Diversity among Old People

Perhaps ironically, a good deal of the current debate about the size, growth, and distribution of public expenditures for the aged results from the significant role that these expenditures have played in improving the well-being of the aged. The role of Social Security has been most notable in this regard. The U.S. Bureau of the Census found that in the absence of social insurance programs, principally Social Security, poverty among the old would be five times the pretransfer rate. By no means can it any longer be said that older people are universally needy or, as was historically nearly the case, singularly needy. Poverty among the old has declined from nearly 40 percent in 1959 to 9 percent in 2006 (U.S. Bureau of the Census, 2008). The broader aging population has also made notable economic progress in recent decades, its average income having risen from $18,133 in 1974 to $28,567 in 2007, an increase of 57 percent (in constant 2007 dollars). In comparison, the incomes of the population at large increased by only 38 percent over the same period (U.S. Bureau of the Census, 2008).

There is also a new twist on the matter of older Americans' ability to work. While it was long common knowledge that older people "couldn't work," in fact they did. As recently as 1950, labor force participation rates among older men were 46 percent, a figure that had fallen to only 16 percent by the early 1990s. The pattern for older women had been largely unchanged during these decades, due to "the combined effects of increased participation by women and decreased participation by the elderly" (Quinn and Burkhauser, 1990, p. 309). Social Security, which had historically been designed not only to support older people not in the workforce but also to encourage them to leave the workforce, has been a major factor this reduced work effort, especially among men. Thus labor force participation has fallen off precipitously at age 62, the age at which workers are eligible for early retirement benefits under Social Security.

Most recently, however, a combination of improved health and well-being among elders and policy enactments have clearly begun to reverse this historical pattern. The percentage of persons aged 60–64 who were in the labor force increased from 43.8 percent in 1985 to 53.3 percent in 2007, and among those aged 65–69, it increased from 18.4 percent to 29.7 percent (U.S. Bureau of Labor Statistics, 2008). Recent years have also seen a gradual increase in older workers engaging in "bridge jobs" (Ruhm, 1995), flexible work schedules (McMenamin, 2007), and phased retirement plans (Morton, Foster, and Sedlar, 2005). For members of these emerging cohorts of older workers, improved health and job opportunities have made work a more rewarding option than was once the case. For growing numbers of workers, the decision to retire (or not) has become more of a choice than was historically the case.

The deep recession of 2008–9, of course, created a stark environment for those older adults wishing to work. In December 2008, the unemployment rate had increased 50 percent from the previous year (Johnson, 2008). The enormous losses many older workers have recently experienced in their retirement plans has made for a yet more precarious situation. The issue here, however, is more one of macroeconomic performance and the need for older people to maintain some form of employment than it is of their interest in working or the ability of many of them to do so.

New work-related opportunities and incentives that have been introduced into public policy in recent years have contributed to the trend toward greater labor force participation. Originating in concerns about a graying population, these moves build as well on assumptions about an improved age-specific health status among the old. The most obvious provision is the rise in the normal retirement age (making a worker eligible for full benefits) from 65 to 67, currently being phased in for workers born after 1938. Elimination of mandatory retirement under the ADEA is also making it possible for more workers, principally white-collar middle-class workers, to choose to remain in the labor force. More important yet has been the elimination of the earnings test under Social Security. Historically, workers aged between 65 and 69 forfeited up to one-third of their Social Security benefits if they continued to work and earn relatively modest amounts. After several years of liberalizing this test, the reduction in benefits was eliminated in 2000, no matter what the level of earnings.

Improvements in well-being among many contemporary elders have led to the development of new constructs capturing the phenomenon, such as "productive aging" (Bass, Caro, and Chen 1993), "the young old" (Neugarten, 1974), and the "third age" (Laslett, 1987). In place of the traditional monolithic view of the old as poor, frail, and unemployable, these categorizations center on the strengths and abilities to be found among many contemporary older people who were not ill and yet were often not working. As we have seen, policy is moving to discourage retirement among a population now argued to be increasingly in good health and around which old age policy can now be notably reconstructed. Additionally, a new composite role being put forth for older Americans is that of civic engagement, encompassing voluntarism, education, and socially minded activities such as environmental protection (Wilson and Simson, 2006).

Yet enormous disparities and imbedded levels of need are lurking just beneath the aggregate improvements in elders' well-being. In addition to differences by race and gender, distinctions at different ages exist within the overall older population. Poverty among older African Americans in 2006 stood at 23 percent, and among older Hispanics at 19 percent, in comparison with 7 percent among older white Americans. At 11.5 percent, the poverty rate among older women is nearly double the 6.6 percent for older men. The average income among people aged 65–69 is $18,249, compared with $13,999 among those aged 80 or older (Congressional Research Service, 2005). The multiple jeopardy associated with these otherwise discrete attributes paints yet a starker picture. Thus median income among young-old (aged 65–74) white men stands at 4.5 percent, compared with the 30.2 percent rate among old-old (aged 75 or older) African American women (Federal Interagency Forum on Aging-Related Statistics, 2008). Were it not for Social Security, these figures would be much more pronounced, because Social Security constitutes 83 percent of the income among the poorest 20 percent of elderly people, but only 18 percent among the most well-off 20 percent (U.S. Bureau of the Census, 2007).

Different sets of vulnerabilities face young-old and old-old populations. For all of the talk in policy circles about the "productive old" and the "able old," millions of workers from their mid-50s to their early 70s struggle, frequently caught in an economic black hole, where they are neither able to work (due to illness and unemployment) nor to retire (due to nonexistent or inadequate pension protection and savings). Involuntary job loss and forced retirement remain especially severe problems for low-income and minority workers (Hayward, Friedman, and Chen, 1996; Flippen, 2005). Concern about these young-old vulnerable workers helped preserve the age-62 early retirement benefit (albeit with a benefit cut) under Social Security when the normal retirement age increases were phased in. However, that age and benefit level will be on the table again if and when moves are made to increase the normal retirement age beyond age 67.

At the other end of the old age spectrum, the plight of the very old has become more rather than less pronounced. The old old are disproportionately women, living alone, often physically or mentally frail, unable to work, and in possession of only meager savings and modest pension benefits. When widowed, women's Social Security benefits decline by one-third. When incapacitated by long-term illness or disability, their needs extend beyond the protections offered by Social Security and Medicare, forcing them to rely on Medicaid's means-tested benefit. And, while evidence is growing that age-specific disability levels are declining modestly, individual and aggregate-level long-term care needs are certain to remain among the most pressing problems of the old.

Overall, we are left with a clear pattern of *structured diversity* among the old. Aggregate improvements in well-being, many of them policy induced, are notable, even historic. Yet, in the face of these overall improvements, clearly identified groups of the old find themselves at social and economic risk. In a time of governmental retrenchment, this diversity poses major questions for public policy and especially for age-based public policy.

Future Costs and Responsibilities

Coloring all discussions of the status of the aged is the question of growing costs of age-based programs and how those costs should be distributed. In the late 1980s and early 1990s, this discussion largely took place in terms of intergenerational transfers. The demographic bulge, represented by the baby boom cohort, brought into question a historic assumption that successive generations of workers would be able and willing to support earlier generations in their old age. Sustaining these programs largely unchecked, critics argued, would be unfair to future workers and would place onerous burdens on the U.S. economy. While acknowledging that the contributions of Social Security and Medicare "deserve our respect," Lamm and Lamm (1996) contended that if these programs continue to go untouched, "with taxes as high as 60 percent of each paycheck, the next generation will have little incentive to work."

The election of George W. Bush and the resurgence of conservative thinking in Washington led many observers to reassess the place of the generational issue in the pressures building on aging policy. Was the concern really one of generations or was it more centrally about a desire to curtail growth in federal social expenditures or, more broadly, to curtail the expectation of Americans that the federal government should be centrally involved in social problem resolution? To these observers, the issue was more one of who should be responsible (Gonyea, 1998; Hacker, 2006) than of are we "consuming our children" to pay for the elderly (Chakravarty and Weisman, 1988). The substitution of defined-contribution for defined-benefit pension plans, the president's effort to partially privatize Social Security, and the growing role of private insurance companies in Medicare Advantage and Part D prescription drug programs appeared to be more about reducing the role of the federal government than worrying about the nation's grandchildren.

As aging programs continue to grow (with that growth to accelerate with baby boomers now entering old age), pressures on the programs will in no way diminish. How they are understood, however, will continue to be of immense importance. Perhaps most germane here is the debate swirling around the future of Medicare. It is now widely held that Medicare represents a greater long-term expenditure burden than does Social Security. This is due largely to the demands of service providers and the place of new technologies that differentiate health care from income maintenance programs and generate very different cost pressures. As a matter of problem definition, the relevant question here is whether Medicare represents an enormous piece of burgeoning entitlement spending for the aged, or whether overall health care spending in the United States, of which Medicare is but one element, is largely out of control.

Other dimensions and definitions may also enter this debate. Thus the issues of aging and of disability among younger populations are increasingly being joined, both conceptually and in program design and administration. And the disproportionate burdens faced by women, due both to their special vulnerabilities in old age and as a result of their disproportionate role as caregivers, are receiving renewed attention. In particular, the pressures on caregivers for the old are being brought increasingly to the fore by both aging-based and women's advocacy organizations, the principal argument being that these often extraordinary efforts must be formally recognized and *monitized*, either in the form of current payments or future Social Security credits.

The latest chapter in this ongoing debate of risk-and-responsibility for the aged is found in the profound U.S. and world-wide recession that began in 2008. The adage that policies change fundamentally only in times of budgetary feast or budgetary famine may well be borne out by the various crises this deep recession has brought with it. Repeated comparisons with problems of the Depression of the 1930s and the responses of Franklin Roosevelt make clear that more than mere hyperbole is at work here. The Obama administration's early efforts to reregulate the financial industry, extend health care to all, and reduce U.S.-generated greenhouse gases, among myriad other undertakings, are remarkable by almost any standard, and certainly by that of the previous eight years.

Yet even while embarking on this host of initiatives, many extending the role of the federal government in momentous ways, President Obama has made clear that he intends to bring new discipline to the expansion of social entitlements. Many of these, of course, focus on older Americans. In a manner reminiscent of "only Nixon could go to China," we may see this Democratic administration bring about spending (if not structural) reforms to Social Security, Medicare, and Medicaid that have eluded earlier administrations, notably those of Ronald Reagan and George W. Bush.

As this debate unfolds, the differential effect of reform proposals on various populations will be of extreme interest. In particular, we may see distinctions and exclusions made among the old in ways that are historically unprecedented. Will taxes and premiums for some elderly be raised and/or will access to benefits for some be limited? Will age become less of a singular eligibility criterion in the name of emphasizing economic or functional needs? There can be no question that the scope of conflict around aging policy has expanded in recent years; the question now arising is, How much more intense will that pressure become?

References

Ball, R. 2000. *Insuring the Essentials: Bob Ball on Social Security*. New York: Century Foundation Press.

Bass, S., F. Caro, and Y.-P. Chen (eds.). 1993. *Achieving a Productive Aging Society*. Westport, Conn.: Auburn House.

Burwell, B., K. Sredl, and S. Eiken. 2007. *Medicaid Long-Term Care Expenditures FY 2006*. HCBS: Clearinghouse for Home and Community Based Services. www.hcbs.org/moreInfo.php/doc/2016/.

Campbell, A. L. 2003. *How Policies Make Citizens: Senior Political Activism and the American Welfare State*. Princeton, N.J.: Princeton University Press.

Chakravarty, S. N., and K. Weisman. 1988. Consuming our children. *Forbes* (Nov. 14): 222–32.

Concord Coalition. 2003. *Seniors Still Come First in the Budget*. Facing Facts Alert 9, No. 2. www.concordcoalition.org/issues/facing-facts/seniors-still-come-first-budget/.

Congressional Budget Office. 2002. www.cbo.gov/showdoc.cfm?index=2300.

Congressional Research Service. 2005. *Topics in Aging: Income and Poverty among Older Americans in 2004*. Washington, D.C.: Congressional Research Service, Library of Congress.

Coughlin, T. A., L. Ku, and J. Holahan. 1994. *Medicaid since 1980: Cost, Coverage, and the Shifting Alliance between the Federal Government and the States*. Washington, D.C.: Urban Institute Press.

Esping-Andersen, G. 1990. *The Three Worlds of Welfare Capitalism*. New York: Cambridge University Press.

Estes, C. L. 1979. *The Aging Enterprise*. San Francisco: Jossey-Bass.

Federal Interagency Forum on Aging-Related Statistics. 2008. *Older Americans, 2008: Key Indicators of Well-Being*. Washington, D.C.: U.S. Government Printing Office.

Flippen, C. 2005. Minority workers and pathways to retirement. Pp. 129–56 in R. B. Hudson (ed.), *The New Politics of Old Age Policy*. Baltimore: Johns Hopkins University Press.

Gonyea, J. G. (ed.). 1998. *Resecuring Social Security and Medicare: Understanding Privatization and Risk*. Washington, D.C.: Gerontological Society of America.

Haber, C. 1983. *Beyond 65: The Dilemmas of Old Age in America's Past*. New York: Cambridge University Press.

Hacker, J. S. 2006. *The Great Risk Shift: The Assault on American Jobs, Families, Health Care, and Retirement—and How You Can Fight Back*. New York: Oxford University Press.

Hartz, L. 1955. *The Liberal Tradition in America*. Cambridge, Mass.: Harvard University Press.

Hayward, M. D., S. Friedman, and H. Chen. 1996. Race inequities in men's retirement. *Journals of Gerontology, Series B: Social Sciences* 51 (1): S1–10.

Himelfarb, R. 1995. *Catastrophic Politics: The Rise and Fall of the Medicare Catastrophic Coverage Act of 1988*. University Park: Pennsylvania State University Press.

Hudson, R. B. 1978. The "graying" of the federal budget and its consequences for old-age policy. *Gerontologist* 18 (5, part 1): 428–40.

———. 1994. The Older Americans Act and the defederalization of community-based care. Pp. 45–75 in P. Kim (ed.), *Services to the Aged: Public Policies and Programs*. New York: Garland.

————. 1999. Conflict in today's aging politics: New population encounters old ideology. *Social Service Review* 73 (3): 358–79.

Huntington, S. 1966. Political modernization: America vs. Europe. *World Politics* 18 (3): 378–414.

Johnson, R. 2008. Older workers and the recession. *San Diego Union-Tribune* (Dec. 8), B7. www.urban.org/publications/901205.html.

Lamm, R., and H. Lamm. 1996. *The Challenge of an Aging Society.* Denver: Denver Center for Public Policy and Contemporary Issues, University of Denver.

Laslett, P. 1987. The emergence of the third age. *Ageing and Society* 7 (2): 133–66.

Marmor, T. R. 1970. *The Politics of Medicare.* Chicago: Aldine.

McMenamin, T. M. 2007. A time to work: Recent trends in shift work and flexible schedules. *Monthly Labor Review* 130 (12): 3–15.

Morton, L., L. Foster, and J. Sedlar. 2005. *Managing the Mature Workforce.* New York: Conference Board.

Neugarten, B. 1974. Age groups in American society and the rise of the young-old. Pp. 187–98 in F. Eisele (ed.), *Political Consequences of Aging.* Annals of the American Academy of Political and Social Science, vol. 415. Philadelphia: American Academy of Political and Social Sciences.

Pear, R. 2003. Medicare plan covering drugs backed by AARP. *New York Times* (Nov. 18), A1.

Quinn, J., and R. Burkhauser. 1990. Work and retirement. Pp. 307–27 in R. H. Binstock and L. K. George (eds.), *Handbook of Aging and the Social Sciences,* 3rd ed. San Diego: Academic Press.

Rimlinger, G. 1971. *Welfare Policy and Industrialization in Europe, America, and Russia.* New York: Wiley.

Rubinow, A. 1934. *The Quest for Security.* New York: Holt.

Ruhm, C. 1995. Secular changes in the work and retirement patterns of older men. *Journal of Human Resources* 30: 362–95.

Samuelson, R. J. 1978. Aging America: Who will shoulder the growing burden? *National Journal* 10: 1712–17.

Schneider, A. L., and H. Ingram. 1993. Social construction of target populations. *American Political Science Review* 87 (2): 253–77.

Skocpol, T. 1985. Bringing the state back in: Strategies of analysis in current research. Pp. 3–43 in P. Evans, D. Rueschemeyer, and T. Skocpol (eds.), *Bringing the State Back In.* New York: Cambridge University Press.

————. 1991. State formation and social policy in the United States. *American Behavioral Scientist* 34 (4/5): 559–84.

Smith, D. G. 2002. *Entitlement Politics: Medicare and Medicaid, 1995–2001.* New York: Aldine de Gruyter.

Upp, M. 1982. A look at the economic status of the aged then and now. *Social Security Bulletin* 45 (March): 16–20.

U.S. Bureau of the Census. 2007. *Current Population Survey, 2007 Annual Social and Economic Supplement.* Washington, D.C.: U.S. Department of Commerce, U.S. Bureau of the Census.

———. 2008. Historical income table P-10: People by median and mean income, 1974–2007. www.census.gov/hhes/www/income/histinc/p10AR .html.

U.S. Bureau of Labor Statistics. 2008. Labor force participation rates for persons aged 60–64, 65–69, and 70–74, 1985–2007. http://data.bls.gov/ PDQ/outside.jsp?survey=ln/.

U.S. Office of Management and Budget. 2009. The 2010 budget: Historical tables; Table 11.3; Outlays for payments for individuals by category and major program, 1940–2014. www.whitehouse.gov/omb/budget/fy2010/ assets/hist11z3.xls.

Walker, L. C., E. H. Bradley, and T. Wetle (eds.). 1998. *Public and Private Responsibilities in Long-Term Care.* Baltimore: Johns Hopkins University Press.

Weaver, R. K. 1988. *Automatic Government: The Politics of Indexation.* Washington, D.C.: Brookings Institution.

Weisberg, J. 2005. Bush's first defeat: The president has lost on Social Security. *Slate* (March 31). www.slate.com/id/2115141/.

Wilson, L., and S. Simson (eds.). 2006. *Civic Engagement and the Baby Boomer Generation.* Binghamton, N.Y.: Haworth Press.

2. Shifting Risk and Responsibility
The State and Inequality in Old Age

Madonna Harrington Meyer, Ph.D.

Who is responsible for taking care of the elderly? For the better part of a century, the U.S. answer has emphasized the model of a three-legged stool. One-third of old age security should come from the welfare state, through universal and poverty-based benefit programs. One-third should come from the corporate sector, through employment-based benefits. The remaining one-third should come from the savings and investments of older individuals themselves. But since the late 1970s and early 1980s, policy makers have restricted supports provided through the welfare state, employers have cut benefits provided through jobs, and many older people and their families have watched their stocks and investments diminish in value. Personal savings are at the lowest rates since the Great Depression, and old age security is once again contested terrain (Zeller, 2007). In this chapter, I explore efforts to shift from collective to individual risk and responsibility in the U.S. old age welfare state. I examine how the ideological debates have shifted as well as how the programs themselves have shifted, increasing both the risk to the individual and the inequality linked to gender, race, class, and marital status. I conclude by contemplating how these trends may be reshaped under President Obama's administration.

Shifting Ideologies about Risk and Responsibility

Historically, most societies placed the burden of any sort of dependency squarely on the family. But between the mid-1800s and mid-1900s, modern welfare states became increasingly involved in taking responsibility for the provision of at least some basic needs, particularly for older people. Welfare states developed health insurance, income security, and various family benefits, partly because officials recognized that filial responsibility had real limits (Harrington Meyer, 1996). The elderly came to be defined as the deserving poor, and policy makers recognized that filial responsibility concentrated risk, privatized cost, and maximized inequality between families.

The United States was reticent in comparison with most other developed Western nations: exceptionally slow to form programs and exceptionally restrictive with the benefits that were offered. Nonetheless, between the 1930s and the 1970s, the United States implemented and expanded poverty-based welfare programs, such as Medicaid and Supplemental Security Income, and two universal programs, Social Security and Medicare. The emergence of these old age policies was based on the notion that welfare state benefits should offset the harsh realities of the market, reduce inequality, and redistribute risk and resources (Yergin and Stanislaw, 1998; Estes and Associates, 2001; Hacker, 2002; Harrington Meyer and Herd, 2007).

A major point of U.S. exceptionalism, however, was the tendency to rely heavily on corporate and market-based, rather than welfare state-based, benefits. Benefits offered by welfare states, especially when universally available, potentially spread risk, share costs, and reduce gender, race, and class inequality (Korpi and Palme, 1998). In contrast, benefits offered through employers or markets tend to help only those who have sufficiently strong links to the labor force to receive those benefits (Harrington Meyer and Pavalko, 1996). To the extent that they have weaker links to the labor force, or are less rewarded for their efforts there, women, minorities, and part-time or low-wage workers are significantly less likely to reap the rewards of employment-based benefits (Korpi and Palme, 1998; Myles and Quadagno, 2000; Harrington Meyer and Herd, 2007).

Though the U.S. welfare state never quite caught up to its peer nations in many programs, attempts to dismantle elements of the welfare state began in the 1980s. As costs for welfare state benefits and employment-based benefits spiraled, cost containment, privatization, and retrenchment became central preoccupations. Neoconservatives and a growing segment of traditionally liberal congressional, administrative, and policy leaders supported a series of proposals aimed at retrenching social welfare, privatizing benefits, and using social policies to bolster markets (Yergin and Stanislaw, 1998; Estes, 2001; Gilbert 2002; Hacker, 2002, 2006; Harrington Meyer and Herd, 2007). The basic premise was that the government should do less because tax-and-spend government is too burdensome on businesses and consumers. Supporters argued that the government should get out of the retirement business and let the market respond to consumer demands for resources such as old age income, health care, and long-term care (Pauly et al., 1991; Hacker, 2006; Harrington Meyer and Herd, 2007). In other words, welfare state benefits should be reduced and privatized in ways that maximize individual choice, risk, and responsibility. Over time, welfare state debates in the United States shifted away from questions about how the nation might best expand social welfare benefits to how it might restrict them in ways that are best for markets (Pauly et al., 1991; Yergin and Stanislaw, 1998; Myles and Quadagno, 2000).

Critics of those market-friendly welfare approaches have cautioned over the last few decades that the emphasis on individual risk and responsibility undermines the philosophy of social risk and collective responsibility (Yergin and Stanislaw, 1998; Gilbert, 2002; Hacker, 2002; Harrington Meyer and Herd, 2007). They warn that a preoccupation with privatization has left many welfare state policies unattended, even though they may have become seriously outdated or remain configured to restrict eligibility and reduce benefits (Herd and Kingson 2005). Failure to develop and implement responsive new welfare policies, coupled with a growing willingness to retrench and privatize existing programs, fuels inequality in old age. While opponents of privatization are optimistic that the tide may have turned with the election of Barack Obama, the extent to which Congress will decide to bolster and update universal old age programs remains unclear.

Economic Security

As ideologies have shifted, welfare state policies have been redefined to varying degrees (Harrington Meyer and Herd, 2007). Those who reach old age with only sparse economic resources generally do so because, across the life course, they have not been well tended by the welfare state nor well rewarded by the market. Thus they have faced cumulative disadvantages with few governmental or corporate supports. Robust universal old age welfare state policies can offset some of the inequalities due to different life-course trajectories (Korpi and Palme, 1998; Harrington Meyer, 2000).

Social Security

When Social Security was enacted in 1935, the elderly were more likely to be poor than other age groups. But by the mid-1980s, primarily because of Social Security, poverty rates for the aged actually dropped below poverty rates for other age groups. Social Security comprises about 40 percent of income for all older people, 60 percent for all older women, and 100 percent for one in five older women (Porter, Larin, and Primus, 1999; U.S. Social Security Administration, 2007). Social Security is particularly important for women, because Social Security alone lifts 60 percent of women beneficiaries out of poverty. Social Security is even more important for older blacks and Hispanics. Because of reduced access to private pensions and private savings, half of older Hispanics and African Americans rely on Social Security for 90 percent or more of their income (Wu, 2004; Torres-Gil, Greenstein, and Kamin, 2005). Social Security comprises almost 80 percent of the income of black and Hispanic women.

The history of Social Security has been primarily one of liberal expansion. Initially, only those who contributed to Social Security were eligible to receive benefits. Over the subsequent half century of the program, benefits were extended to wives and widows, formulas were made gender neutral, strict earnings tests were eliminated for all but early retirees, and the program's progressive benefit structure redistributed resources from high to low lifetime earners (Harrington Meyer, 1996; Century Foundation, 1998; U.S. Social Security Administration, 2007) Supporters of the program have called for additional expansions that would help families juggle work and children and that acknowledge the presence of unmarried couples (see Harrington Meyer and Herd, 2007). But critics have argued that with the aging of the baby boom generation, the country can no longer afford such universal and redistributive polices, and that the time has come to shift greater amounts of risk and responsibility away from the government and markets and onto older people and their families (Pauly et al., 1991; Yergin and Stanislaw, 1998; Myles and Quadagno, 2000; Hacker, 2002).

One policy change that has already shifted risk and responsibility to individuals concerns the age for full retirement. Beginning in 2003, the age of eligibility for full benefits has been gradually increasing from age 65 to age 67, where it will be in 2027. The age for early retirement remains at age 62, but the penalty for taking early benefits, which most men and nearly all women take, has increased from 20 to 30 percent (U.S. Social Security Administration, 2007). Hardest hit are those who are unable to continue working due to poor health or unemployment. Women and blacks and Hispanics are more likely to be affected by both (Harrington Meyer, 1996; Moon with Herd, 2002).

The privatization of Social Security would be a move that would shift even more risk and responsibility onto individuals. President Bush declared privatization as his number one domestic priority in his second inaugural speech. The proposal gained considerable traction, but that effort fell by the wayside in 2006 without formal legislation ever having been introduced. Privatization would have allowed workers to divert at least part of their contributions to individual accounts. Supporters of privatization continue to point out that even though the Social Security program now has a $2 trillion surplus, the surplus will begin to dwindle as more and more of the baby boomers make claims (U.S. Social Security Administration, 2007). It is estimated that these reserves will be gone by 2041 and the Federal Insurance Contributions Act (FICA) payroll tax receipts then being generated by current workers will cover only 80 percent of the paid benefits.

This budget shortfall, predicted to appear in three decades, has been used as a rationale for partially dismantling Social Security, but there are many other ways to address the shortfall (AARP, 2005; Harrington Meyer and Herd, 2007). One option is to raise the FICA tax by 1 to 2 percent. Another is to raise the annual cap on taxable earnings from its current value, $102,000, to $140,000 and then index it to inflation (AARP 2005; U.S. Social Security Administration, 2007). During the 2008 campaign, presidential candidate Obama proposed increasing the payroll tax for those earning over $250,000 a year, but no legislation to that effect has yet been introduced. Steps such as these would ease the financial pressures generated by the aging of baby boomers without privatizing this historically universal program.

Preoccupation with privatization has led to a great deal of what might be termed benign neglect regarding Social Security. Unlike most European countries, the United States has not seriously entertained policy changes that would help families juggle paid and unpaid work, such as care credits or a generous minimum benefit (see Harrington Meyer and Herd, 2007; U.S. Social Security Administration, 2007). Nor has it acknowledged the growing legions of cohabitating couples, whether gay or straight. U.S. policy makers need to attend to these and other modest adjustments if they wish to make the Social Security system more responsive to changing sociodemographic trends. Such adjustments would broaden the program's capacity to shore up economic security in old age and to reduce the inequality linked to gender, race, class, and marital status.

Supplemental Security Income

Supplemental Security Income (SSI) has provided monthly cash benefits to the aged, blind, and disabled poor since it was created in 1972. Because women live longer and are more likely to be poor, nearly two-thirds of elderly SSI recipients are women (U.S. Social Security Administration 2007). SSI benefits have been indexed to cost-of-living increases since the implementation of the program and have risen steadily each year. Federal maximum benefits in 2006 were $623 a month for a single person and $934 for an aged couple (U.S. Social Security Administration, 2007). Maximum benefits are about 77 percent of the federal poverty line for single beneficiaries and 87 percent for older couples (U.S. Social Security Administration, 2007). However, the size of the maximum benefit is somewhat moot because most people do not receive the maximum. The average monthly payments to single, poor older people in 2006 were just $316 (U.S. Social Security Administration, 2007). States are permitted to supplement these benefits and many do, though few supplements enable their recipients to come close to or reach the federal poverty line.

As with most poverty-based programs, SSI is underused. Moreover, SSI use among the elderly has dropped from 10 percent in 1975 to an all-time low of 3 percent in 2006 (U.S. Social Security Administration, 2007). Some of the decline is due to the expansion of Social Security coverage and benefits over this period of time, but some is due to features of the SSI program itself (Harrington Meyer and Herd, 2007). Older people who are eligible for SSI might not apply because they are either unaware of the benefits, or overwhelmed by the cumbersome eligibility forms, or too stigmatized by the means-test. Others are dissuaded by strict earnings and asset tests that have not been updated in decades. For example, even though they are poor, less than 2 percent of SSI recipients report earnings, in part because the earnings test is so strict (U.S. Social Security Administration, 2007). Unlike Social Security, SSI considers all earned and unearned income in calculating benefits. Under federal guidelines, the first $65 in earned income, along with an additional $20, is disregarded each month. Any additional earnings decrease benefits by $1 for every $2 earned. Assets, excluding a house, a car, and burial funds under certain conditions, must be below $2,000 for individuals and $3,000 for couples. Additionally, SSI reduces payments by one-third if the recipient lives with someone, sharing food and shelter. Benefit reductions due to co-residence become increasingly problematic as people age and face declining incomes and health.

SSI has had the effect of shifting risk and responsibility onto poor older people, not by privatization, but by failing to upwardly adjust earnings and asset limits (Harrington Meyer and Herd, 2007). SSI's modest income disregards have been in place since 1981; the asset maximums have been in place since 1989 (U.S. Social Security Administration, 2007). Neither has been linked to the cost of living and neither can be raised except by congressional legislation. By failing to adjust the income disregard and the asset maximums to take into account more than 20 years of inflation, SSI has been retrenched more by default than by explicit policy changes. But the overall effect of many SSI policies in the last few decades is to disqualify some individuals, lower benefits for others, and shift risk and responsibility back onto these poorer individuals and their families (Harrington Meyer and Herd, 2007).

Private Pensions

Private pensions, which historically have helped to determine who would and who would not be poor in old age, are the second-largest income stream for older people. We think of these pensions as exclusively private, but in fact they are funded in part through government subsidies, or *tax expenditures*, to individuals and corporations. Nonetheless, private pensions contribute to inequality in old age because not all workers receive them, particularly those individuals who work in low-wage occupations. Thus, among older people in the top earnings quartile, 63 percent have private pensions; among those in the lowest earnings quartile, only 20 percent are covered (Employee Benefit Research Institute, 2004).

Historically, most workers with private pensions were covered by defined-benefit plans. Under these plans, employees received a benefit amount that increased with hours, salaries, and years of service. Recently, however, most companies have shifted to defined-contribution plans for their workers. In fact, between 1979 and 2004, the proportion covered only by defined-benefit plans dropped from 62 to 10 percent, while the proportion covered only by defined-contribution plans rose from rose from 16 to 63 percent (Employee Benefit Research Institute, 2004; Harrington Meyer and Herd, 2007). Defined-contribution plans differ markedly because they shift the responsibility and risks associated with private pension accumulation, and often much of the cost, from employers to employees. Because participation is not compulsory or automatic, employees are more readily able to opt out, reduce contributions, or withdraw money before retirement for expenses such as health costs, children's educations, or weddings. Women are significantly more likely than men to do all three (Munnell and Sundén, 2004; Shuey and O'Rand, 2006). Defined-contribution plans concentrate rather than spread the risk of unfortunate investment strategies, as the deep recession beginning in 2008 has made abundantly clear. The resulting shortfalls are, of course, much harder to absorb for those with lower incomes. What was once a strong leg of the three-legged income-security stool is now shaky because with each passing year, employers are contributing less to these plans and making employees even more responsible for their own pension accumulations (Employee Benefit Research Institute, 2004; Munnell and Sundén, 2004; Shuey and O'Rand, 2006).

Health Care

Risk and responsibility are being shifted in the health care arena as well. The United States devotes a higher proportion of resources to health care on both a gross domestic product (GDP) and per capita basis than any other industrial nation, yet its health status, by a number of measures, does not rank among the leading nations. This is due in part, but not exclusively, to the United States having left 17 percent of its population uninsured (Britt, 2004; Holtz-Eakin, 2004). For the most part, nonelderly Americans rely on corporate or employment-based health insurance coverage. Employers and employees receive tax incentives aimed at encouraging the provision of health insurance through jobs. These tax breaks amounted to well over $100 billion in revenues lost to the government in 2006 alone (Selden and Gray, 2006). Yet the already-spotty health insurance coverage provided by employers has been declining steadily for two decades. Between 1979 and 2004, the proportion of working men of all ages with insurance through their own jobs declined from 65 to 51 percent, while the proportion of women with insurance through their own jobs declined from 47 to 39 percent (Employee Benefit Research Institute, 2004).

The distribution of these heavily subsidized benefits is far from equal (Harrington Meyer and Herd, 2007). Whites, men, full-time, and higher-paid workers are most likely to have health insurance; while blacks and Hispanics, women, part-time, and low-wage workers are more likely to be uninsured or to rely on poverty-based programs (Employee Benefit Research Institute, 2004; Harrington Meyer and Herd, 2007). As employees struggled with disappearing employee health benefits, the health insurance industry celebrated banner years. Between 2001 and 2005, health insurance premiums rose 60 percent and profits and salaries for top executives doubled (Britt, 2004; Holtz-Eakin, 2004). Reliance on market-based health insurance is increasingly risky as access and coverage shrink; the net effect is increased health and economic inequality throughout the life course.

Medicare

On turning 65, nearly all older Americans turn to Medicare. Since 1965, Medicare has provided universal health care benefits to the aged and the disabled, and it has done a remarkable job of increasing access to many types of acute health care for the aged. Before the program began, just 56 percent of the aged had hospital insurance, compared with 97 percent in 2007 (Harrington Meyer and Herd, 2007; U.S. Social Security Administration, 2007). But other kinds of health care coverage, most notably long-term care, remain out of reach for many. The entire system operates at high costs, and recent policy initiatives have shifted many risks and responsibilities back onto individuals and families.

Costs began rising dramatically from the moment Medicare was implemented, and as a result cost containment has been on the front burner for decades (Harrington Meyer and Herd, 2007). In 2008, Medicare expenditures were $428 billion, or $10,500 per beneficiary (MedPAC, 2008). Various cost-cutting mechanisms have been explored over the years. In an early effort to curb runaway costs in 1984, policy makers implemented a prospective payment system (PPS) aimed at reducing unnecessary medical treatment and cutting costs. This legislation changed the way Medicare paid for services—from a retrospective cost-plus-profit system to a system that paid a preset amount per person per primary diagnosis. Hospital stays shortened dramatically and the rate at which total costs were rising slowed measurably (Estes, 1989; Estes and Associates, 2001). But hospitals and clinics then shifted unprofitable care to families (Glazer, 1990; Estes and Associates, 2001). Both the quantity and the quality of care work changed as hospitals discharged patients quicker and sicker and Medicare and Medicaid coverage for home care dried up. With little training, families were suddenly expected to take on highly techni- cal work including chemotherapy, apnea monitoring, phototherapy, oxygen tents, tubal feedings, dressing changes, and more. Estes (1989) calculated that in the first five years of Diagnostic Related Groupings (DRGs), more than 21 million days of care work had been transferred from hospitals to families.

In the wake of PPS, the demand for post-acute home care rose dra- matically, but Medicare was slow to respond. Then, in the late 1980s, a series of court cases by families desperate for Medicare home health services challenged the restricted interpretation of these Medicare pol- icies (Moon with Herd, 2002; Harrington Meyer and Herd, 2007). Consequently, throughout the 1990s home care and skilled nursing care grew quickly (MedPAC, 2008). But the relief that families re- ceived in the 1990s was short lived. Concerned by rapid Medicare cost increases, legislators pushed through a Balanced Budget Act in 1997 that reduced payments to hospitals, shifted home health care from Medicare Part A to Part B, restricted access to home health and other services, and shifted costs and care work to the aged and their families (Moon with Herd, 2002; MedPAC, 2008). Total home health expenditures have crept back up slowly, but the overall share of the Medicare budget devoted to home health care dropped from 8 per- cent in 1994 to just 4 percent in 2007 (MedPAC, 2008). There are now fewer licensed providers, fewer persons receiving home health care, fewer visits provided per person, and fewer types of care covered (Harrington Meyer and Herd, 2007; MedPAC, 2008).

Medicare costs have also been cut by shifting expenses onto older beneficiaries. In addition to premiums and copayments, or *copays*, Medicare recipients pay deductibles, a coinsurance of 20 percent, any costs above the allowable rate, and all costs for uncovered goods and services such as long-term care, preventive care, dental care, vision, and eyeglasses (Harrington Meyer, 2000; Employee Benefit Research Institute, 2004; U.S. Social Security Administration, 2007). All of these out-of-pocket expenses have risen dramatically and are expected to continue rising at rates much higher than the cost of living. The Medicare trustees predict that by 2030, the Medicare Part B premium will increase to $150 in 2004 dollars (Johnson and Penner, 2004). Because the Part B premium is deducted from Social Security benefits before the checks are mailed, the net effect is smaller Social Security benefits across the board. One consequence of recipients being responsible for deductibles, copays, premiums, and uncovered medical goods is that Medicare covers only about 45 percent of old age health care costs (Moody, 2002).

In yet another effort to shift costs away from the government, Congress has turned periodically to Health Maintenance Organization (HMO) and Preferred Provider Organization (PPO) managed care options for Medicare beneficiaries. As early as 1982, the Tax Equity and Fiscal Responsibility Act (TEFRA) developed HMO or PPO options under Medicare. Many providers targeted the healthiest enrollees and then used the difference between costs and reimbursement rates to make benefits—and profits—more generous. Enrollments rose from just 6 percent of all Medicare beneficiaries to 11 percent between 1994 and 1996 (Biles, Nicholas, and Guterman, 2006). Participation fell after Congress then lowered Medicare reimbursements to managed care providers, only to increase once again in the wake of passage of the Balanced Budget Act of 1997. This act created Medicare+Choice (M+C), leading to an escalation in enrollment that soon reached 16 percent of Medicare beneficiaries. But by 1998 reduced federal payments once again undermined HMO and PPO popularity (Moon with Herd, 2002; Kaiser Family Foundation, 2005), with many plans simply pulling out of M+C service areas, cutting benefits, or raising premiums. As a result, enrollment dropped again (Kaiser Family Foundation 2005).

Then, to reverse declining enrollments, the 2003 Medicare Modernization Act increased reimbursements and redubbed the program Medicare Advantage (MA); enrollments rose to their current high of 18 percent (MedPAC, 2007; U.S. Social Security Administration, 2007). Critics warn that while costs under Medicare Advantage are lower for those in good health, out-of-pocket costs are often higher than they would be under traditional Medicare for the sickest beneficiaries (Biles, Nicholas, and Guterman, 2006). They also point out that cutting costs by shifting to HMOs has not worked (Herd, 2005; Harrington Meyer and Herd, 2007); the government was paying an extra $546 per enrollee in private plans in 2005, compared with those in traditional Medicare. Biles, Nicholas, and Guterman (2006) reported that in 2005, every MA plan paid more for every Medicare plan enrollee than the average of fee-for-service costs. The Congressional Budget Office estimated that Medicare Advantage would add $14 billion in new Medicare costs over its first ten years (Congressional Budget Office 2005). In response to these concerns, in early 2009 the Obama administration proposed cutting back MA payments.

The growing preference among conservative policy makers for privatization was evident in the design of the Medicare Part D prescription drug program, enacted in 2003. Historically, the absence of prescription drug coverage was a particularly problematic aspect of Medicare, because both the use and price of prescription drugs have risen sharply. While many older people had drug coverage through supplemental policies, MA, or Medicaid, 25 percent had no prescription coverage at all (Hoadley, 2006). Congress responded not by offering a single, universal benefit through Medicare, but by requiring older people enrolled in Part D to select and pay premiums to one private drug plan from a sea of complex and ever-changing private plan options (Hoadley, 2006; Harrington Meyer and Herd, 2007). The prescription drug benefit is complex and costly, with beneficiaries paying a monthly premium, an annual deductible, a copayment, and then the full amount of any costs inside what has been dubbed "the donut hole." A catastrophic benefit kicks in only after annual drug costs exceed $5,100 (Kaiser Family Foundation, 2004). Given that out-of-pocket expenses may be as high as $3,600 a year for prescriptions alone, the policy shifted risk and costs from the government onto older people and helped to underwrite the efforts of insurance and pharmaceutical companies (Waxman, 2006; Harrington Meyer and Herd, 2007).

The outlook for Medicare—and many Medicare recipients—is troubling. Total costs are rising sharply and the number of enrollees is expected to double between 2000 and 2030 (MedPAC, 2008). Meanwhile, much of the cost and much of the work associated with old age health care is shifted back onto the elderly and their families. Four decades into the Medicare and Medicaid programs, the costs of health care for the aged are, in fact, a greater burden than before the programs began. Out-of-pocket expenses for elderly people rose from 15 percent of their annual income in 1965 to 22 percent in 1998. By 2025, out-of-pocket health care expenses are expected to reach 30 percent (Moon with Herd, 2002).

The effect of shifting unpaid long-term health care work back onto families may have been even more pronounced (Harrington Meyer and Herd, 2007; U.S. Social Security Administration, 2007; MedPAC, 2008). Stone (2000) points out that there are 40 unpaid informal care workers for every paid formal care worker. The total value of annual care work, which often has adverse impacts on the economic, physical, emotional, and social health of those doing that care work, is now estimated to be between $50 billion and $103 billion (Stone, 2000; National Alliance for Caregiving and AARP, 2004; Holtz-Eakin, 2005).

Retiree and Medigap Supplemental Insurance

Retiree reliance on employment-based health insurance dropped significantly in recent years. Even among large employers, the proportion who offer retiree health benefits has dropped from 66 percent in 1988 to just 36 percent in 2004 (MedPAC, 2008). White, male, full-time, and higher-paid workers are more likely to accrue these retiree health benefits, but even for those groups, coverage is on the decline. Moreover, the diminishing pool of employers who still offer retiree coverage are pushing more of the costs onto the retirees themselves and tightening restrictions on benefits. The Employee Benefit Research Institute (2004) reports that most employers have tightened eligibility requirements, capped benefits, and increased cost-sharing for those covered by retiree benefits.

While reliance on retiree health insurance is waning, reliance on private Medigap policies is growing. Because Medicare leaves many costs uncovered, the majority of Medicare beneficiaries pay out-of-pocket premiums on supplemental insurance policies that cover Medicare premiums, copays, deductibles, and exclusions such as long-term care, eye exams, and hearing aids (Centers for Medicare and Medicaid

Services, 2005b). Whites are more likely to have supplemental coverage, particularly among low-income populations. While 48 percent of poor whites had Medigap coverage, only 17 percent of poor blacks and Hispanics had such coverage (Centers for Medicare and Medicaid Services, 2005a, 2005b; Harrington Meyer and Herd, 2007). Access may become increasingly difficult because supplemental insurance premiums have risen significantly and are expected to continue to do so (Moon with Herd, 2002).

Navigating the market for privately purchased Medigap policies is tricky. From their inception, these private-market insurance policies have been criticized for denial of coverage, duplicate coverage, severance of coverage, fraud, and price gouging. Despite broad Congressional regulation of the market, problems persist (Moon with Herd, 2002). In addition, a reliance on private supplemental policies shifts responsibility for the aged out of both the welfare state and the corporate-benefits sector and into the private market. Thus the expense and the risk fall on older individuals and their families. Those with the fewest resources, who often have the poorest health, are least likely to be able to obtain and retain private insurance and are increasingly likely to do without insurance and, at times, needed care (Harrington Meyer and Herd, 2007).

Medicaid

Since 1965, Medicaid has provided free and comprehensive health care coverage for many of the aged and disabled poor. The proportion of older people relying on Medicaid has decreased from 16 percent in 1970 to 13 percent in 2006, in part because eligibility criteria are strict. The federal income maximum is set at just 73 percent of the federal poverty line, and the federal asset maximum has been frozen for decades at just $2,000 per individual and $3,000 per couple (Kaiser Family Foundation, 2003; Congressional Budget Office, 2005; U.S. Social Security Administration, 2007). Participation is also low because the process of applying is arduous and stigmatizing, and the rules of participation are restrictive. In fact, only one-half of those who are eligible actually receive Medicaid (Moon with Herd, 2002; Kaiser Family Foundation, 2003). Nonetheless, total Medicaid expenditures for the aged rose from $21 billion in 1990 to $39 billion in 2006 (Congressional Budget Office, 2005; U.S. Social Security Administration, 2007). Per person expenditures for the aged have risen from $3,000 in 1975 to more than $13,000 in 2004. The majority of older Medicaid users are also covered by Medicare. For these *dual-eligible* beneficiaries, Medicaid covers costs Medicare does not, including the Medicare Part B premium, nursing home care, and Medicare copays and deductibles (Harrington Meyer, 2000; Kaiser Family Foundation, 2003; U.S. Social Security Administration, 2007). Because full coverage is so comprehensive for these enrollees and because health care providers are prohibited from charging costs above the allowable rates to Medicaid recipients, full Medicaid coverage reduces out-of-pocket expenses from 20 percent to just 5 percent of their annual income for this low-income older population (Kaiser Family Foundation, 2003).

A subset of dual Medicare and Medicaid enrollees receive limited coverage under new rules that relax eligibility guidelines. Since 1998, Medicare recipients with incomes below 100 percent of the federal old age poverty line and assets up to $4,000 for an individual and $6,000 for a couple may be eligible for the Qualified Medicare Beneficiary (QMB) program, which covers their Medicare Part B premium and most deductibles and copays. Those with incomes between 100 and 120 percent of the poverty line, and assets up to $4,000 for an individual and $6,000 for a couple, may be eligible for the Specified Low Income Medicare Beneficiary (SLMB) program, which covers their Part B premiums. For those who are enrolled, QMB and SLMB benefits help by reducing out-of-pocket costs to 13 percent of their total annual incomes (Kaiser Family Foundation, 2003). QMB and SLMB also involve complex application procedures. Only 55 percent of those who qualify for QMB actually participate, and only 16 percent of those who qualify for SLMB do (Moon with Herd, 2002; MedPAC, 2008).

For those older Americans who rely on Medicaid for their health care, access to that care can be problematic (Harrington Meyer and Herd, 2007). As a poverty-based program, Medicaid generally prohibits health care providers from charging patients any amount over the Medicaid assignment, even though Medicaid reimbursement rates to providers are notoriously low. One consequence is that many doctors, clinics, labs, hospitals, and nursing homes either cap the number of Medicaid patients or refuse to treat them (Harrington Meyer, 2000; Congressional Budget Office, 2005; MedPAC, 2008). Thus, among primary care physicians in the United States in 2002, 85 percent were accepting new private payers, 83 percent were accepting new Medicare recipients, and only 66 percent were accepting new Medicaid patients (MedPAC, 2008). Many providers discriminate on the basis of payer source; because they are more likely to be on Medicaid, older women, blacks, Hispanics, and unmarried persons are more likely to face denial of or delays in treatment or admission (Wallace et al., 1998; Harrington Meyer, 2000).

Those who hope to bypass paying for long-term care out of pocket or through Medicaid can purchase private long-term care insurance. Despite considerable governmental regulation, prices for policies are expensive and volatile, the market has experienced mismanagement and fraudulent behavior, and individuals with pre-existing conditions are often denied policies or saddled with high premiums (Harrington Meyer and Herd, 2007). Though about 40 percent of elders could reasonably afford a policy, only about 7 percent in fact have one (Moon with Herd, 2002; Congressional Budget Office, 2005; Holtz-Eakin, 2005).

In recent years, to cut costs, many states have introduced Medicaid copayments for prescription drug coverage and services, reduced the scope of coverage, eliminated dental and vision care, or limited the number of prescriptions, physician visits, or the amount of medical equipment per year. As a result, out-of-pocket expenses have risen at twice the rate of incomes, and older Medicaid recipients now spend 2.4 percent of their annual income on out-of-pocket medical costs (Ku and Broaddus, 2005). While Medicaid does provide comprehensive health care services to poor older persons and reduces some out-of-pocket expenses, it nonetheless shifts risk and responsibility onto individuals through a stringent gate-keeping mechanism. Income and asset requirements, as well as provider reimbursement rates, have not kept pace with cost-of-living increases, and the overall effect is to minimize the proportion of older people who are eligible for Medicaid as well as to minimize access to benefits among beneficiaries.

Conclusion

Preoccupation with shifting risk and responsibility from the government onto individuals has prompted U.S. policy makers to reshape the old age welfare state. Policy makers have raised the age of eligibility for full Social Security benefits and increased the financial penalty for taking early retirement benefits. Moreover, policy makers have focused so single-mindedly on cost containment and privatization that few have seriously considered more incremental changes within the existing framework that would make this program more responsive to families juggling paid and unpaid work, to cohabitating couples, and to lower-income recipients. In terms of SSI for elderly people, policy makers have neglected the program, freezing income disregards and asset maximums for decades. As for private pensions, companies have reduced access and coverage dramatically, most notably by shifting from defined-benefit to defined-contribution plans. With regard to Medicare, policy makers have focused on shifting costs and thereby raising out-of-pocket expenses for older people, pushing care work out of the benefit plan and onto the shoulders of families, directing the provision of benefits into the market, and forfeiting the government's buying-power capacity to use leverage to negotiate lower costs. Access and coverage are drying up quickly for retired-employee health insurance. Many older people turn to private Medigap and long-term care policies, but those market-based solutions are rife with problems and leave many older people exposed to a great deal of risk. Finally, Medicaid coverage for the aged is highly constrained because income and asset guidelines have not kept pace with inflation and because more of the costs are being shifted onto poor beneficiaries as states struggle to meet rising costs. Taken together, these policy changes all shift responsibility for economic and health security in old age from the government onto individuals, diluting the protective features of welfare state programs and increasing the inequality linked to gender, race, and marital status.

It is ironic that policy makers have been retrenching and privatizing old age programs at a time when the vast majority of Americans think the nation is doing too little for the elderly. Between 70 and 90 percent of poll respondents report that they would be willing to pay higher taxes to keep universal old age benefits and that they favor universal health insurance for all (Century Foundation, 1998; AARP, 2005; Public Agenda, 2005; Street and Sittig Cossman, 2006). These popular public opinions now have the opportunity to be translated into welfare policy under the guidance of the Obama administration. The welfare state can again be redefined with the objective of reducing inequality in old age. And if the goal truly is to reduce inequality in old age, then policy reforms should be more *responsive*, focusing on policies that match family demographics in the twenty-first rather than the nineteenth century; *redistributive*, emphasizing universal policies that constrain rather than escalate the inequalities linked to gender, race, class, and marital status; and *collective*, focusing on policies that spread the risks and responsibilities of old age dependency across families rather than concentrating them within families. The welfare state represents a great opportunity to ameliorate inequalities.

References

AARP. 2005. *Public Attitudes toward Social Security and Private Accounts.* Washington, D.C: AARP Knowledge Movement.

Biles, B., L. Nicholas, and S. Guterman. 2006. Medicare beneficiary out-of-pocket costs: Are Medicare Advantage plans a better deal? *Issue Brief* (May). Commonwealth Fund Publication 927.

Britt, R. 2004. Insurers get bigger health dollar cut: Profits up, premiums up, but medical spending lags. *CBS.MarketWatch.com* (Oct. 15). www.marketwatch.com/story/health-insurers-getting-bigger-cut-of-medical-dollars/.

Centers for Medicare and Medicaid Services. 2005a. *Medicare Aged and Disabled Enrollees by Type of Coverage, All Areas, as of July 1, 1966–2003.* Washington, D.C.: U.S. Department of Health and Human Services.

———. 2005b. *Your Medicare Coverage.* Washington, D.C.: U.S. Department of Health and Human Services.

Century Foundation. 1998. *The Basics: Social Security Reform.* New York: Century Foundation.

Congressional Budget Office. 2004. *Administrative Costs of Private Accounts in Social Security.* Washington, D.C.: Congressional Budget Office.

———. 2005. *The Long-Term Budget Outlook.* Washington, D.C.: Congressional Budget Office.

Employee Benefit Research Institute. 2004. Health insurance coverage of individuals ages 55–64. *Notes* 25 (3): 15.

Estes, C. 1989. Aging, health, and social policy: Crisis and crossroads. *Journal of Aging and Social Policy* 1 (1–2): 17–32.

Estes, C., and Associates. 2001. *Social Policy and Aging: A Critical Perspective.* Thousand Oaks, Calif.: Sage Publications.

Gilbert, N. 2002. *Transformation of the Welfare State: The Silent Surrender of Public Responsibility.* New York: Oxford University Press.

Glazer, N. Y. 1990. The home as workshop: Women as amateur nurses and medical care providers. *Gender and Society* 4 (4): 479–99.

Hacker, J. S. 2002. *The Divided Welfare State: The Battle over Public and Private Social Benefits in the United States*. New York: Cambridge University Press.

———. 2006. *The Great Risk Shift: The Assault on American Jobs, Families, Health Care, and Retirement—and How You Can Fight Back*. New York: Oxford University Press.

Harrington Meyer, M. 1996. Making claims as workers or wives: The distribution of Social Security benefits. *American Sociological Review* 61 (3): 449–65.

——— (ed.). 2000. *Care Work: Gender, Labor, and the Welfare State*. New York: Routledge Press.

Harrington Meyer, M., and P. Herd. 2007. *Market Friendly or Family Friendly? The State and Gender Inequality in Old Age*. New York: Russell Sage Foundation.

Harrington Meyer, M., and E. Pavalko. 1996. Family, work, and access to health insurance among mature women. *Journal of Health and Social Behavior* 37 (4): 311–25.

Herd, P. 2005. Universalism without the targeting: Privatizing the old-age welfare state. *Gerontologist* 45 (3): 292–98.

Herd, P., and E. R. Kingson. 2005. Selling Social Security. Pp. 183–204 in R. B. Hudson (ed.), *The New Politics of Old Age Policy*. Baltimore: Johns Hopkins University Press.

Hoadley, J. 2006. *Medicare's New Adventure: The Part D Drug Benefit*. Commonwealth Fund Publication No. 911. New York: Commonwealth Fund, Commission on a High Performance Health System.

Holtz-Eakin, D. 2004. *Health Care Spending and the Uninsured*. Statement of the Director before the Committee on Health, Education, Labor, and Pensions, U. S. Senate, January 28. Washington, D.C.: Congressional Budget Office.

———. 2005. *The Cost and Financing of Long-Term Care Services*. Statement of Douglas Holtz-Eakin, Director, before the Subcommittee on Health, Committee on Ways and Means, U.S. House of Representatives, April 27. Washington, D.C.: Congressional Budget Office.

Johnson, R. W., and R. G. Penner. 2004. *Will Health Care Costs Erode Retirement Security?* Issue in Brief No. 23. Chestnut Hill, Mass.: Center for Retirement Research, Boston College.

Kaiser Family Foundation. 2003. *Dual Enrollees: Medicaid's Role for Low-Income Medicare Beneficiaries*. Fact Sheet 4091. Menlo Park, Calif.: Henry J. Kaiser Family Foundation.

———. 2004. *Summaries of the Medicare Prescription Drug Improvement and Modernization Act of 2003*. Publication No. 6120. Menlo Park, Calif.: Henry J. Kaiser Family Foundation.

———. 2005. *Medicare Advantage*. Fact Sheet 2052-08. Menlo Park, Calif.: Henry J. Kaiser Family Foundation.

Korpi, W., and J. Palme. 1998. The paradox of redistribution and strategies of equality: Welfare state institutions, inequality, and poverty in the Western countries. *American Sociological Review* 63 (Oct.): 661–87.

Ku, L., and M. Broaddus. 2005. *Out-of-Pocket Medical Expenses for Medicaid Beneficiaries Are Substantial and Growing*. Washington, D.C.: Center on Budget and Policy Priorities.

MedPAC. 2007. *The Medicare Advantage Program and MedPAC Recommendations*. Testimony before the Committee on Finance, U.S. Senate, April 11. Washington, D.C.: Medicare Payment Advisory Commission.

———. 2008. *A Data Book: Health Care Spending and the Medicare Program*. Washington, D.C.: Medicare Payment Advisory Commission.

Moody, H. R. 2002. *Aging: Concepts and Controversies*. Newbury Park, Calif.: Pine Forge Press.

Moon, M., with P. Herd. 2002. *A Place at the Table: Women's Needs and Medicare Reform*. New York: Century Foundation.

Munnell, A. H., and A. Sundén. 2004. *Coming Up Short: The Challenge of 401(k) Plans*. Washington, D.C.: Brookings Institution Press.

Myles, J., and J. Quadagno. 2000. Envisioning a third way: The welfare state in the twenty-first century. *Contemporary Sociology* 29 (1): 156–67.

National Alliance for Caregiving and AARP. 2004. *Caregiving in the U.S.* Washington, D.C.: National Alliance for Caregiving and AARP.

Pauly, M., P. Danzon, P. Feldstein, and J. Hoff. 1991. A plan for "responsible national health insurance." *Health Affairs* 10 (1): 5–25.

Porter, K. H., K. Larin, and W. Primus. 1999. *Social Security and Poverty among the Elderly: A National and State Perspective*. Washington, D.C.: Center on Budget and Policy Priorities.

Public Agenda. 2005. Medicare: Results of survey question re. federal budget. *PublicAgenda.org Issue Guides* (Apr. 18–22). New York: Public Agenda.

Selden, T., and B. Gray. 2006. Tax subsidies for employment-related health insurance: Estimates for 2006. *Health Affairs* 25 (6): 1568–79.

Shuey, K. M., and A. M. O'Rand. 2006. Changing demographics and new pension risks. *Research on Aging* 28 (3): 317–40.

Stone, R. I. 2000. *Long-Term Care for the Elderly with Disabilities: Current Policy, Emerging Trends, and Implications for the Twenty-First Century*. Washington, D.C.: Milbank Memorial Fund.

Street, D., and J. Sittig Cossman. 2006. Greatest generation or greedy geezers? Social spending preferences and the elderly. *Social Problems* 53 (1): 75–96.

Torres-Gil, F., R. Greenstein, and D. Kamin. 2005. *Hispanics' Large Stake in the Social Security Debate* (June 28). Washington, D.C.: Center on Budget and Policy Priorities.

U.S. Social Security Administration. 2007. *Annual Statistical Supplement 2006 to the Social Security Bulletin*. SSA Publication No. 13-11700. Washington, D.C.: Department of Health and Human Services. www.socialsecurity.gov/policy/docs/statcomps/supplement/2006/.

Wallace, S. P., L. Levy-Storms, R. S. Kington, and R. M. Andersen. 1998. The persistence of race and ethnicity in the use of long-term care. *Journals of Gerontology, Series B: Social Sciences* 53 (2): S104–12.

Waxman, H. A. 2006. *Analysis: Pharmaceutical Industry Profits Increase by Over $8 Billion after Medicare Drug Plan Goes into Effect*. U.S. House of Representatives, Committee on Government Reform (Sept.). http://oversight.house.gov/documents/20060919115623-70677.pdf

Wu, K. B. 2004. *African Americans Age 65 and Older: Their Sources of Income*. Fact Sheet 100. Washington, D.C.: AARP Public Policy Institute.

Yergin, D., and J. Stanislaw. 1998. *The Commanding Heights: The Battle between Government and the Marketplace That Is Remaking the Modern World*. New York: Simon & Schuster.

Zeller, T., Jr. 2007. Savings rate at Depression-era lows . . . Does it matter? *New York Times News Blog* (Feb. 1).

3. Aging Policy and Structural Lag

Janet M. Wilmoth, Ph.D.

Societies like the United States that experience demographic and social changes along various dimensions are subject to rapid social change. Under these conditions, social institutions are unable to effectively meet the basic needs of society and its members. The ways in which social institutions operate, and the assumptions on which those operations rest, lag behind the social "reality" experienced by the individuals who occupy roles in those institutions (Riley and Riley, 1994). This structural lag is exacerbated by public policies that were designed to address the needs of individuals and families during an earlier historical time, when demographic and social circumstances were different.

Given this, one might expect policy makers to take into account demographic shifts in the population when evaluating and (re)creating policy. But, as noted by Hudson (2005, p. 13), "the contemporary social policy debate is more about political ideology than it is about population dynamics." This is unfortunate, given that population dynamics drive social changes that create structural lag, making certain features of public policy outdated. Thus bringing public policies in line with current demographic and social circumstances is essential, not only for alleviating structural lag but also for ensuring that public funds are being expended on programs and services that are designed to meet the current needs of the population, as opposed to maintaining policies that are responsive to historical circumstances that no longer exist and social dynamics that have changed form.

In this chapter, I explain the concept of structural lag in detail. Its theoretical grounding in sociology is discussed and its relevance to old age policy is explained. I then identify key demographic and social trends in the following areas that have contributed to structural lag in the United States: retirement; morbidity, disability, and life expectancy; marriage and families; women's labor force participation; and racial/

ethnic composition. I describe how the intersection of these trends creates structural lag that influences engagement among retirees, later-life financial security among working women, and health among racial and ethnic minorities. Particular attention is given to the role of public policy in generating and alleviating lag in each of these areas. Finally, I discuss the challenges of crafting policy that effectively alleviates the structural lag experienced by various segments of society.

Structural Lag

The concept of structural lag is grounded in the age-stratification framework, a sociological perspective that emerged out of structural functionalist theory during the latter half of the twentieth century (Merton, 1957, 1995; Riley, Johnson, and Foner, 1972; Riley, Foner, and Waring, 1988; Riley, Kahn, and Foner, 1994). To understand structural lag, one must first be familiar with five basic sociological concepts from structural functionalism: stratification, social status, roles, norms, and opportunity structures. *Stratification* is a system through which individuals are grouped into categories, or strata, according to their social status. *Status* is based on a position in society that is located in a particular social institution and associated with a certain set of behaviors (i.e., *roles*) that reflect socially constructed rules of conduct for the role occupants (i.e., *norms*). However, the status associated with specific roles varies, which influences one's location in the stratification system. One's location in the stratification system, in turn, determines access to *opportunity structures*, which shape the probability of achieving socially desirable outcomes such as educational attainment, economic success, and good health.

The age-stratification framework builds on these concepts by arguing that society is stratified by age just as it is stratified by race, gender, and class (Riley et al., 1968; Riley, 1971, 1987; Riley, Johnson, and Foner, 1972). This age-stratification system allocates individuals to the appropriate age-graded roles. While these age-graded systems are institutionalized, they are not immutable. The age-stratification system can be influenced by the movement of successive cohorts through the system. Each birth cohort is unique because its members experience historical events at a particular developmental point in the life course. These historical events differentially influence the perceptions and values of each cohort's members, which in turn influence how roles are enacted by individuals. As individuals within a specific cohort age, their collective enactment of age-graded roles can reshape social structures that generate the age-stratification system.

From the age-stratification perspective, social change is occurring on two levels. Micro-level change occurs in people's lives, which is collectively represented in age-related experiences across cohorts. Macro-level change occurs across historical time, as age-related roles and norms shift in response to internal pressures from individuals who occupy these roles and to external pressures generated by the changing social and cultural climate. Riley and Riley (1994) referred to the first type of change as the "dynamism of changing lives" and the second type of change as the "dynamism of structural change." They argue that these dynamisms are distinct but interdependent processes. More importantly, they are asynchronous. The first proceeds along the time dimension of age, whereas the second proceeds along historical time. Given this, changes in people's lives can outpace structural changes, which is known as *structural lag*. Conversely, structural changes can outpace changes in people's lives, which is known as *person lag*. The mismatch between women's increasing rates of labor force participation and the dearth of low-cost, high-quality child care is an example of structural lag. An example of person lag is when rapid advances in technology make workers' training obsolete, leaving them lacking the skills that are necessary to do their jobs and be competitive in the job market.

Riley and Riley (1994, p. 24) argue that in most modern societies structural lag is more prevalent than person lag, because "many structures (such as summer vacations for schoolchildren to work on the farm, or 65 as the expected age of retirement) tend to retain their earlier form." It is interesting to note that the examples they provide are not structures per se, but instead are policies that are enacted by a government and implemented within a social institution (e.g., local school boards setting policies regarding the school year and the federal government establishing age-based eligibility criteria for receiving Social Security). These policies create structure that shapes social norms and individual behavior. Thus public policy is a critical component of structural lag.

The actions of policy makers have been cited as a potential mechanism for reducing structural lag (Foner, 1994). Indeed, policy can prompt structural changes that help to move a society from being age

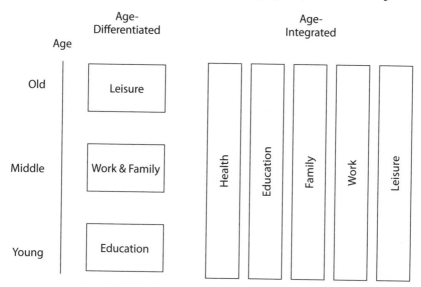

Figure 3.1. Expanded Model of Riley and Riley's Age-Integration Theory.
Source: O'Rand, 2005, figure 6.1.

segregated to age integrated. Age segregation is based on the tripartition of roles across the life course: educational roles tend to be allocated to the young, work and family roles to the middle age groups, and leisure to the old (Kohli, 1986; Riley and Riley, 1994). This age segregation of roles, which is organized around the principle of work, limits opportunity structures and creates various pressures for different age groups, because the available social roles at a given age may not be consistent with the roles an individual might want to assume. For example, middle-aged adults experience substantial time squeezes meeting the demands of work and family that make it difficult to gain additional education or have serious leisure pursuits. And older adults are limited primarily to leisure activities and nonpaid volunteer opportunities, even though most are sufficiently healthy to participate in work and educational roles. O'Rand's (2005) expanded model of Riley and Riley's (1994) age-integration theory illustrates the limited opportunity structures in an age-differentiated society (figure 3.1).

This figure also shows how roles could be restructured so that they are more accessible across the life course. This would create an age-integrated society in which individuals have more equal access to opportunity structures and are able to strike a balance between various available roles across the entire life course. Given the centrality of work in organizing roles in an age-segregated society, moving toward an age-integrated society requires restructuring work-related opportunity structures (Settersten, 1999) and the domains that shape work behavior across the life course (including education, family, and health). This restructuring comes about through structural changes that are prompted by policy that allows for life-course flexibility. As noted by O'Rand (2005, p. 113), policies based on the notion of age integration support "social and market institutions sensitive to age-variant patterns of role incumbency and status transition across the life course."

As this discussion demonstrates, *public policy can generate and alleviate structural lag and person lag.* Given that structural lag is currently more common in the United States than person lag, the remaining portions of this chapter will focus on issues related to structural lag.

Key Demographic and Social Trends Contributing to Structural Lag

As it is well known, the absolute number and percentage of the U.S. population aged 65 or older is growing rapidly, the age-sex structure in the United States is becoming more rectangular shaped, and old age dependency ratios are steadily increasing (Himes, 2001). Despite these demographic facts, there are ongoing debates about the various implications of these shifts in the population structure. Since Samuel Preston's (1984) presidential address to the Population Association of America on the divergent well-being of children and older adults, there has been extensive discussion about whether increased spending on public programs for older adults jeopardizes the well-being of younger generations. Another related issue, based in the generational accounting construct (Kotlikoff, 1996; Smetters and Gokhale, 2004), is the increased burden that will be placed on future working-age cohorts if current public programs for older adults are sustained or expanded. These debates focus attention primarily on fiscal concerns while largely ignoring issues related to the appropriateness of current age-related policies, given the following recent demographic and social trends.

Retirement

During the mid- to late twentieth century, age at retirement declined dramatically (Gendell and Siegel, 1996; Gendell, 2001). However, there is disagreement regarding the extent to which these trends will continue. Some economists indicate that the trend toward early retirement, which had been flat since 1985, is starting to reverse due to changes in private and public sector policies (Clark and Quinn, 2002). Recent Census Bureau reports indicate labor force participation among adults ages 62 or older has increased over the past ten years, particularly among older Hispanic men, black men, and black women (O'Rand, 2005; Purcell 2007). However, others make the case that the average retirement age is continuing to decline even in the presence of increasing labor force participation rates by older adults (Gendell, 2001) and that early retirement will continue to be an attractive and affordable option for more affluent segments of the older adult population (Costa, 1998). Demographers speculate that even if age at retirement were to remain stable or increase somewhat, the average length of retirement is likely to increase, due to projected improvements in life expectancy (U.S. Bureau of the Census, 2000).

Morbidity, Disability, and Life Expectancy

There have been substantial improvements in life expectancy as death rates, particularly among the oldest old, have continued to decline (National Vital Statistics Reports, 2004). In 2005, life expectancy at age 65 was 17.2 years for men and 20.0 years for women, and at age 75 it was 10.8 years and 12.8 years for men and women, respectively (Centers for Disease Control and Prevention, 2007). However, heart disease, cancer, and stroke, which are the leading causes of death in the United States, continue to be common health conditions (Centers for Disease Control and Prevention, 2003). In addition, the prevalence of Alzheimer's disease and other chronic conditions is increasing (Sloane et al., 2002). Serious and chronic conditions increase the risk that older adults will have functional limitations that make it difficult to perform instrumental and physical activities of daily living. Although recent research suggests that disability among older adults is declining, it is unclear whether the observed trends will continue for future cohorts (Freedman, Martin, and Schoeni, 2002).

One recent trend that could affect both morbidity and mortality among future cohorts is the increasing rate of obesity among middle-aged adults (Himes 2000; Center on an Aging Society, 2003; Peters et al., 2003). However, the extent to which obesity will affect the health status and disability rates of future older adult cohorts will depend on aggregate changes in diet and exercise, the development of medical treatments for obesity, and the extent to which assistive devices are available for obese individuals.

Given the uncertainty about disability trends, we do not have a clear understanding of recent or future changes in active life expectancy. Estimates of active life expectancy vary across studies, but there is agreement that the percentage of inactive life (1) increases with age, (2) is higher for women than men, and (3) varies between and within race/ethnic groups (Manton and Stallard, 1991; Crimmins, Hayward, and Satio, 1996; Hayward and Heron, 1999; Geronimus et al., 2001). Future trends in active life expectancy will depend on the pace of improvements in life expectancy and changes in disability prevalence.

Marriage and Family

The traditional U.S. family, which is composed of a married-couple family with only the male working in the labor force, is increasingly rare. In fact, only 7 percent of all U.S. households fit this definition in 2002, and only 13 percent of married-couple households are families in which only the husband is in the labor force (Population Reference Bureau, 2003). Two primary demographic trends have contributed to these fundamental changes in the U.S. family. The first is the overall retreat from marriage. The percentage of the population that is married has been consistently declining, particularly among black females, due to increasing age at first marriage and the percentage of the population that is never married or divorced (U.S. Bureau of the Census, 2003a, 2003b). The second trend that has reshaped the family is related to changes in fertility. Although the total fertility rate has hovered around 2 children per woman since 1970 (Kent and Mather, 2002), there have been substantial changes in the characteristics of mothers giving birth. Delayed childbearing and births to unwed mothers are increasingly common (Heck et al., 1997; Ventura and Bachrach, 2001).

Women's Participation in the Labor Force

Women's participation in the labor force not only has influenced U.S. families, but also has implications for later-life financial security. The rising labor force participation of women has been well documented, but the variation in participation is often overlooked. For example, labor force participation rates historically have been higher among black than among white women, whereas Hispanic women tend to have lower labor force participation than either black or white women (U.S. Bureau of Labor Statistics, 2001). Married women, particularly those with children under the age of 6, are less likely to be in the labor force than unmarried women. Even when women are in the labor force, they are more likely than men to be working part-time (DiNatale and Boraas, 2002). Women continue to experience considerable social pressure to reduce working commitments when bearing and rearing children (Treas and Widmer, 2000), which has serious consequences for women in terms of wages. Gender wage gaps remain a persistent feature of the U.S. workforce (U.S. Bureau of Labor Statistics, 2001). This is due in part to continued occupational sex segregation in which women are more likely to be employed in lower-wage occupations. However, the wage penalty for motherhood also contributes to the wage gap (Budig and England, 2001).

Racial and Ethnic Composition

Although the older adult population is less racially and ethnically diverse than the population as a whole, it will become increasingly diverse over the next fifty years. In 2006, 81 percent of the older adult population was non-Hispanic white, but this percentage is projected to be approximately 61 percent by 2050 (Federal Interagency Forum on Aging-Related Statistics, 2008). This increasing diversity is due in part to the rapid growth in the Hispanic population, which is the fastest-growing minority group in the United States (Administration on Aging, 2009; Federal Interagency Forum on Aging-Related Statistics, 2008). This growth in the older Hispanic population, as well as in the older Asian population, is fueled by changing immigration patterns among younger and middle-aged adults. In addition, the number of immigrants who are age 60 or older has risen steadily over the last thirty years (U.S. Immigration and Naturalization Service, 1993; U.S.

Citizenship and Immigration Services, 2004). These changes in immigration patterns will affect the composition of the U.S. elderly population, especially minority elderly populations and the older adult populations of geographic areas with a disproportionate number of immigrants, both through the aging of currently young immigrants and through an increase in immigrants age 60 or older at the time of their arrival.

The changing racial and ethnic composition of the older adult population is important, because later-life outcomes vary substantially across racial and ethnic groups. Part of the variation across these groups in later life can be attributed to socioeconomic status. Older minorities are often overrepresented among low-status groups along various dimensions, including education, income, and wealth, and there is mounting evidence that the economic disparities across groups are increasing (U.S. Bureau of the Census, 2002, 2008; Utendorf, 2002; Federal Interagency Forum on Aging-Related Statistics, 2008).

Intersecting Trends and Old Age Policy

As noted by Friedland and Summer (1999), "demography is not destiny," but demographic trends and related changes in social dynamics do set the stage on which public policy decisions will play out. Although each of the previously discussed trends has independent implications for structural lag, it is the intersecting effects of these trends that are the most salient for policy debates. Particularly relevant for old age policy is the way in which these demographic and social trends shape engagement among retirees, later-life financial security for working women, and health among racial and ethnic minorities.

Engagement among Retirees

Considerable structural lag is generated by the intersection of early retirement age and longer, healthier lives. Together, these trends have resulted in a larger portion of the life course being spent in what has been called the *roleless role* (Burgess, 1960). In 1995–2000, the average age at retirement for men was 62, with 18 expected years in retirement (6 years longer than in 1950–55), and for women it was 61.8, with 21.7 retirement years (8 years longer than in 1950–55) (Gendell, 2001). The lack of roles available to retirees is due in large part to the organization of social roles around work, which creates age segregation that allocates leisure roles to older adults and curtails other types of social engagement.

Recent policy changes are reorganizing work by recognizing the existing variation in retirement age among recent cohorts, which has opened up more opportunities for older adults to stay in the workforce. For example, the Senior Citizens' Freedom to Work Act of 2000 eliminated the Social Security annual earnings test for older adults who are at or past full retirement age. This means that the Social Security benefits received by older adults who are at full retirement age are not reduced when they have earnings from paid employment. The 1983 Social Security Amendments, which included a provision for increasing the full retirement age from 65 for cohorts born before 1938 to 67 for cohorts born in 1960 or later, is another example of a policy change that promotes labor-force participation among older adults. A final set of incentives within the Social Security system for adults continuing to work are policies that reduce the benefit for retiring early (i.e., between age 62 and the full retirement age); provide delayed retirement credit, in which the benefit is increased (between 3% and 8%, depending on one's birth cohort) for each year retirement is delayed up to age 69; and include earnings past the full retirement age in the benefit formula calculation, which can increase the Social Security benefit (see www.ssa.gov for details regarding these policies).

However, many policies continue to support traditional notions of work as an activity that is pursued primarily by middle-aged adults. These policies discourage substantial paid employment among older adults by providing disincentives to work. Examples include the Social Security earnings test that is applied to individuals who retire before the full retirement age (which reduces the benefit that is received if employment earnings exceed an annual limit; in 2008 that limit was $13,560 for the years before the full retirement age and $36,120 for the year full retirement age is attained) and taxing Social Security benefits when total income exceeds a minimum threshold (in 2008 the threshold was $25,000 for individual returns and $32,000 for joint returns). In addition, there are few policies that explicitly encourage engagement in non-work-related roles. One notable exception is the community-based programs funded by the Older Americans Act. But chronic underfunding of those programs limits their availability, particularly to middle- and upper-income older adults (Gelfand, 2006).

Policies that generate incentives to work and promote nonwork role options in later life, such as providing tax incentives to companies that permit workers to establish flexible hours or allowing older adults to claim continuing education costs as tax deductions, would promote age integration. This would enable older adults to stay engaged longer and use the additional years of life to make meaningful contributions to society. In an age-integrated society, older adults would not be caught in a roleless role because they would have access to more opportunities to participate in society.

Later-Life Financial Security for Working Women

In many respects, public policy related to the U.S. pension system is out of sync with the lived experience of many women and their families. This structural lag is the product of policies that do not recognize or address the variation across women regarding the time allocated to educational, work, and family roles. The Social Security program is based on the one-breadwinner model that privileges married couples in which one spouse—usually the male—is employed. Yet the traditional U.S. family (i.e., a married-couple family with only the male working in the labor force) is increasingly rare, due to the demographic trends that were previously discussed. Consequently, an increasing proportion of women are *dually entitled* to Social Security, on the basis of their own earnings records and the earnings records of their husbands (Street and Wilmoth, 2001). Dually entitled women's Social Security benefits are based on the spouse's average lifetime earnings that produces a higher benefit. Given the persistent gender wage gap and time spent out of the labor force due to care work, women who are dually entitled typically receive Social Security benefits that are based on their husband's earning record (because the 50% benefit based on the husband's earnings record is larger than the 100% benefit based on the wife's earnings history). These women are essentially receiving the exact same benefit that they would have received if they had never worked (and never made FICA contributions to Social Security).

In addition to these issues related to dual entitlement, it is important to note that a growing proportion of women will qualify for Social Security benefits solely on the basis of their own earnings. This is particularly true for African American women, whose declining marriage rates mean fewer of them will be able to meet the eligibility criteria for receiving spousal benefits, which is being currently married or having had a ten-year marriage (Harrington Meyer, Wolf, and Himes, 2005). Women who qualify for Social Security on their own earning records are likely to receive fewer benefits than men with comparable work histories, due to wage discrimination. One might argue that these women can compensate by participating in private pension plans. However, lower wages decrease the likelihood that an employee will participate in defined-contribution pension plans and tax-deferred retirement savings plans. Despite the increasing popularity of defined-contribution plans among employers, particularly in industries dominated by women, few women participate in these plans, and the women who do participate tend to make lower contributions and are more risk averse (O'Rand, 2001). Consequently, a smaller percentage of women receive occupational pensions than men and, among those who receive some income from occupational pensions, women receive a lower amount than men. These dynamics place women, particularly minority women, at substantial risk of financial insecurity in later life.

One way to alleviate this structural lag is to change the basis for qualifying for and calculating benefits received from the public pension system, so that changes in the U.S. family are taken into account and women's undervalued and unpaid contributions to society are recognized. For example, the minimum number of years one needs to be married to qualify for spousal benefits could be reduced. Similarly, the 35 best years of earnings that are used to calculate Social Security benefits could be reduced to the 30 or 25 best years. This would eliminate multiple zero earnings years that many women have because of time out of the labor force due to child care. Other options would be to eliminate zero (or low) earning years if they are spent pursuing higher education, or to alter replacement rates so that low-income workers receive even higher replacement rates. Such policy changes would make the formula for calculating Social Security benefits more responsive to the lived experiences of current and future female cohorts.

Health Care among Racial and Ethnic Minorities

The structural lag between the health needs of older minority adults and the programs and services that are designed to meet those needs has historical roots in the segregated health care that existed prior to the civil rights movement. The legacy of this legal health care segregation and discrimination continues in a de facto form through the separate and unequal tiers of the health care system, which relegates Native Americans, African Americans, and many immigrant groups to lower tiers with poorer-quality services and worse health outcomes (Smedley et al., 2002).

There is ample evidence that, compared with non-Hispanic whites, African Americans, and Hispanic Americans have higher rates of disease and disability but are less likely to use health care services (Smedley et al., 2002). Financial barriers to access, including higher rates of being uninsured among minorities (Barnes and Schiller, 2006), contribute to the lower rate of health care use. The one exception to the general lower use of health care services among minorities is nursing home use, which is likely due to Medicare and Medicaid coverage of nursing home stays. Nursing homes lagged behind other health care sectors in providing services to minorities because they were insulated from civil rights enforcement until Medicare and Medicaid were enacted. Despite this, by 2000 the rates of nursing home use among African Americans were higher than among whites, although disparities in the quality of nursing homes used by African Americans and whites continue to exist (Smith et al., 2008).

In terms of general health care use, studies based on populations covered by Medicare and Medicaid suggest that enrollment in managed care can reduce racial disparities in the use of health care (Balsa, Cao, and McGuire, 2007; Le Cook, 2007). However, the evidence is mixed regarding whether managed care improves the quality of care received by, or health outcomes among, minorities. Research suggests that the performance of health care organizations in serving minority populations could be further enhanced by initiating comprehensive policies that encourage cultural competency training for health care providers and staff, reduce administrative and linguistic barriers, offer targeted educational programs about the importance of routine preventative care and the role of patients as active participants in the care process, and establish best-practice programs for the conditions that disproportionately affect minorities (Langwell and Moser, 2002; Smedley et al., 2002).

Improving access to and the quality of health services received by minority groups will help reduce racial and ethnic disparities in health outcomes. The federal government and other nonfederal organizations have initiated various programs and collaborations to address these health disparities (see appendix C in Smedley et al., 2002, for a detailed discussion). Nonetheless, this structural lag is likely to continue and perhaps magnify as the older population grows in size and diversity. Increased demand for health programs and services may reinforce existing barriers to access if the supply is not expanded, and the quality of the services received may be inadequate if the unique circumstances of minority populations are not taken into account during health care program planning and implementation.

Challenges of Designing Policy Reforms to Alleviate Structural Lag

The previous discussion demonstrates how certain aspects of policy are not consistent with the lived experiences of many Americans, creating the structural lag that limits access to opportunity structures in ways that increase social, economic, and health inequalities among older adults. It also points to the importance of altering policy to alleviate structural lag and maximize access to opportunities across the life course. But what is the best approach for altering old age policy? This chapter has argued that altering public policy to be more responsive to the changing demographic characteristics of, and the resulting social dynamics in, the population is crucial not only to alleviating structural lag experienced by specific groups, but also to ensuring that public funds are spent on programs that will benefit all segments of society.

The demographic and social pressures to strengthen public and private sector programs for older adults come at a time when support for social insurance programs has been waning. Over the past thirty years, the burden of risk for life's uncertainties has been shifting from the federal government to state and local governments, from public sector to private sector institutions, and from institutions to individuals (Harrington Meyer, 2005; Hacker, 2006). In this climate, policies that take a micro-level approach, which focuses on individual solutions that place the burden on risk on individuals and their families, are politically popular. However, such policies are not as effective in alleviating structural lag, because ultimately structural lag is grounded in macro-level processes. Given this, macro-level solutions—which aim to alter social institutions through a mix of programs that place the burden of risk primarily on the governmental and corporate sectors—are necessary.

In crafting macro-level solutions, policy makers need to consider a broader range of issues than are typically discussed in public discourse. Simply responding to the projected increase in the older adult population is not an adequate approach. The various demographic and social trends that are creating structural lag, and the challenges of designing policy reforms that will effectively alleviate that lag for various segments of the population, must also be considered.

One such challenge is recognizing that policy changes aimed at a given age group can have substantially different implications for individuals within that group, depending on their social location. For example, longer life expectancy had placed added pressure on social insurance programs like Social Security. This pressure could be reduced by increasing the minimum age for receiving early Social Security benefits from 62 to 65 and raising the age for receipt of full Social Security benefits beyond the scheduled increase to age 67. However, given that there are substantial differences in life expectancy across race, ethnicity, gender, and social class, such changes in Social Security policy would further disadvantage portions of the older adult population.

A second challenge is being able to identify the intergenerational repercussions of various policy reforms. For example, in response to recent changes in the U.S. family, one might advocate for policies that provide more support for dual-earner couples in midlife, such as providing expanded family leave benefits and subsidized child care programs that are comparable to other developed countries. Such policies would facilitate women's labor force participation and could potentially generate a higher proportion of women who are dually entitled to Social Security or entitled to those benefits on the basis of their own earnings records. However, in the absence of changes to the formula for calculating Social Security benefits and expanded tax incentives for retirement savings, these women would likely experience compromised financial security in later life. As this example demonstrates, policy designed to minimize structural lag for one age group could lead to worsening conditions for another age group.

A final challenge is that making public policy more responsive to demographic and social trends could exacerbate solvency issues, at least in the short term. A prime example of this would be implementing more flexible policies that reflect the reality of U.S. families, such as lowering the number of years one must be married to an individual to qualify for the receipt of Social Security benefits on the basis of his or her earnings record; allowing individuals in civil unions to qualify for benefits based on the earnings record of a domestic partner; setting a cap on the number of zero earning years that can be used to calculate Social Security benefits; and establishing a standard care work credit so that the benefit amounts for family care providers are not discounted due to time spent out of the paid labor force. Such policies would minimize the structural lag experienced by members of U.S. families, but they would also increase the costs of public programs because these reforms involve expanding coverage and benefits. Thus policy makers have to strike a balance between the social necessity of eliminating outdated policies and the fiscal viability of proposals that alleviate structural lag.

Ultimately, given current economic conditions, policy makers' concerns about the fiscal implications of these demographic and social trends are likely to trump the desire to alleviate the structural lag that is created by these trends. The Congressional Budget Office (2005, 2008) projects that by 2035, Social Security spending will represent more than 6 percent of the gross domestic product (GDP). Similarly, spending on Medicare and Medicaid could increase to anywhere from 6 percent to almost 15 percent of the GDP, depending on assumptions about the growth in medical costs per beneficiary. However, it is not clear how these projections will be influenced by the recent recession that sent shock waves throughout the U.S. and world economies.

The best course of action for addressing these projected fiscal demands is difficult to determine, due to a variety of factors. The first of those factors is the political climate, which is shaped by the political party that holds key government offices, the efforts of lobbying groups, and grassroots action on the part of citizens. Shifts in political power have a profound effect on the course of public policy, even in the face of pressing demographic and economic concerns (for example, see Rothman's [2001] discussion of national health care). The second unpredictable factor is the projected characteristics of the population, because the range of potential demographic outcomes is much wider than is suggested by the middle-series projections that are typically cited. The extent of the fiscal pressure generated by the aging of the U.S. population will depend on future trends in fertility, mortality, morbidity, and migration (Lee and Skinner, 1999; Lee, 2000). The third unpredictable factor is economic growth, which has been seriously undermined by the recent economic recession. Even under the best-case scenario, economic growth alone is unlikely to resolve the nation's fiscal imbalances over the long term (Congressional Budget Office, 2003). Therefore, the nation faces difficult policy choices regarding government expenditures and sources of revenue.

Conclusion

Despite these challenges in determining the best course of action for old age policy reforms, it is imperative that action be taken sooner rather than later. Delaying any action is tempting when there are so many pressing fiscal concerns. But delayed action is likely to force larger cuts in spending and/or more substantial tax increases, inhibit the government's ability to deal with future events (e.g., war, economic recession), and make it more difficult for individuals to plan for policy changes (Congressional Budget Office, 2003). It could also increase the burden placed on younger generations in correcting the impending fiscal imbalance and exacerbate gender, racial, and socioeconomic disparities among future cohorts. Therefore, taking early action to develop macro-level reforms that are responsive to recent demographic and social trends—and mindful of issues related to structural lag—will minimize the impact of policy changes while maximizing potential beneficial outcomes, which include enhancing the ability of social institutions to effectively meet the basic needs of society and improving the well-being of all segments of society.

Acknowledgments

Part of this chapter, in an earlier form, appeared as Janet Wilmoth and Charles Longino, 2006, Demographic trends that will shape U.S. policy in the 21st century, *Research on Aging* 28 (3): 269–88. Available online at http://roa.sagepub.com/cgi/reprint/28/3/269/.

References

Administration on Aging. 2009. A statistical profile of Hispanic older Americans aged 65+. www.aoa.gov/AoARoot/Aging_Statistics/Minority_Aging/Facts-on-Hispanic-Elderly-2008.aspx [retrieved September 18, 2009].

Balsa, A. I., Z. Cao, and T. G. McGuire. 2007. Does managed health care reduce health care disparities between minorities and whites? *Journal of Health Economics* 26 (1): 101–21.

Barnes, P., and J. S. Schiller. 2007. Early release of selected estimates based on data from the 2006 National Health Interview Survey (June). www .cdc.gov/nchs/nhis/released200706.htm.

Budig, M., and P. England. 2001. The wage penalty for motherhood. *American Sociological Review* 66 (2): 204–25.

Burgess, E. W. (ed.). 1960. *Aging in Western Societies*. Chicago: University of Chicago Press.

Center on an Aging Society. 2003. *Obesity among Older Americans: A Risk for Chronic Conditions*. Data Profile Series 2, No. 10. Washington, D.C.: Center on an Aging Society, Georgetown University.

Centers for Disease Control and Prevention. 2003. *[Health, United States, 2003:] Chartbook on Trends in the Health of Americans*. National Center for Health Statistics. www.cdc.gov/nchs/data/hus/hus03cht.pdf [retrieved April 6, 2004].

———. 2007. *Health, United States, 2007: With Chartbook on Trends in the Health of Americans*. National Center for Health Statistics. www .cdc.gov/nchs/data/hus/hus07.pdf#027 [retrieved January 29, 2009].

Clark, R., and J. Quinn. 2002. Patterns of work and retirement for a new century. *Generations* 26 (2): 17–24.

Congressional Budget Office. 2003. *The Long-Term Budget Outlook*. www.cbo.gov/doc.cfm?index=4916/ [retrieved April 21, 2004].

———. 2005. *The Long-Term Budget Outlook*. www.cbo.gov/doc.cfm? index=6982/ [retrieved February 6, 2009].

———. 2008. *Updated Long-Term Projects for Social Security*. www.cbo .gov/ftpdocs/96xx/doc9649/08-20-SocialSecurityUpdate.pdf [retrieved February 6, 2009].

Costa, D. 1998. *The Evolution of Retirement*. Chicago: University of Chicago Press.

Crimmins, E., M. Hayward, and Y. Saito. 1996. Differentials in active life expectancy in the older population of the United States. *Journals of Gerontology, Series B: Social Sciences* 51 (3): S111–20.

DiNatale, M., and S. Boraas. 2002. The labor force experience of women from 'Generation X.' *Monthly Labor Review* 125 (3): 3–15.

Federal Interagency Forum on Aging-Related Statistics. 2008. *Older Americans, 2008: Key Indicators of Well-Being*. Washington, D.C.: U.S. Government Printing Office.

Foner, A. 1994. Endnote: The reach of an idea. Pp. 263–80 in M. W. Riley, R. L. Kahn, and A. Foner (eds.), *Age and Structural Lag*. New York: Wiley.

Freedman, V., L. Martin, and R. Schoeni. 2002. Recent trends in disability and functioning among older adults in the United States: A systematic review. *JAMA: Journal of the American Medical Association* 288 (24): 3137–46.

Friedland, R., and L. Summer. 1999. *Demography Is Not Destiny*. Washington, D.C.: National Academy on an Aging Society.

Gelfand, D. E. 2006. *The Aging Network: Programs and Services*, 6th ed. New York: Springer.

Gendell, M. 2001. Retirement age declines again in the 1990s. *Monthly Labor Review* 124 (10): 12–21.

Gendell, M., and J. Siegel. 1996. Trends in retirement age in the United States, 1955–1993, by sex and race. *Journals of Gerontology, Series B: Social Sciences* 51 (3): S132–39.

Geronimus, A., J. Bound, T. Waidmann, C. Colen, and D. Steffick. 2001. Inequality in life expectancy, functional status, and active life expectancy across selected black and white populations in the United States. *Demography* 38 (2): 227–51.

Hacker, J. 2006. *The Great Risk Shift: The Assault on American Jobs, Families, Health Care, and Retirement—and How You Can Fight Back*. New York: Oxford University Press.

Harrington Meyer, M. 2005. Decreasing welfare, increasing old age inequality: Whose responsibility is it? Pp. 65–89 in R. B. Hudson (ed.), *The New Politics of Old Age Policy*. Baltimore: Johns Hopkins University Press.

Harrington Meyer, M., D. A. Wolf, and C. L. Himes. 2005. Linking benefits to marital status: Race and Social Security in the U.S. *Feminist Economics* 11 (2): 145–62.

Hayward, M. D., and M. Heron. 1999. Racial inequality in active life among adult Americans. *Demography* 36 (1): 77–91.

Heck, K., K. Schoendoft, S. Ventura, and J. Kiely. 1997. Delayed childbearing by education level in the United States, 1964–1994. *Maternal and Child Health Journal* 1 (2): 81–88.

Himes, C. 2000. Obesity, disease, and functional limitation in later life. *Demography* 37 (1): 73–82.

———. 2001. *Elderly Americans*. Population Bulletin 56, No. 4. Washington, D.C.: Population Reference Bureau.

Hudson, R. B. 2005. Contemporary challenges to age-based policy. Pp. 1–22 in R. B. Hudson (ed.), *The New Politics of Old Age Policy*. Baltimore: Johns Hopkins University Press.

Kent, M. M., and M. Mather. 2002. *What Drives U.S. Population Growth?* Population Bulletin 57, No. 4. Washington, D.C.: Population Reference Bureau.

Kohli, M. 1986. Social organization and subject construction of the life course. Pp. 271–92 in A. B. Sorsense, F. E. Weinert, and L. R. Sherrod (eds.), *Human Development and the Life Course: Multidisciplinary Perspectives.* Hillsdale, N.J.: Lawrence Erlbaum Associates.

Kotlikoff, L. 1996. Generational accounting. *Public Policy and Aging Report* 7 (4): 4–6, 17.

Langwell, K. M., and J. W. Moser. 2002. Strategies for Medicare health plans serving racial and ethnic minorities. *Health Care Financing Review* 23 (4): 131–47.

Le Cook, B. 2007. Effect of Medicaid managed care on racial disparities in health care access. *Health Services Research* 42 (1): 124–45.

Lee, R. 2000. Long-term population projections and the U.S. Social Security system. *Population Development and Review* 26 (1): 137–44.

Lee, R., and J. Skinner. 1999. Will aging baby boomers bust the federal budget? *Journal of Economic Perspectives* 13 (1): 117–40.

Manton, K., and E. Stallard. 1991. Cross-sectional estimates of active life expectancy for U.S. elderly and oldest old populations. *Journal of Gerontology* 46 (3): S170–82.

Merton, R. K. 1957 [1968]. Continuities in the theory of social structure and anomie. Pp. 215–48 in R. K. Merton, *Social Theory and Social Structure.* New York: Free Press.

———. 1995. Opportunity structure: The emergence, diffusion, and differentiation of a sociological concept. Pp. 3–78 in F. Adler and W. S. Laufer (eds.), *The Legacy of Anomie Theory.* Advances in Criminological Theory 6. New Brunswick, N.J.: Transaction.

National Vital Statistics Reports. 2004. Table 12. Estimated life expectancy at birth in years, by race and sex. www.cdc.gov/nchs/data/dvs/nvsr52_14t12.pdf [retrieved April 6, 2004].

O'Rand, A. 2001. Perpetuating women's disadvantage: Trends in U.S. private pensions, 1976–1995. Pp. 142–57 in J. Ginn, D. Street, and S. Arber (eds.), *Women, Work and Pensions: International Issues and Prospects.* Philadelphia: Open University Press.

———. 2005. When old age begins: Implications for health, work, and retirement. Pp. 109–128 in R. B. Hudson (ed.), *The New Politics of Old Age Policy.* Baltimore: Johns Hopkins University Press.

Peeters, A., J. Barendregt, F. Willekens, J. Mackenbach, A. A. Mamun, and L. Bonneux. 2003. Obesity in adulthood and its consequences for life expectancy: A life table analysis. *Annals of Internal Medicine* 138 (1): 24–32.

Population Reference Bureau. 2003. Traditional families account for only 7 percent of U.S. households. www.prb.org/Articles/2003/TraditionalFamiliesAccountforOnly7PercentofUSHouseholds.aspx [retrieved April 9, 2004].

Preston, S. 1984. Children and the elderly: Divergent paths for American's dependents. *Demography* 21 (4): 435–57.

Purcell, P. 2007. *Older Workers: Employment and Retirement Trends.* CRS Report for Congress. Washington, D.C.: Congressional Research Service, Library of Congress.

Riley, M. W. 1971. Social gerontology and the age stratification of society. *Gerontologist* 11 (1): 29–87.

———. 1987. On the significance of age in sociology. *American Sociological Review* 52 (1): 1–14.

Riley, M. W., A. Foner, M. E. Moore, B. Hess, and B. L. Roth. 1968. *An Inventory of Research Findings.* Vol. 1 of *Aging and Society.* New York: Russell Sage Foundation.

Riley, M. W., A. Foner, and J. Waring. 1988. Sociology of age. Pp. 243–90 in N. Smelser (ed.), *Handbook of Sociology.* Newbury Park, Calif.: Sage Publications.

Riley, M. W., M. Johnson, and A. Foner. 1972. *A Sociology of Age Stratification.* Vol. 3 of *Aging and Society.* New York: Russell Sage Foundation.

Riley, M. W., R. L. Kahn, and A. Foner (eds.). 1994. *Age and Structural Lag: Society's Failure to Provide Meaningful Opportunities in Work, Family, and Leisure.* New York: Wiley.

Riley, M. W., and J. W. Riley, Jr. 1994. Structural lag: Past and future. Pp. 15–36 in M. W. Riley, R. L. Kahn, and A. Foner (eds.), *Age and Structural Lag.* New York: Wiley.

Rothman, O. 2001. A century of failure: Health care reform in America. Pp. 266–74 in P. Conrad (ed.), *The Sociology of Health and Illness: Critical Perspectives,* 6th ed. New York: Worth.

Settersten, R. A., Jr. 1999. *Lives in Time and Place: The Problems and Promises of Developmental Science.* Amityville, N.Y.: Baywood.

Sloane, P., S. Zimmerman, C. Suchindran, P. Reed, L. Wang, M. Boustani, and S. Sudha. 2002. The public health impact of Alzheimer's disease, 2000–2050: Potential implication of treatment advances. *Annual Review of Public Health* 23: 213–31.

Smedley, B. D., A. Y. Stith, A. R. Nelson, and Institute of Medicine Committee on Understanding and Eliminating Racial and Ethnic Disparities in Health Care. 2002. *Unequal Treatment: Confronting Racial and Ethnic Disparities in Health Care.* Washington, D.C.: Institute of Medicine.

Smetters, K., and J. Gokhale. 2004. *Fiscal and Generational Imbalances: New Budget Measures for New Budget Priorities.* Washington, D.C.: AEI Press.

Smith, D. B., Z. L. Feng, M. L. Fennell, J. Zinn, and V. Mor. 2008. Racial disparities in access to long-term care: The illusive pursuit of equity. *Journal of Health Politics and Law* 33 (5): 861–81.

Street, D., and J. Wilmoth. 2001. Social insecurity? Women and pensions in the United States. Pp. 20–141 in J. Ginn, D. Street, and S. Arber (eds.), *Women, Work, and Pensions*. Philadelphia: Open University Press.

Treas, J., and E. Widmer. 2000. Married women's employment over the life course: Attitudes in cross-national perspective. *Social Forces* 78 (4): 1409–36.

U.S. Bureau of the Census. 2000. *Projections of the Total Resident Population by 5-Year Age Groups, Race, and Hispanic Origin with Special Age Categories: Middle Series, 1999 to 2070*. www.census.gov/population/www/projections/natsum-T3.html [retrieved April 8, 2004].

———. 2002. Table 3. Poverty status of people, by age, race, and Hispanic origin: 1959–2002. www.census.gov/hhes/www/poverty/histpov/hstpov3.html [retrieved April 9, 2004].

———. 2003a. Table MS-1: Marital status of the population age 15 and over, by sex and race; 1950 to present. www.census.gov/population/socdemo/hh-fam/tabMS-1.pdf [retrieved April 9, 2004].

———. 2003b. Table MS-2: Estimated median age at first marriage, by sex; 1890 to present. www.census.gov/population/socdemo/hh-fam/tabMS-2.xls [retrieved April 9, 2004].

———. 2008. Table P-10 (a, b, c, and d): Age—people (both sexes combined) by median and mean income: 1974 to 2008. www.census.gov/hhes/www/income/histinc/incpertoc.html [retrieved September 18, 2009].

U.S. Bureau of Labor Statistics. 2001. *Highlights of Women's Earnings in 2000*. Report 952. www.bls.gov/cps/cpswom2000.pdf [retrieved April 2, 2004].

U.S. Citizenship and Immigration Services. 2004. *Fiscal Year 2001 Statistical Yearbook*. www.dhs.gov/files/statistics/publications/archive.shtm [retrieved April 9, 2004].

U.S. Immigration and Naturalization Service. 1993. *Statistical Yearbook of the Immigration and Naturalization Service*. Washington, D.C.: U.S. Immigration and Naturalization Service.

Utendorf, K. 2002. The upper part of the earnings distribution in the United States: How has it changed? *Social Security Bulletin* 64 (3): 1–11.

Ventura, S., and C. Bachrach. 2000. *Nonmarital Childbearing in the United States, 1940–99*. National Vital Statistics Reports, Vol. 48, No. 16 (revised). Hyattsville, Md.: Centers for Disease Control and Prevention, National Center for Health Statistics. www.cdc.gov/nchs/data/nvsr/nvsr48/nvs48_16.pdf.

4. What Justice Requires
Normative Foundations for U.S. Pension Reform
John Myles, Ph.D.

It is hardly surprising that retirement systems designed under conditions of high fertility and sustained growth in the labor force might require some serious tweaking once those conditions have disappeared. Prudence suggests that we should do something about the social policy legacy we leave to our children now that we are having so few of them. But because there is much uncertainty about the imputed second-order effects of population aging on both the economy (what will happen to wages, prices, and capital markets?) and the polity (will retirees really control the political agenda?), even the most socially responsible reformer risks doing too much as well as too little. So what is to be done?

Schokkaert and Van Parijs (2003) propose a noncontroversial starting point: a minimal requirement of intergenerational justice is that we leave future generations a stock of physical, human, and environmental capital at least as valuable as the one at our disposal. But our legacy to future generations also includes the real welfare gains embedded in the social institutions inherited from the past. As Schokkaert and Van Parijs highlight, our income security systems for both the old and the young are among these institutions: the traditional family structure in which parents care for children when they are too young to work and children support their parents when they are too old and frail to work are important characteristics of the human species, probably with deep biological roots. Contemporary historiography (Haber and Gratton, 1994) confirms that the emergence of mandatory public pensions were as important for the children of the elderly as for the elderly themselves, a form of risk-sharing not only against the risk of one's *own* longevity but also against the risk of *one's parents'* longevity and the imperative of supporting parents financially through an extended old age. For a species motivated by filial piety, old age insurance is also insurance for the young. Rising Social Security costs may lead our children to complain about high taxes or to ask us to retire later. It is unlikely, however, that they will be grateful if we expose them to the risk of supporting us directly to the age of 95. Just as intergenerational justice requires us to leave them with a sustainable environment, it also requires us to leave them with sustainable pension systems at least as good as those we have had to care for our parents in their old age.

My goal in this chapter is to identify reform strategies that satisfy standards of both intergenerational equity *between* workers and retirees and intragenerational justice *among* workers and retirees. To deal with intergenerational equity, I advocate an expanded variant of the *Musgrave rule* elaborated by Richard Musgrave at the beginning of the 1980s (Musgrave, 1986). The idea is simple: fair or proportional sharing *between* workers and retirees of the *additional* retirement costs that result from demographic change. Unlike Musgrave, however, whose main concern was the political viability of public pay-as-you-go pension schemes, I conclude that satisfying the principle of intergenerational equity requires application of the rule to both sides of the retirement income ledger, to private as well as to public pensions. With respect to intragenerational justice, I begin from a normative position that is broadly Rawlsian in inspiration—changes to the status quo should be of most advantage to the least advantaged—and propose two complementary strategies inside public sector schemes: greater reliance on interpersonal transfers, on the one hand, and, on the other, a shift from payroll taxes toward greater reliance on general revenue financing in public sector plans.

The origins of this discussion lie in earlier work written mainly for a European audience.[1] Unlike the United States, large-scale pension reforms have been commonplace in Europe since the 1980s, and my comments were written in part as a reflection on these reforms. I do not pretend to have worked out all of the implications of these proposals for the very different institutional environment of the U.S. retirement system. Lest they appear utopian (i.e., normatively desirable but practically unfeasible) within the U.S. context, however, I hasten to add that the strategies advocated here are not presented as proposals for an instantaneous grand redesign of existing institutions, but as guidelines, or *litmus tests*, against which *particular* reforms introduced incrementally can be evaluated. Pension reform in the United States, though hotly contested for several decades now, still gives no clear indication of its likely destination. My purpose here is an effort to highlight some of the normative implications—what justice requires—of alternative pathways toward that destination. Some of the flaws I perceive on both sides of the U.S. debate are taken up in the conclusion.

The Economics of Population Aging: Three Dilemmas in Search of Solutions

Following Thompson (1998), we can highlight the problems facing societies with aging populations with a simple accounting identity. The economic cost of supporting the retired population is simply the fraction of each year's economic activity given over to supplying the goods and services the retired consume or:

$$\text{Cost of Supporting the Retired} = \frac{\text{Consumption of the Retired}}{\text{Total National Production}}$$

which in turn, following Hicks, can be written as:[2]

$$\text{Cost of Supporting the Retired} = \frac{\text{Number of retirees}}{\text{Number of employees}} \times \frac{\text{Average consumption of retirees}}{\text{Average production per employee}}$$

Assuming all else remains fixed, population aging raises total retirement costs. A 10 percent increase in the ratio of retirees to workers results in a 10 percent increase in the cost of supporting the retired. Higher retirement costs are not a problem per se. In a stable population (with no population aging), we might expect future generations to behave much like earlier ones and take some of the gains that result from higher productivity (the *wealth effect*) in the form of more retirement. Population aging, however, acts as a *multiplier*, raising the cost for the same amount of leisure over each person's life course.

Cost shifting to the private sector does not change this scenario per se.[3] Public and private pensions are simply alternative ways for working-age individuals to register a claim on future production (Barr, 2001). The share of total consumption by the retired rises, irrespective of whether it is financed with state pensions or with investment returns from bonds and equities. Indeed, as Thompson (1998) observes, proposals to shift toward group or personal advance-funded accounts are often made on the grounds that retirees will receive higher returns from their contributions. If this turns out to be true, the effect of change will be to *raise* future retirement costs.

The most obvious strategy is an extension of the working life. Simulations for a stylized OECD country (Organisation for Economic Cooperation and Development, 2001) indicate that the impact of a *5 percent reduction* in the number of beneficiaries—equivalent to an effective increase of 10 months in the average retirement age—is equivalent to a *10 percent reduction* in average retirement benefits. The reason for the difference can be understood by referring to the accounting equation introduced above. An increase in the retirement age changes both the numerator and the denominator of the retiree/employee ratio. A reduction in benefits affects only the numerator of the ratio between the average consumption of the retired and average productivity per worker. The combination of more work among young and old alike would, in the abstract, also conform to a basic standard of intergenerational equity, according to Musgrave's principle to fixed proportional shares (see below). Finally, the potential welfare loss that might otherwise result from a longer working life will be offset, on average, by increased longevity. Because people are (and will be) living longer, *more* working years does not mean *fewer* retirement years.

Policy makers, however, face a formidable political obstacle to implementing later retirement ages. Most workers in most countries look forward to retirement, and raising the age of eligibility for retirement benefits is among the least popular reform options. Because the relevant policy lever is not the normal retirement age (age 65 or 67), but the age at which retirement benefits can first be accessed (62 for Social Security), such a strategy raises difficult equity issues (discussed below) and posits regulation of the age at which private as well as public retirement wealth can be accessed (Myles, 2002). Later retirement is likely to be part of the solution, especially given anticipated increases in labor demand, but it is unlikely to be the whole solution.

Another strategy is to leave the problem of cost allocation to markets and families.[4] In a totally privatized system based on advance funding and other personal assets, the business cycle and changes in the demand for labor and capital that are uniquely attributable to population aging would solve the problem of cost allocation by producing lucky and less-lucky generations (Thompson, 1998). Some cohorts and individuals would benefit from favorable wage histories and returns on their capital and so be in a position to retire early in relative comfort. Other cohorts and individuals would be less fortunate and would be required to work longer to avoid an impoverished retirement. Families would decide about the intergenerational transmission of wealth so that (perversely), *within* generations, children from wealthy families and with few siblings would be the winners.

For most nations, however, relinquishing the problem of cost allocation to markets and families is not a feasible option for both political and economic reasons and, hence, is utopian. Even if one believes such a choice to be desirable, it is simply not on the menu of feasible options available to most countries, because they are not starting from a tabula rasa.[5] The possible choices available today are, in the jargon of political economy, *path dependent*, constrained by choices made in the past. For example, because of the high transition costs associated with moving from a mature pay-as-you-go to a private advance-funded design, the public pension systems now in place will endure well into the future, so policy makers have no option but to make choices about cost allocation. Even in the absence of this economic constraint, however, the past decade has shown that popular support for established retirement income programs is both broad and deep, so truly radical reform of this sort faces an equally daunting political constraint (Myles and Pierson, 2001).

There are also sound normative reasons for a public role in allocating the transition costs arising from changes in population structure. The rising retirement costs produced by the current baby dearth and increased longevity are a collective risk, like other exogenous shocks (e.g., natural disasters, recessions), and hence an appropriate target for intercohort risk sharing. Sinn (2000) raises an alternative possibility: cohorts that have reduced their fertility, and hence are the "cause" of the problem, should be held accountable for their fertility behavior and have their pensions reduced accordingly. In philosophy, the logical form of this argument is known as the problem of the *any* and the *all* (Hernes, 1976). Fertility rates, like prices, are aggregative outcomes that depend on decisions made by *all* individuals but not on the decision of *any* particular individual.[6] Because only individuals, not collectivities (e.g., cohorts or generations), are moral agents, it is difficult ex post facto to sustain Sinn's claim and others that take this form.

To throw into relief the core issues facing policy makers, it is helpful to begin from an imaginary starting point—a useful fiction—in which all of the consumption of the retired (including health care and other service costs) comes from pensions financed from payroll taxes on the wages of the nonretired, assumptions that can be relaxed once the main elements of the story are in place.

Intergenerational Equity and the Musgrave Rule

Following Musgrave (1986),[7] the challenge facing policy makers in pay-as-you-go systems is, first, an intergenerational dilemma that can be illustrated by contrasting two ideal/typical pay-as-you-go designs. In the standard defined-benefit model with a fixed replacement rate (FRR) common to the majority of developed countries, retirees are entitled to a given fraction of their earnings in the form of benefits plus an adjustment factor to reflect productivity gains and higher wages in the subsequent generation. When the ratio of retirees to workers changes, workers must adjust their contribution rates accordingly. In effect, benefits drive taxes (so that taxes are the dependent variable) and *all of the costs associated with demographic change fall on contributors and their dependants.*

An alternative to a fixed replacement rate is a pay-as-you-go design based on a fixed contribution rate (FCR).[8] The working population is required to contribute a fixed fraction of its income for the support of retirees. In this design, taxes drive benefits, so that benefits are the dependent variable. As the ratio of retirees to workers rises, benefits must decline and *all of the costs associated with demographic change fall on retirees.* Traditionally, U.S. Social Security has been based on the FRR design. A decision to freeze current contribution rates and allow benefits to fall proportionately would produce a de facto shift to the FCR model.

How might a three-generation household faced with the prospect of demographic aging but committed to intergenerational risk-sharing resolve this dilemma? Assuming they are satisfied with the status quo (i.e., current consumption levels of the generations relative to one another are neither too high or too low), the solution would undoubtedly approximate the fixed ratio or fixed relative position (FRP) model advocated by Musgrave (1986, chapter 7).[9] Contributions and benefits are set so as to *hold constant* the ratio of per capita earnings of those in the working population (net of contributions) to the per capita benefits (net of taxes) of retirees. Once the ratio is fixed, the tax rate is adjusted periodically to reflect both population and productivity changes. Both it and the fixed contribution method obviate the need for projections but, in addition, the FRP model allows for a proportional sharing of risk. As the population ages, the tax rate rises but benefits fall, so that both parties "lose" at the same rate (i.e., both net earnings and benefits rise more slowly than they would in the absence of population aging).[10]

The FRP principle says nothing about what the relative position of retirees to workers and their dependants *should* be. It simply provides a rule for allocating the *additional* costs of demographic change between generations once an acceptable ratio is established.[11] From the perspective of a multigenerational household facing the prospect of fewer workers and more retirees in the near future, it reflects a joint commitment to maintaining the status quo in relative terms. In the same way that pension benefits are usually indexed so that wages and benefits will rise together with increases in productivity, the Musgrave rule indexes *both* contributions *and* benefits to population aging.[12]

Our hypothetical three-generational household faces a *point-in-time* decision concerning the allocation of costs between generations already alive. Such a situation is close to the real-life political choices facing policy makers both now and in the future: should they raise payroll taxes on younger workers, reduce benefits for retired workers (or those about to retire), or some combination of the two? This perspective is useful because, in an important sense, all politics are point-in-time politics (i.e., in the hands of those currently alive). If payroll taxes rise significantly relative to pension benefits for retirees (the FRR solution), policy makers can anticipate the displeasure of workers and their employers. If, alternatively, real benefits are falling year after year relative to national living standards (the FCR solution), retirees and those near retirement will be unhappy.

If we shift our perspective from a point-in-time to a life-course framework, however, the case for the Musgrave rule is even more persuasive. What are the implications of the three designs from the point of view of the *entire* life course of cohorts born in the future, the legacy that we will leave to our children and grandchildren?

Under FCR, the living standards of future generations would be preserved during childhood and over their working years, but they would experience a sharp decline in living standards in retirement. Under FRR, in contrast, successive cohorts would experience declining living standards in childhood and during the working years but a relatively affluent old age. FRP, in contrast, effectively smoothes the change across the entire life course and maintains the status quo with respect to the lifetime distribution of income. In this respect, FRP is a conservative strategy based on the assumption that, on average, the lifetime distribution of income available to current generations should be preserved more or less intact into the future. Future generations may of course disagree with our judgments and conclude that they want a different allocation of income over the life course. It would seem presumptuous however, for the current generation to lock in future generations in advance by adopting either the FRC or the FRR design.[13]

The core of Musgrave's (1986) life-course argument, however, rests on practical, political grounds. His main rationale for the FRP model is based on the assumption that neither of the alternatives, FRR or FCR, are *politically* sustainable under conditions of population aging. They are based, in his terms, on an intergenerational contract that either cannot be kept or at least generates great uncertainty about its future. As opinion polls make clear, under the prevailing FRR model, young, working-age contributors are skeptical that future generations will continue to support a system in which the active population bears all of the retirement costs associated with population aging. The result is a sense of injustice and cynicism rampant among many young adults, the outcome of their being required to contribute to a system that "won't be there for me."

Under FRP, taxes/contributions will undoubtedly increase as a result of demographic aging, though less quickly than under the FRR design. Thus the FRP principle runs counter to the notion that a hard budget line should be established for contribution levels or that there is an upper ("acceptable") limit to tax levels associated with sound public finance. The assumption of an upper limit implies a level of taxation that will automatically trigger a general application of the FCR model ("no new taxes") in response to changes in the retirement dependency ratio. Thus far, empirical evidence and historical experience makes me skeptical, or at least agnostic, concerning claims that there are "natural" limits to taxation levels that can be known a priori. Consequently, I see no sound reason for locking in specific upper limits as long-term policy targets; such a determination should be left to future generations. As taken up below, however, I do think there is good reason for reconsidering the *mix* of taxes used to finance pay-as-you-go pension schemes.

In a dynamic context of change, fixed replacement (FRR), fixed contribution (FCR), and fixed relative position (FRP) can be thought of as alternative principles for the intergenerational allocation of the *change* in retirement costs attributable to changes in the retiree dependency ratio. Moreover, the choice of which principle is applied is a matter of degree. The choice is a normative one that will be determined via politics, and it is conceivable, perhaps even desirable, that the mix of choices might change over time in response to changing circumstances.[14] One reason for expecting future departures from the FRP principle is that *proportional* sharing measured in income terms does not guarantee *fair* sharing measured in terms of consumption. Proportional sharing may be unfair if there are large changes in the relative prices for essential goods and services consumed by the old and the young (e.g., long-term care versus education and training). Hence I advocate the Musgrave rule as a litmus test, not as an iron law. I propose the FRP principle as a benchmark, or litmus test, for intergenerational equity, in the sense that the burden of proof falls on the would-be reformer who would allocate the costs that result from demographic change in ways that depart from FRP.

Although application of the Musgrave rule is relatively straightforward in nations in which all or most of the consumption of retired people comes from pensions financed with payroll taxes on the wages of nonretired people, it is decidedly messier in mixed systems, such as the U.S., in which occupational plans and personal retirement accounts provide a large share of retirement income. As noted above, to satisfy the requirements of intergenerational equity and to bequeath a sustainable pension regime to the next generation, the Musgrave rule must be applied to the entire retirement budget, to the private as well as to the public (= *total social*) costs that result from demographic change. The important implication of this conclusion is that in mixed-pension regimes, where both public and private sources provide a large share of retirement income, the future share of public pensions in the retirement budget is indeterminate. Application of a Musgrave-like strategy means that whether or not total *public* expenditures should be allowed to rise or fall is contingent on future levels of retirement income from private retirement savings. Applying the Musgrave rule (or any other standard of intergenerational equity) to the increase in retirement costs that results from demographic change by reference to the public budget alone (e.g., for Social Security and Supplemental Security Income, or SSI) would, justifiably, erode any public trust in the policy process. Moreover, the favorable tax regime available to occupational plans and to personal retirement accounts clearly warrants that they, too, be charged with social goals.

Analytically, the major difficulty is to provide the appropriate accounting frameworks so that the intergenerational allocation of costs associated with any *specific* reform to either side of the public/private ledger (and their interaction) is transparent to the political process. A full accounting scheme of the allocation of retirement costs among working and retired populations also requires estimates of likely second-order behavioral response to policy changes. Thus when policy changes intended to induce greater personal saving for retirement are made, the intended (or probable) effect of such changes on the intergenerational allocation of retirement costs (including the possibility that retirement costs could rise) needs to be established.

Intragenerational Justice

As Wolfson et al. (1998) have shown, the enormous heterogeneity *within* generations (or cohorts) swamps differences between generations with respect to the distribution of winners and losers that result from population aging. The upshot is that the *intergenerational* dilemma is compounded by at least two *intragenerational* dilemmas, one among retirees (beneficiaries), and a second among the working-age population (contributors). The notion of justice adopted here is broadly Rawlsian in inspiration: changes to the status quo should be of most advantage to the least advantaged.

When Pension Systems Contract: Intragenerational
Justice among Retired People

The problem on the benefit side (i.e., among retired people) can be
highlighted by comparing a pension system that is expanding with
one that is contracting. Expansion/contraction can take two forms:
(1) an increase or decrease in the number of years of retirement; and
(2) an increase or decrease in the benefits received during retirement.
When retirement ages are falling, the social welfare gains in additional
leisure and free time tend to go disproportionately to the least well
off. An additional year of retirement, for example, represents a larger
proportional gain for someone with a 7-year life expectancy than for
someone with a 12-year life expectancy. But the reverse is also true:
an additional year of employment represents a proportionately greater
loss for those with shorter life expectancies. Raising the retirement age
for public sector benefits has the greatest effect on those without sufficient means to finance early retirement on their own and the least impact on those who do. Because health (e.g., life expectancy, disability)
and wealth tend to be correlated, the equity problem is compounded.

As with changes in retirement age, the more disadvantaged tend to
gain most when public pension benefits are expanding, because they
are less able or likely to provide income security for themselves. But,
conversely, they stand to lose the most when income security systems
are contracting. The standard result from studies of savings behavior is that the savings-to-permanent-income ratio rises with permanent income and does so in a sharply nonlinear fashion (Diamond
and Hausman, 1984). The implication is that behavioral response to
lower mandatory pensions will be a function of income level: low-
income families are less likely to compensate for this reduction with
more savings than high-income families. If a proportional share of the
costs of population aging is to be transferred to retirees, how can this
be done so that it does not fall disproportionately on the least advantaged among them?

Financing Pensions: Intragenerational
Justice among the Working Population

On the contribution side, pay-as-you-go pensions are financed with
a tax on wage income—the payroll tax—while income from capital

and transfers are exempt.[15] The payroll tax is a flat tax, often with a wage ceiling that makes it regressive. Unlike income taxes, there are no exemptions and no allowances for family size. Low-wage workers, and especially younger families with children, typically bear a disproportionate share of the cost as a result. These effects are compounded to the extent that high payroll taxes discourage employment, especially at the lower end of the labor market where the social safety net, minimum wages, or industrial relations systems make it difficult for employers to pass such costs on to employees.

Application of the Musgrave rule, however, implies that a proportional share of the increased retirement costs that result from population aging will fall on the working-age population (i.e., that worker contributions will rise). Clearly, however, allocating these costs based on a flat-rate tax without deductions for children or other circumstances (i.e., flat-rate payroll taxes) is inconsistent with the notion that these costs should be of greatest advantage (or the least disadvantage) to the least well off within the working-age population. In effect, charging the costs of this transition to the working-age population via a payroll tax creates a huge problem of intragenerational justice among the working-age population, because the distribution of the additional costs in no way reflects their ability to pay. Not surprisingly, the main target of European pension reform in the 1990s was to slow or freeze the rate of growth in payroll contribution rates, an objective embraced not only by employers and governments but also by labor organizations.

Redesigning Benefits: Intragenerational Justice for Retired People

If a proportional share of the costs of population aging is to be transferred to retirees, how can this be done so that these costs do not fall disproportionately on the least advantaged among them? Clearly, reforms that simply cut all pensioner benefits by a proportional amount (e.g., by reducing all pensions by 5%) do not satisfy this standard. Moreover, the behavioral response to such reductions can be expected to increase inequality among the retired. As mentioned earlier, the standard result from studies of savings behavior is that the savings-to-permanent-income ratio rises with permanent income and does so in a sharply nonlinear fashion (Diamond and Hausman, 1984). The implication, then, is that the behavioral response to reduced *mandatory* pensions will be a function of income level: lower-income families are less likely to compensate with more *voluntary* retirement savings than higher-income families.

The notion that the costs of restructuring should be born by those most able to afford it and that the weakest members of society should be protected is hardly novel. But how to implement it? We propose two forms of targeting public sector benefits to meet this challenge, both drawn from the real-world experience of contemporary affluent democracies.

Eliminating Old Age Poverty. Building or enhancing generous basic security schemes with a minimum guarantee above the poverty line goes a long way toward addressing the Rawlsian problem identified above. It establishes a floor beyond which the most disadvantaged pensioners bear *none* of the additional costs of population aging and so meets at least a minimal requirement of intragenerational justice for retired people.

Declining poverty rates among the elderly have been a distinguishing feature of all OECD countries since the 1960s. Old age poverty rates below 10 percent are now relatively common, and some countries have achieved rates close to 5 percent or less (Hauser, 1997; Smeeding and Sullivan, 1998; table 4.1). The major flaw in the U.S. design is that it lacks such a plan; hence old age poverty rates remain high by international standards.

The most effective antipoverty systems are not necessarily the most costly. Both high-spending Sweden and low-spending Canada achieve poverty rates of less than or close to 5 percent (see also Smeeding and Sullivan, 1998), a result of the fact that both countries provide guaranteed minimum benefits that raise the vast majority above standard poverty lines. Canada provides a guaranteed annual income to the elderly, and Sweden a guaranteed minimum pension. Both make benefits conditional on the presence or absence of other economic resources (i.e., they are *targeted*), but in a way that departs significantly from traditional *means-tested* programs such as SSI. To distinguish traditional means-testing from these modern variants, it is useful to provide some definitions.

- *Means-testing*: Individuals qualify for benefits on the basis of a test for both income and assets, requiring individuals to spend

Table 4.1 Poverty Rates among the Population 65+

< 5%	5%–9%	10%–14%	15%–19%	> 20%
Sweden	Canada	Austria	Belgium	Australia
	Denmark	Germany	Switzerland	Spain
	France	Italy		United States
	Norway			
	United Kingdom			

Source: Data from LIS Key Figures, Luxembourg Income Study, 2008 (www.lisproject.org).

their way into poverty to qualify. *Tax-back rates* (i.e., the rate at which benefits are cut as other income rises) are typically high and can be in excess of 100 percent. Supplemental Security Income (SSI) in the United States is an example. Usually the aim is to restrict benefits to a small fraction of the population (the poor), and such benefits are modest. Because of the intrusiveness of the means-test, there is often considerable stigma attached to accepting benefits, so that take-up rates tend to be low. Poverty rates among seniors remain high as a result.

• *Income-testing*: As the term suggests, income-testing is based on a test of income but not of assets, so there is no requirement to spend oneself into poverty to qualify. Interest or dividends from investments are included in the test, but not the underlying capital that generates the income. Tax-back rates are always *much* less than 100 percent, so that benefits are not "for the poor alone"; they often extend well into middle-income groups, albeit at declining rates. The implicit model is closer to Milton Friedman's design for a negative income tax (NIT), or a guaranteed annual income (GAI), than traditional means-tests for the poor (see Myles and Pierson, 1997). Canada's Guaranteed Income Supplement for seniors is the exemplar.[16] Because such plans are administered through the tax system, any stigma is minimal and take-up rates are high. In the United States, the Earned Income Tax Credit (EITC) provides one model for such a strategy.

• *Pension-testing*: As practiced in Sweden and Finland, pension-testing is a yet more restricted type of test, including only income that comes from *public* pension programs in those countries. Unlike a guaranteed annual income scheme, it functions to provide a guaranteed annual pension. Individuals with earnings histories and contributions below the minimum are provided with pension supplements on a sliding scale. Where all or most of the income of retirees comes from the public pension system, of course, the distinction between income-testing and pension-testing is merely a formal one.

Providing all elderly citizens with a minimum guarantee above a poverty line indexed to national living standards is well within the reach of most rich democracies, because the poverty gap—the difference between family income and the poverty line—of poor elderly people is typically modest compared with that of working-age families (table 4.2).

Providing retirees with a high guaranteed annual income or a minimum pension is less problematic than providing such benefits to working-age families, because the issue of work incentives does not arise.[17] Over some range of the earnings distribution, a high guarantee level may have an impact on savings behavior, but this is likely to occur over a short time period, relatively late in the work career, when the impact of more or less savings on retirement income is known.

Building or enhancing generous basic security schemes with a minimum guarantee above the poverty line goes a long way toward addressing the Rawlsian problem identified above. It establishes a floor beyond which the most disadvantaged pensioners bear *none* of the additional costs of population aging and so meets at least a minimal requirement of intragenerational justice among retirees. Because a guaranteed annual income or a minimum pension involves interpersonal redistribution, there is a strong case for general-revenue taxes (e.g., from income, consumption, and other taxes) rather than payroll taxes as the source of financing for these schemes. Payroll taxes impose all of the cost on the working-age population, with perverse distributional effects within that population. A large or rising share of general-revenue financing provides a powerful tool for reallocating the costs of population aging based on one's ability to pay among the retired as well as the working-age population because, like the young, the old are also subject to income and consumption taxes.

The cost of eliminating poverty among the elderly will be higher in nations like the United States, with a greater earnings inequality over

Table 4.2 The Cost of Eliminating Old Age Poverty, 1990s Estimates

Country (year)	No. of poor households with old people (1,000s)	Poverty gap (local currency)	Extra cost as % of GDP
Canada (1994)	118	1,591	0.025
Finland (1995)	21.7	3,708	0.015
France (1994)	664.1	8,083	0.073
Germany (1989)	633.8	3,617	0.080
Netherlands (1991)	36.9	5,312	0.036
Norway (1995)	60.6	6,612	0.043
Sweden (1995)	27.2	10,524	0.017
United States (1997)	5,565.9	2,931	0.201

Source: Data from Luxembourg Income Study databases (www.lisproject.org) and Organisation for Economic Cooperation and Development national accounts (www.oecd.org/std/national -accounts/).
Note: Extra cost as % of GDP = number of poor households × poverty gap/GDP. Estimates are based on the objective of bringing families containing persons 65 or older up to 50 percent of the median adjusted disposable income line. This exercise ignores the fact that this, in itself, will alter the overall distribution and, thus, also the median.

the working life, because there will be more retirees who are eligible for such benefits. One might think of these additional costs as an *inequality tax*, the cost of which must be evaluated on the basis of one's prior assumptions concerning the effects of wage inequality during the working life on employment and labor market flexibility.

Rationalizing Redistribution in Earnings-Related Schemes. The modern institution of retirement rests on much more than a promise that retirees will not fall into poverty. Postwar retirement patterns reflect the development of institutions that promised much more, namely, that the majority would be able to maintain living standards not unlike those reached during their working years. All of this suggests that the main challenge, once an adequate basic security scheme is in place, is the probable impact of reform on workers with average and below-average earnings who, under current provisions, would have retirement incomes well above the guaranteed minimum. The challenge, moreover, is not gender neutral. The distribution of income security losses that can result from lower public pensions will have a greater impact on women, because they typically have lower lifetime earnings and longer life expectancies than men.

Although earnings-related pension schemes ostensibly reflect individual work histories and contributions, all systems have traditionally incorporated design features that produce significant interpersonal transfers and cross-subsidies. Eliminating transfers and cross-subsidies that could be identified as "inequitable," "perverse," or "outdated" (such as special privileges for public employees) provided many European countries with an effective means of cost reduction during the 1990s. At the same time, some of the savings were used to provide new cross-subsidies that were considered to be socially desirable, such as pension credits for child and elder care. This rationalization of the redistributive design features to achieve equity or to more clearly realize socially desirable distributive outcomes offers policy makers a potent tool for solving the Rawlsian problem among the non-poor.

The 1995 Swiss reform is especially striking (and relevant for the United States), because this reform was about introducing gender equality and was subject to a national referendum (Bonoli, 1997). As in the United States, a married man with a dependent spouse was eligible for a *couple pension* corresponding to 150 percent of his own pension entitlement, a practice that disproportionately benefits higher-income families (Harrington Meyer, 1996). Women's organizations successfully took the lead in demanding the end of the couple pension. In the new design, all contributions paid by the two spouses while married are added together, divided by two, and counted half each. Strikingly, however, couples with children below the age of 16 now receive additional credit, equal to the amount of contributions payable on a salary three times the minimum pension (56% of the average wage). Compensation is provided for years spent in child-rearing but, unlike the previous formula, not for providing housekeeping services to a spouse. The result is a cross-subsidy to families with children from those who remain childless.

An Appropriate Role for General-Revenue Financing

As discussed above, a rising share of general-revenue financing in the retirement budget provides a powerful tool for reallocating the costs of population aging based on ability to pay not only among the working-age population, but also among the retired. While retirees are not subject to payroll taxes, they do pay income and consumption taxes.[18] Assuming the more affluent among both retirees and the active working population pay higher taxes, their share of the additional costs associated with demographic change rises proportionately with increases in the share of retirement costs financed from general-revenue sources.

General revenue is the appropriate financing mechanism for all retirement benefits that involve interpersonal transfers, whether inside Social Security (e.g., the spousal benefit, benefit formulas that favor lower-income workers) or outside of it (SSI). Changes of this sort to the financing mechanism have been a common strategy in the European reforms of the 1990s, and Bonoli's (1996) interviews with party officials and labor leaders in France and Germany provide striking evidence for the self-conscious character of this strategy. In the words of a French trade unionist, "the financing of contributory benefits . . . must be done through contributions based on salaries. In contrast, non-contributory benefits must be financed by the public purse." Tuchszirer and Vincent (1997) highlight a similar logic underlying the 1995 Toledo Pact, an all-party agreement on the framework for reforming the Spanish social security system.

If pursued aggressively, if only incrementally, the criteria for reform outlined above implies a strategy that potentially alters the traditional social insurance model of old age security, at least in the long term. On the benefit side, any reductions required by the Musgrave rule are offset by new or expanded interpersonal transfers for less-advantaged retirees. On the contribution side, these additional costs are met not through higher payroll taxes, but with general-revenue financing raised among both the retired and the nonretired, based on their ability to pay. The implication on the benefit side is that, over time, the earnings-replacement function of the public sector insurance scheme diminishes somewhat for higher-income families (which may be made up for by second- and third-tier savings).[19] And, with time, the share of general-revenue financing for the income security system as a whole rises. The exact mix at the end of the process will vary from country to country, because we assume that there is a wide variety of initial starting points and that the strategy is applied incrementally only to the allocation of the *change* in retirement costs that results from population aging.

Conclusion

In the U.S. context, critics of the status quo often appeal to intergenerational equity to justify reforms, but only within the context of addressing the public finance (i.e., Social Security) implications of population aging. Concerns over intergenerational equity can be mostly resolved in such a framework by pension regimes where all or most retirement income is from publicly financed sources, but not in mixed systems such as the one in the United States. Supporters of the status quo, in contrast, often highlight the fact that reducing Social Security benefits has the largest impact on the least advantaged among the retired, but such proponents have largely overlooked the implications of rising payroll taxes for the least advantaged among the working population. Allowing payroll taxes to rise solves the public finance problem, but financing the transition to a society increasingly composed of older individuals on the backs of lower-income and especially younger workers does not satisfy the principle of intragenerational justice. The one-sided focus on long-term public finance issues posed by Social Security has also distracted attention from the equally pressing point-in-time challenge of constructing an adequate basic security system for retirees. By international standards, Social Security and SSI perform poorly in protecting the least advantaged, despite their redistributive features.

Notes

1. Specifically, this chapter draws on material from Myles (2002), originally written as part of a larger report on welfare state reform for the European Union, and a subsequent exchange (Myles, 2003) with Erik Schokkaert and Philippe Van Parijs (2003) in the *Journal of European Social Policy*. For reasons of space, I only briefly allude to the discussions of gender equality and later retirement contained in these papers.

2. Peter Hicks, personal communication (Dec. 2001).

3. Advocates for privatization typically argue that the result would be higher investment and hence larger gains in productivity under a privatized system, but, as discussed later, this is a result over which there is considerable skepticism.

4. On this, see the exchange between Richard Epstein and David Braybrooke in Laslett and Fishkin (1992).

5. The important distinction between tabula rasa choices and transformation choices is developed by Orszag and Stiglitz (1999). As they note,

the social effects of *transforming* a mature pension system into a system of individual accounts may be substantially different from the social effects of the initial choice between a public defined-benefit system and individual accounts.

6. Aggregative outcomes such as prices or fertility rates, Hernes (1976, p. 516) writes, "are partly under human control and partly the result of chance processes; in part they can be affected by conscious action but to a considerable extent they are unintended."

7. In the context of the issues addressed in this chapter, the principle of *equity* should be understood as referring to fair burden sharing, that is, an equitable sharing between citizens of the costs (or benefits) of demographic transition. Still, every parent who has tried to explain to younger children why it is fair that they are put to bed before their older siblings knows that determinations of what is equitable are often highly contested. It is not surprising, then, that the contemporary notion of intergenerational equity and its range of application should also be contested (Laslett and Fishkin, 1992). In some contexts, the concept is used to discuss point-in-time differences between generations or cohorts currently alive (the old, the young), while in other contexts it pertains more to the legacy that one generation (all those now living) will leave to future generations (those not yet born). Here, I make use of both senses of the term (see text below). The range of outcomes considered also varies. Should policies aimed at effecting equity between generations be applied only to the activities of government or to the entire social, economic, and natural infrastructure left to future generations?

8. It is important to recall that I am describing a fixed contribution model in a pay-as-you-go design, not to be confused with a fixed contribution model in a funded scheme, where benefits reflect contributions plus (or minus) realized gains (or losses) on invested contributions. Few readers outside of France will be familiar with the pay-as-you-go FCR model.

9. The FRP principle, however, would not satisfy a concept of fairness defined by the notion that each generation ought to pay the same proportion of their salaries to get the same level of pension rights during retirement. On a three-generational family farm, for example, the *share* or proportion of output required to support aging parents in retirement under FRP will be larger when there are two producers in the working-age generation than when there are four.

10. This is not the place to engage in an in-depth discussion of the normative merits of reciprocity and equiproportional burden sharing. Rather, in line with Musgrave's original approach, stated in terms of the political viability of Social Security arrangements, I note that proportionality indeed often acts as a focal point in negotiation problems (thus lending support to

FRP as a benchmark). *Political viability*, or a policy's sustainability, is not an intrinsic feature of an ideal normative conception of justice. But it is a desideratum, and an important one, when pragmatically implementing a theory of justice.

11. It should be clear that implementation of FRP does not preclude passing judgment on the current distribution (e.g., that it is too high or too low), making adjustments accordingly, and applying FRP thereafter.

12. Hence, the FRP design can be distinguished from solutions that index benefits but not contributions to the higher retirement costs that result from increased longevity, the latter being essentially an FCR strategy.

13. As Musgrave (1986) observes, at any given point in a cohort's life course, those motivated by their immediate (i.e., myopic) self-interest are likely to make choices that depart from the FRP design. For young workers entering the labor force with foreknowledge that the population is aging, a self-interested response from a cohort concerned mainly with its immediate living standards (i.e., a myopic choice) would lead to a preference for a model based on a fixed contribution rate, because their contributions to support the retired would not rise during their working years. These preferences, however, would undoubtedly change as they approach retirement, because now they would face an impoverished old age relative to earlier retiree cohorts.

14. The choice of principles might well vary according to the *source* of change in retirement costs. Thus the FRP principle might be applied to distribute the costs that result from demographic change (i.e., past changes in fertility), while the FCR principle might be adopted to accommodate any decline in retirement ages, and some mix of the two might be employed for changes that result from greater longevity.

15. For the purposes of this discussion, I adopt the standard assumption that payroll taxes, even when borne by the employer, are additions to labor costs which are ultimately born by labor, typically in the form of lower wages.

16. Every NIT model is defined by three parameters: the *guarantee level* (the level of benefit provided to people with no other income); the *tax-back rate* (the rate at which benefits are reduced as the recipient gains income); and the *break-even point* (the income level at which benefits disappear). A high guarantee level is desirable to provide people with adequate incomes and a low tax-back rate is desirable to encourage people to work. But such a combination means that the break-even point is high and so are the costs. In practice, virtually all NIT proposals are broken into two tiers to contain costs and maintain work incentives. One tier is intended for people who are not expected to work (such as the elderly), with a high guarantee level,

a high tax-back rate, and a low break-even level. The second tier, for those expected to work, typically has a lower tax-back rate and a higher relative break-even point, but a lower guarantee level.

17. For working-age families, the level at which social benefits affect work incentives is a function of wage distribution. When wage inequality is in the lower end of the distribution curve (e.g., when low-paid workers earn about 40% of the median wage), a high guarantee level will have more disincentive effects than when wage inequality is more modest (e.g., where low-paid workers earn about 70% of the median).

18. I do not preclude the possibility that there may be significant advantages to a system of earmarked Social Security contributions, so long as such contributions are based on total income and provide for some degree of progressivity, especially in the lower tail of the distribution, and for adjustments for family size.

19. I hasten to add, however, that there is no intrinsic reason why second-tier employer pensions cannot incorporate interpersonal transfers to achieve desirable social objectives.

References

Barr, N. 2001. *The Welfare State as Piggy Bank: Information, Risk, Uncertainty, and the Role of the State.* Oxford: Oxford University Press.

Bonoli, G. 1996. Politics against convergence? Current trends in European social policy. Presented at the Distributive Dimension of Political Economy Conference, Centre for European Studies, March 1–3, Harvard University, Cambridge, Mass.

———. 1997. Switzerland: Institutions, reforms, and the politics of consensual retrenchment. Pp. 109–29 in J. Clasen (ed.), *Social Insurance in Europe.* Bristol, U.K.: Policy Press.

Diamond, P., and J. Hausman. 1984. Individual retirement and savings behavior. *Journal of Public Economics* 23 (1–2): 81–114.

Haber, C., and B. Gratton. 1994. *Old Age and the Search for Security: An American Social History.* Bloomington: Indiana University Press.

Harrington Meyer, M. 1996. Making claims as workers or wives: The distribution of Social Security benefits. *American Sociological Review* 61 (3): 449–65.

Hauser, R. 1997. *Adequacy and Poverty among the Retired.* Paris: Organisation for Economic Cooperation and Development.

Hernes, G. 1976. Structural change in social processes. *American Journal of Sociology* 82 (3): 513–47.

Laslett, P., and J. Fishkin (eds.). 1992. *Justice between Age Groups and Generations.* New Haven, Conn.: Yale University Press.

Musgrave, R. 1986. *Fiscal Doctrine, Growth, and Institutions.* Vol. 2 of *Public Finance in a Democratic Society.* New York: New York University Press.

Myles, J. 2002. A new social contract for the elderly? Pp. 130–72 in G. Esping-Andersen, D. Gallie, A. Hemerijck, and J. Myles, eds., *Why We Need a New Welfare State.* Oxford: Oxford University Press.

———. 2003. What justice requires: Pension reform in aging societies. *Journal of European Social Policy* 13 (3): 264–69.

Myles, J., and P. Pierson. 1997. Friedman's revenge: The reform of liberal welfare states in Canada and the United States. *Politics and Society* 25 (4): 443–72.

———. 2001. The comparative political economy of pension reform. Pp. 305–33 in P. Pierson (ed.), *The New Politics of the Welfare State.* Oxford: Oxford University Press.

Organisation for Economic Cooperation and Development. 2001. *Aging and Income: Financial Resources and Retirement in 9 OECD Countries.* Paris: Organisation for Economic Cooperation and Development.

Orszag, P., and J. Stiglitz. 1999. Rethinking pension reform: Ten myths about Social Security systems. Presented at the World Bank's New Ideas about Old Age Security Conference, September 14–15.

Schokkaert, E., and P. Van Parijs. 2003. Social justice and the reform of Europe's pension systems. *Journal of European Social Policy* 13 (3): 245–63.

Sinn, H-W. 2000. Why a funded pension system is useful and why it is not useful. *International Tax and Public Finance* 7 (4/5): 383–410.

Smeeding, T., and D. Sullivan. 1998. Generations and the distribution of economic well-being: A cross-national view. LIS Working Paper No. 173, Luxembourg Income Study Working Paper Series. Luxembourg and New York: Luxembourg Income Study.

Thompson, L. 1998. *Older and Wiser: The Economics of Public Pensions.* Washington, D.C.: Urban Institute.

Tuchszirer, C., and C. Vincent. 1997. Un consensus presque parfait autour de la réforme du système du retraite. *Chronique Internationale de l'IRES* 48 (special issue): 26–30.

Wolfson, M., G. Rowe, X. Lin, and S. Gribble. 1998. Historical generational accounting with heterogeneous populations. Pp. 107–26 in M. Corak (ed.), *Government Finances and Generational Equity.* Ottawa: Statistics Canada.

5. Political Power and the Baby Boomers

Frederick R. Lynch, Ph.D.

The potential for economic strain and age-based politics caused by 78 million aging baby boomers was becoming the focus of increasing research, commentary, and alarm even before the recent economic turmoil. Analyses such as those of Peter Peterson (1999, 2004), Kotlikoff and Burns (2004), and Rivlin and Sawhill (2007), magnified by the news media and through the Internet, launched anxious political debates over health care, Social Security, and Medicare reforms.

Since 2008, the urgency and scope of these policy debates have intensified in the wake of a record-setting decline in home values, a stock market meltdown, and a subsequent deep recession. These dramatic events dimmed retirement prospects for a great number of aging boomers—a majority of whom were inadequately prepared financially for retirement *before* 2008. In addition, the Obama administration is attempting to overhaul the entire health care system, and proposals for entitlement changes will likely follow.

Aging baby boomers will actively shape—and be shaped by—these political and policy dialogues. Will they respond as an age-based, program-driven voting bloc, determined to resist entitlement cutbacks? What factors might facilitate generational consensus, convergence, and collective action to defend entitlements and boomers' longstanding, center-stage social status?

Grim financial scenarios for Medicare and Social Security illustrate rising societal strains, and financial turmoil and a recession provide the sense of crisis that collective behavior theorist Neil Smelser (1962) posited as the primary source of social and political movements. A significant number of boomers may respond politically to any threats to these programs because (1) some two-thirds of boomers are financially unprepared for retirement; (2) their self-directed, defined-contribution retirement plans (IRAs, 401[k]s), jobs, and health insurance have been jeopardized by economic instability; (3) boomers are increasingly at risk for illness and chronic disease; (4) they are encountering age discrimination in the workplace; (5) they face rising costs of employer-based health insurance; and (6) their generational identity is being molded and reinforced by marketers, advertisers, and news media profiles.

Age-based consciousness and conflict over entitlements are also being driven by deeper demographic developments: (1) an aging, largely white, well-educated population demanding a larger share of the national budget; (2) a burgeoning, young, increasingly nonwhite, multicultural population facing fierce job competition and rising inequalities in a globalizing economy; (3) declining family, interpersonal, and institutional loyalties; and (4) a nation-state with its national identity, boundaries, civic society, and budgets eroded by globalization, mass immigration, and rugged "supercapitalism" (Reich, 2007).

Boomers are not merely a demographic cohort, they are a generation with a shared history, culture, and identity. To deepen this distinction, I briefly review Mannheim's (1952) seminal essay on this concept. I then discuss the concept and criticisms of senior voting power. Using a basic social movements framework, I next assess qualitative and quantitative evidence for boomers' senior power potential. By *senior power*, I mean increased generational consciousness and age-based political action by significant numbers of boomers through voting blocs, or through more active participation in preexisting senior advocacy networks, or through the formation of new, web-based political and social movements.

Mannheim's Concept of Generations

Mannheim (1952) located the study of generations within the wider enterprise of the sociology of knowledge, that is, how identity is forged through shared experiences and interpretations of events and processes within specific historical and sociocultural contexts. He likened generational identity to the Marxian concept of class and class consciousness: "The fact of belonging to the same class, and that of belonging to the same generation or age group, have this in common, that both endow the individual sharing in them with a common location in the social and historical process, and thereby limit them to a specific range of potential experience, predisposing them for a certain characteristic mode of thought and experience, and a characteristic type of historically relevant action" (p. 291). The drama of youth shapes each generation's perspective differently. The salience and distinctiveness of generational consciousness varies, and subgroups, or *generational units*, may interpret the same historical processes differently.

Mannheim's concept of generations has been neglected formally, though informally it has been increasingly and indiscriminately mingled with the related concept of *age cohort* in analyses of baby boomers. Alwin, McCammon, and Hofer (2007) cited a lack of conceptual clarity among several terms: *cohort* (people born during a specific time period who share the experience of the life cycle), *cohort effects* (individual change produced by the unique intersection of biography and history), *generation* (when cohorts become collective actors who jointly construct social reality and share a distinctive culture or identity), *aging* and *life cycle dynamics* (common to all individuals), and *period effects* (when all members of a society respond to and are affected by historical events or processes such as war, disaster, or economic depression).

I define boomers both as a birth cohort and as a self-conscious generation shaped by shared general responses to a common history and life cycle passage, sharpened by the biology, psychology, and economics of aging. Boomers' senior citizen identity is also an increasingly media-molded one, accelerated by the mainstream news media focus on generational themes of the recent presidential campaign and, especially, via coverage of imperiled retirement prospects in the wake of the 2008 market meltdowns.

When discussing aging baby boomers, I am primarily referring to the first of two mini-cohorts in this vast generation: the *older boomers*, born from 1946 to 1955, as opposed to *younger boomers*, born from 1956 to 1964 (see Metlife Mature Market Institute, 2009).

The Senior Power Model and Its Critics

Several analysts have offered dramatic predictions of boomers' senior power potential. Dychtwald (1999) portrayed aging boomers as the newest, most powerful gerontocracy, as did a *Time Magazine* cover story on aging boomers (Okrent, 2000). Kotlikoff and Burns (2004) depicted older boomers' future economic demands on the young as "fiscal child abuse," while Peterson (2004) charged that the major political parties and two boomer presidents "have declared war on the future" by failing to address looming entitlement problems. Likewise, Keating (2004, p. 48) warned that "as they assume the role of our country's elders, boomers will mobilize to protect their interests." Although McManus (1996) found modest generational differences across a range of attitudinal and behavioral variables, she, too, predicted future us-against-them generational polarization on public policies.

These senior power predictions are premised on older citizens' higher rates of political participation—attributed to increased leisure time in retirement, long-term residence, and increased attention to news media. Campbell (2003, p. 2) offered a more provocative cause: older voters' higher participation rates reflect their stake in maintaining entitlement programs, especially Social Security and Medicare. "An otherwise disparate group of people were given a new political identity as program recipients, which provided a basis for their mobilization by political parties, interest groups and policy entrepreneurs." Campbell did not demonstrate distinctive age-based voting patterns, but she did credit the role of senior citizens' advocacy groups and the growing "aging policy bureaucracy" in the government's shaping of congressional activity.

Binstock (2000, 2007) and Schulz and Binstock (2006) challenged this popular senior power model that presumes age-based self-interest, homogeneous political attitudes, and the effectiveness of "gray lobby" advocacy groups. They demonstrated that among major influences on voting behavior, age is usually eclipsed by socioeconomic status, gender, race, ethnicity, religion, health status, and the like. Schulz and Binstock remained skeptical of boomers' senior power potential, noting that young and middle-aged boomers have not been a cohesive voting bloc—thus far. However, they have always qualified their senior power model critique by noting that Social Security and Medicare reform had not been actively discussed political threats. But entitlement reform is high on the agenda of the administration of President Barack Obama.

A Basic Social Movements Framework

Political or social movements mobilize to promote or resist change, often in response to a sense of rising frustration or urgency. Tensions arising from the inability or unwillingness of established authorities to deal effectively with social strains or problematic trends are an especially potent source of large-scale reform and protest movements. Mature political and social movements develop leadership and structure, especially when the movements arise in response to major economic or societal trends (Marx and McAdam, 1994).

Two basic social psychological processes facilitate mobilization. First, preexisting or socially constructed *consensus* among movement members on basic values, attitudes, and norms facilitates communication, interaction, and cohesion. Second, mobilization and movement building are greatly enhanced when there is *convergence* on similar interests reinforced by shared background characteristics—such as age, race, class, gender, and the like (see Turner and Killian, 1987).

The chief external factor stimulating collective mobilization is growing societal strain or conflict, such as economic conflicts or value incongruence. In his *Theory of Collective Behavior*, Smelser (1962) emphasized the primacy of social strain in a value-added model that posits a synergistic combination of factors. In addition to mounting societal strain, there must also be *structural conduciveness* (free speech, freedom of assembly, markets) permitting collective recognition and debate about these social strains. Next, a *generalized belief* arises that identifies and characterizes sources of the strain and suggests appropriate action. *Group mobilization* is subsequently furthered by a dramatic confirmation of the generalized belief via a specific event or *crisis*. Smelser's final factor is *reaction* by the state or other authorities. Proportionately measured reaction may quell a nascent movement; insufficient response may embolden collective protest; a heavy-handed response may spark outrage and reinforce a movement's mission and cohesion.

The transition from modern to postmodern society is also a factor in the rising structural strain and crisis over age-based entitlements. Twentieth-century social movements responded to industrial capitalism and to a nation-state framework where a liberal, inclusive value system nourished politics, an expanding civic society, and welfare state programs. Postmodern society is characterized by a globalization of markets, religious fundamentalists' challenge to Western rationalism and science, and fading geographical borders, national identity, and sovereignty (Garner 1996).

The current turmoil in financial markets and the subsequent recessions are worldwide, and they reflect the instabilities and uncertainties of this new postmodern order. This crisis, of course, fits into Smelser's sequential model. The question is, Will these changes and events produce sufficient generational convergence or consensus for age-based bloc voting, or more active, generationally conscious political mobilization by economically vulnerable aging baby boomers?

Generational Convergence

Boomers' senior power potential is most strongly rooted in the growing convergence of shared biological, economic, and sociological vulnerabilities. For nearly thirty years, aging boomers have witnessed what Jacob Hacker termed *The Great Risk Shift* (2006), the shifting of retirement and health insurance risk from institutions to individuals. Boomers have seen the decline of defined-benefit pensions (professionally managed lifetime income) and the rise of defined-contribution systems of individually funded and managed 401(k) accounts and individual retirement accounts (IRAs). This transformation has been a formula for generational disaster. The lasting consequences of the 2008–9 stock market decline and recession will mean that many boomers' only hope for some sort of economic security in retirement will be to work longer. "People who got caught in this downdraft in their 50s simply don't have time to increase their savings by an amount that would be sufficient. Your savings rate would have to be so high that you wouldn't have enough to live on. The only option is to stay in the labor force longer" (Munnell, 2009).

Risk Shift: Retirement and Recession

U.S. workers have long exhibited overconfidence, ignorance, and little policy awareness about retirement planning. Many assume retirement benefits that, in fact, they do not have; they know little about long-term care or the levels of Social Security benefits (Helman, VanDerhei, and Copeland, 2007). Two major surveys by AARP (1999, 2004a) and by Merrill Lynch (2005) found that approximately 40 percent of boomers felt inadequately prepared for retirement. An economic risk assessment model (Munnell, Webb, and Delorme, 2006) confirmed such perceptions, estimating that 36 percent of older boomers and 43 percent of younger boomers are at risk of having inadequate retirement income. A revised model, adding in health care liabilities, boosted those figures to 50 percent and 61 percent, respectively (Munnell et al., 2008).

Boomers oft-reported intentions to remedy inadequate retirement preparation by working until or beyond age 65 appear to be unrealistic. Two recent surveys found that 40 percent of preretired boomers planned to work beyond age 65, but only 13 percent of current retirees had actually done so (Rotenberg, 2006; Employee Benefit Research Institute, 2007). Nearly 40 percent of current retirees had been forced to retire primarily because of health reasons or job loss. Indeed, 46 percent of respondents in a "Boomers Turning 60" survey had *already* retired (AARP, 2006). Even if increased numbers are both able and willing to work longer, a long recession will likely limit their chances of doing so. This transfer of retirement saving and planning from institutions to individuals basically magnified existing economic inequalities among aging boomers—and may ultimately fragment any age-based political responses.

Wealth among boomers has been highly concentrated—as much, if not more so, than in the general population. Before the 2008 recession, Lusardi and Mitchell (2006) found that the average boomer had a modest net worth. The median total net worth for older boomers (born from 1946 to 1953) was just $151,500. Subtract housing and business assets, and this figure declined to a paltry $48,000; for the top 10 percent, the figures were $888,010 and $536,700, respectively. According to a boomer demographic profile (Metlife Mature Market Institute 2004), older boomers' average household income before taxes was $58,889; for younger boomers, it was $54,149; approximately 36 percent of all boomers had a household income of $75,000 or higher. Most boomers' primary asset has been their house (see also Gist and Wu, 2004).

About 71 percent of older boomers (aged 48–57) have indicated some form of retirement coverage (Verma, 2006). Coverage varies considerably by income, education, and job tenure. Lower-income boomers tend to have only one retirement plan or none; 36.8 percent of boomers earning more than $80,000 have both defined-benefit and defined-contribution plans. For boomers who participate in 401(k) plans, savings vary widely by age and job tenure. In 2006, boomers in their fifties had an average 401(k) balance of $148,927, ranging from $80,465 (for those on the job for 5–10 years) to $192,003 (with

20–30 years on the job). Those in their forties had an average of balance $108,262 and ranged from $74,075 (for those on the job for 5–10 years) to $146,489 (for those in a position for 20 or more years). Nearly two-thirds of 401(k) assets were invested in stocks. The median account balance for boomers was approximately $111,000 (Helman, VanDerhei, and Copeland, 2007). These amounts were obviously inadequate for pending retirement needs. As the 2008 recession took hold, the number of workers who were "very confident" that they had saved enough for retirement fell from 27 to 18 percent in one year, the sharpest one-year decline in 18 years (Helman, Greenwald, and VanDerhei, 2008).

The 2008–9 financial meltdown and recession confirmed these grim scenarios. Ironically, the stock market decline has had something of leveling effect in terms of retirement account inequities; those with the most to lose suffered the greatest losses. Older employees (aged 55–64) with the longest job tenure and largest 401(k) balances lost the most: approximately 25 percent of their account value. Conversely, those with shortest tenure and lowest balances experienced modest gains—provided they maintained monthly contributions (VanDerhei, 2009). Home values fell 40 to 50 percent in housing markets that had experienced the greatest gains—especially on the East and West coasts. Nationally, according to the Case-Shiller housing index, home values in 2008 fell a record 17 percent.

Health Anxieties and Age Discrimination

In addition to deep declines in the values of their homes and retirement accounts, aging boomers encounter rising costs and deductibles for employer-sponsored health insurance—they are coping with their own, their spouse's, or their parents' chronic diseases and deaths—as well as age discrimination and downsizing.

Preliminary studies indicate that aging boomers have health problems equal to or worse than those of their parents at the same age (Stein, 2007). Yet between 2000 and 2005, the percentage of retirees without health insurance rose to 25 percent (Smolka, Purvis, and Figueiredo, 2007). That figure has surely increased since the onset of the 2008 recession, as suggested by the massive Economic Stimulus Act passed by Congress in early 2009, which contained extensions on unemployment insurance and financial assistance for those trying to maintain health insurance policies with previous employers through COBRA programs. More generally, only half of the boomers expect to have health insurance that will meet their needs in retirement (AARP, 2004a; Merrill Lynch, 2005). Millions more boomers are likely as unaware of postretirement medical expenses as they are about their future financial needs (see Fidelity Research Institute, 2007).

In addition to coping with biological signs of aging and health insurance difficulties, older workers also face age discrimination (see Cohen, 2003; Baldas, 2007; Dennis and Thomas, 2007), which is now being exacerbated during one of the worst recessions since the Great Depression. Data on the recession's full impact on older (and younger) boomers are still preliminary, but there has been a sharp rise in age discrimination complaints to federal agencies (see Levitz and Shishkin, 2009). Rix (2004, 2006) had long predicted reemployment frustration, due to a mismatch between the types of jobs available and the training and desires of older, educated workers.

Generational Labeling, Civic Activism, and Political Recruitment

The collective consciousness of aging boomers is increasingly being stimulated by mass-media advertising campaigns mounted by AARP, the news media, and by corporate marketers in finance, travel, the pharmaceutical industries, and other health-related industries. Especially during 2008–9, numerous news media features on the recession's impact on boomers' retirement prospects have increased boomer angst, if not a full-blown generational consciousness. The entertainment media is boosting boomers' cultural nostalgia by recycling the music and television programs of their youth.

Web sites premised on boomers' self-identity—such as Eons.com—have not been very successful, but savvy entrepreneurs are mapping boomers' collective concerns by researching which Web site topics they frequent (such as finance and health). (As a result of caring for his own dying mother, aging boomer Andy Cohen discovered burgeoning boomer interest in elder care and founded Caring.com, a thriving web-based business [Cohen, 2009].)

Whatever the role of the mass media in stoking generational consciousness, a recent Metlife Mature Market Institute (2009) study found that nearly 82 percent of older boomers "like" or "somewhat like" being described as a baby boomer; on the other hand, nearly half of younger boomers "don't like" the boomer label and approximately one-third prefer to be identified as "Generation X." For younger boomers, this rejection of boomer identity no doubt reflects popular, negative boomer stereotypes as the greedy, spendthrift, self-centered, self-indulgent "Me generation" (Wolfe, 1980). (For examples of boomer identity rejection, see Lang, 2007; Schmich, 2007.) Thus the term "boomer" is never used in age-directed advertising by pharmaceutical, health care, and financial services. (Well-known television advertisements by Ameriprise and Fidelity Investments refer to "generation" when targeting boomers' "active adult" retirement interests with a background of music and imagery of the 1960s.)

Boomers' cultural preference for "bowling alone" rather than maintaining their parents' levels of civic and volunteer activities (Putnam, 2000) is also being targeted by nonprofit and government campaigns that seek to boost boomers' civic involvement (see, for example, the Corporation for National Community Service, 2007). Thus far, the response to these campaigns appears minimal—in part because the severe economic downturn has kept more boomers working full time. However, increased participation in civic activities has been associated with increased political consciousness and activity (see Galston and Lopez, 2006).

Boomers' identity as aging Americans is also being reinforced by active solicitations from the 40-million-member AARP, which anchors the Leadership Council of Aging Organizations, an umbrella organization for 51 other senior, nonprofit service or advocacy groups (see Schulz and Binstock, 2006; Binstock, 2007). The role of AARP in fostering—or diluting—boomers' political consciousness and activism will be crucial.

Demographic Change and Generational Tensions

One source of aging boomer political consciousness may arise from competition for public sector priorities and resources with an increasingly multiethnic, multicultural younger America. High immigration levels for thirty years have fueled a racial generation gap between an older, slower-growing, non-Hispanic white population and a rapidly growing population of younger Hispanics, blacks, and Asians (Roberts, 2007; U.S. Bureau of the Census 2007; see also Frey 2006, 2008).

This age and race gap overlaps an economic one; Cauchon (2007) found a growing wealth gap between younger and older Americans. Angel and Angel (2006, p. 97) warned that "these data make it clear that the potential for serious intergenerational conflict fueled further by racial and ethnic tensions is . . . quite real."

Hayes-Bautista (2004), Schrag (2006), and Myers (2007) explored immigration's role in fueling generational, ethnic and political divisions in California. The still heavily white electorate favors low taxes and has curtailed spending increases for public infrastructure and services, especially schools. Voting patterns based on age, class, and race have been reinforced by demographic sorting trends in California and elsewhere that encourage the formation of geographically and sociologically homogeneous communities (Galston and Nivola, 2008; see also Frey, 2008, Teixeira, 2009). Myers (2007, 2009) optimistically proposed "rediscovering the intergenerational social contract" between aging boomers and immigrants by stressing mutual interdependence. Ultimately, however, prospects for cooperation or conflict between these two populations will heavily depend on the length and depth of the recession and whether age-conscious boomers suspect that their age-based entitlements might be redistributed to other programs geared to growing numbers of immigrants and their children.

Mixed Findings on Generational Consensus

Boomers' shared history and collective identity have been chronicled by numerous authors (see Jones, 1980; Light, 1988; Strauss and Howe, 1991; Dychtwald, 1999; Gross, 2000; Macunovich 2002; Gillon, 2004; Steinhorn, 2006; Stewart and Torges, 2007). They identify the following set of shared generational experiences: childhood and family culture shaped by a "procreation ethic" that idealized marriage and children; a large and ethnically homogeneous cohort; a relatively affluent and competitive childhood and adolescence; optimism, idealism and great expectations heavily nourished by television; an increasingly mobile, automobile-centered lifestyle; rock music culture; competitive adult job markets; a decline in male wages (relative to those of their fathers); women's liberation and changing family structures; and a series of galvanizing events and passages: the civil rights movements, the Vietnam War, the two Kennedy and King assassinations, and the Watergate scandal.

During the 1960s, a vocal minority of educated older boomer youth established a generational political and cultural tone, mixing emphases on community and institutional change with "do-your-own-thing" individualism. Though this cultural revolution may not have had broad-based generational support, it nonetheless propelled long-term social policy and legal and cultural changes, especially with regard to race, ethnic, and gender discrimination.

Fiercely competitive job markets dampened their youthful idealism and counterculture. Light (1988) emphasized boomers' emerging market-driven, free agent outlook and waning faith in government action during the 1980s. Alwin (1998) and Williamson (1998) described the emergence of boomers' antigovernment voting patterns in the 1990s, and a more recent AARP study of boomers' political attitudes (2004c) confirmed a generational preference for individualized, issue-specific, and nontraditional "politics of tailored engagement," somewhat outside the boundaries of the two-political-party system.

In surveys and focus groups, boomers have consistently registered an optimistic, resilient, individualistic, can-do ideology that attributes individual success—or lack thereof—to personal factors such as motivation, confidence, or willpower. One-third of the respondents stated that "nothing" is keeping them from achieving their goals (AARP, 2002a, 2004b; see also AARP, 2006). On the other hand, Howe and Strauss (2007) restated their earlier prediction that many boomers' strong and abiding idealism, moralism, and concern for the common good will trump their fierce individualism and transcend any potential politics centered on age-based self-interest.

Boomers remain wary of major institutions. In the 1970s, 3 percent of boomers believed government was telling the truth; in 2002, 6 percent agreed. Only 16 percent of boomers in the 1970s had a great deal of confidence in Congress, and even fewer (13%) did in 2002. Levels of confidence in education and in organized religion were cut in half. While confidence levels fell slightly toward the Supreme Court, confidence in corporations, the presidency, and the military rose somewhat (AARP, 2002b). In a recent Pew Research Center (2007, p. 51) survey of political attitudes, 69 percent of boomers agreed that "when something is run by the government, it is usually inefficient and wasteful."

CNN exit polls found a slight majority of boomers voted for George W. Bush in 2000 and 2004. (In 2004, younger boomers gave Bush a somewhat larger 53%–46% margin than the 51%–48% given by older boomers.) One year later, however, boomers were among those most strongly opposed to Bush's Social Security reforms (Greenberg, Quinlin, Rosner Research, 2005). And by 2007, a survey of political trends suggested that boomers are part of a five-year "dramatic shift" toward identification with the Democratic Party and increased support of government programs (Pew Research Center, 2007).

In 2008, the boomer vote was evenly split between Republican John McCain and Democrat Barack Obama. But this general finding masked considerable race, class, and educational divisions within this giant generation. (For example, white voters aged 45–64—a rough boomer demographic—voted for McCain over Obama, 56% to 42%.) Thus, although boomers seem to share a broad, somewhat paradoxical commitment to both rugged individualism, on the one hand, and transcendent social idealism, on the other, age-based mobilization based on these outlooks may be undermined by more salient sociological divides.

Fractured Consensus or Convergence

Light (1988) forecast many of the same factors later seen by Binstock (2000) as fracturing generational political consensus or convergence: (1) age—older and younger boomers have had different life experiences, (2) gender, (3) education, (4) ethnicity, (5) socioeconomic status, (6) marital status, (7) geographic splits, and (8) lingering divisions over the Vietnam War.

Class differences among aging boomers are the most likely barriers to consensus and convergence. Changes in inequality among boomers reflect broader social and cultural trends. Boomer women closed or even reversed gender gaps in education, but differences in educational attainment by race and ethnicity increased. (Among older baby boomers, 25% of the whites were college graduates, 45% of U.S.-born Asians, and about 15% of blacks and U.S.-born Hispanics.) Hughes and O'Rand (2004) saw changing family structure reinforcing these trends: stable, highly educated, white and Asian two-income families pulled further away from others with less education, such as immigrant Hispanics, and there were especially larger numbers of one-parent families among blacks.

Boomers' diverse family structures also fragment their culture and voting behavior. Seventy-one percent are married, and 15.2 percent are divorced; 56 percent have children at home (Metlife Mature Market Institute, 2004). Married couples with children have typically been the most reliably conservative or Republican—especially those who attend church regularly. Those not in traditional relationships are among the most secular. Approximately one-third have either no children or only one. Nearly 13 percent of boomers have never married. Children, or the absence thereof, could strongly divide aging boomers' outlooks: those with children will care more about loading entitlement costs on future generations.

Differences in class, education, family structure, and religious orientation are among the key variables at work in the oft-discussed, boomer-based culture wars. These divisions among boomers emerged strongly in the 2008 presidential elections. Many state Democratic primaries fractured along the lines of age, race, and class—that is, classic generational politics—in which older, white, working- and middle-class voters (especially women) backed Hillary Clinton, while Barack Obama generally obtained his largest majorities among blacks and among younger and higher-income, well-educated whites (Seelye, 2008; see also Abramowitz and Teixeira, 2008; Teixeira, 2009). In one of the most detailed analyses of the factors shaping Democratic primary voting, Cost (2008) emphasized that among older and middle-aged white voters, "socioeconomic status permeates the Obama v. Clinton contest."

By mid-2008, pollster Charlie Cook (*Political Wire*, 2008) correctly prophesized that "[white] baby boomers may decide the next presidential election . . . Obama is losing white voters born between 1944 and 1958 by 18 percentage points." In the November general election, according to the CNN exit polls (2008), whites aged 45–64 (boomers) voted for McCain over Obama 56 percent to 42 percent; this differed little from other white age groups except for those aged 18–29, who preferred Obama to McCain, 54 percent to 44 percent. Nearly 95 percent of blacks in all age groups voted for Obama, while Obama received almost two-thirds of the Latino vote—with the curious exception of Latino boomers, who only gave Obama a 58 percent majority.

Conclusion

Aging baby boomers are beginning to realize that they will be far more dependent on Social Security and Medicare than they once assumed, and they regard those programs with a growing sense of entitlement. Boomers' age consciousness is also being reinforced by corporate advertisers, outreach by advocacy groups, and the mainstream news media.

The stock market decline and the recession have revealed the inherent flaws in the system of individually based retirement accounts, which are increasingly the foundation of many boomers' retirement finances. A devastating assessment of this system was offered by economist and stock market expert Edward Yardeni (Petrumo, 2008): "There's just no way you can really save out of the median income in this country and retire comfortably." He predicted that many people who know they're already far behind in building a nest egg for retirement are going to simply give up, realizing that trying to catch up is practically impossible. Yardeni's words echoed a report by Ernst and Young (2008) that warned: "Many of the 77 million baby boomers retiring over the next few years will face unprecedented challenges in maintaining their standard of living in retirement."

Despite their collective economic jeopardy, however, boomers' continuing optimistic individualism and lingering mistrust of government may continue to fragment any coherent, organized, age-based response to this problem. Incredibly, a recent Focalyst survey (2006) found that 75 percent of boomers remained optimistic about their present and future. The high degree of inequality and other demographic divisions among boomers also inhibit any economic and sociological convergence.

Thus far, and somewhat paradoxically, the greatest barrier to an aroused, age-conscious, senior voting bloc or social movement is politicians' fear of it. The "sleeping giant" of senior activism has remained a "latent constituency," because politicians have largely avoided active discussions of Social Security or Medicare reforms (Binstock, 2007).

There are signs that a more unified boomer political response as a potential program constituency could crystallize if present or future Social Security or Medicare benefits are threatened. AARP surveys (2004a, 2004c) found boomers had increasingly favorable attitudes toward Social Security and Medicare and a rising sense of entitlement: 71 percent of respondents reported at least a "somewhat favorable" view of Social Security—up from 56 percent in 2002. Nearly 90 percent of boomer respondents in a Merrill Lynch (2005) survey agreed that their generation is fully entitled to Medicare and Social Security.

Boomers' senior power potential is still just that. But the theoretical precursors are percolating. Smelser's (1962) premobilization stages of communication, structural strain, and rising anxiety and urgency are increasingly visible on a daily, if not hourly, basis on Internet news sources. The financial and institutional crises are confirming these fears. New forecasts of Social Security's and Medicare's deteriorating fiscal futures, in combination with multiple financial crisis and a deep recession, are forcing politicians and policy makers to provide a new definition of the situation and to undertake both remedial action and fundamental reforms. Massive financial bailouts for banks and other industries and healthcare reform proposals are examples of these new and urgent responses to rising economic and structural strains.

The essential catalyst that is lacking for boomer senior power is leadership. In nearly nine years of field research and interviewing on this topic, I constantly asked, "Is there a Claude Pepper for the boomers?" (referring to the late U.S. senator from Florida who was widely recognized as senior citizens' legislative champion). Virtually everyone answered, "No one I can think of." (Significantly, few, if any, perceived AARP as the potential champion.)

Still, crises tend to produce leaders. And the financial crises and recession will leave permanent and widely shared psychological scars as large boomer majorities contemplate the actual or potential loss of jobs, health insurance, and retirement savings. A considerable followership base is being built among aging boomers for an individual, organization, or movement that will vigorously defend their interests and articulate their hopes and fears.

References

AARP. 1999. *Baby Boomers Envision Their Retirement: An AARP Segmentation Analysis.* Washington, D.C.: AARP.

———. 2002a. *Boomers at Midlife: The AARP Life Stage Study.* Washington, D.C.: AARP.

———. 2002b. *Tracing Baby Boomer Attitudes Then and Now.* Washington, D.C.: AARP.

———. 2004a. *Baby Boomers Envision Their Retirement II.* Washington, D.C.: AARP.

————. 2004b. *Boomers at Midlife: The AARP Life Stage Study, Wave 3.* Washington, D.C.: AARP.

————. 2004c. *A Changing Political Landscape as One Generation Replaces Another.* Washington, D.C.: AARP.

————. 2006. *Boomers Turning Sixty.* Washington, D.C.: AARP.

Abramowitz, A., and R. Teixeira. 2008. The decline of the white working class and the rise of a mass upper class. Pp. 109–46 in R. Teixeira (ed.), *Red, Blue, and Purple America: The Future of Election Demographics.* Washington, D.C.: Brookings Institution Press.

Alwin, D. F. 1998. The political impact of the baby boom: Are there persistent generational differences in political beliefs and behavior? *Generations* 22 (1): 46–54.

Alwin, D. F., R. J. McCammon, and S. M. Hofer. 2007. Pp. 45–74 in S. K. Witbourne and S. L. Willis (eds.). *The Baby Boomers Grow Up: Contemporary Perspectives on Midlife.* Mahwah, N.J.: Lawrence Erlbaum Associates.

Angel, R. J., and J. L. Angel. 2006. Diversity and aging in the United States. Pp. 94–110 in R. Binstock and L. George (eds.), *Handbook of Aging and Social Sciences*, 6th ed. San Diego: Academic Press.

Baldas, T. 2007. Age bias suits on the rise with older employees working longer. *National Law Journal* (Mar. 16). www.law.com/jsp/article .jsp?id=1173949426492#/ [retrieved March 16, 2007].

Binstock, R. H. 2000. Older people and voting participation: Past and future. *Gerontologist* 40 (1): 18–30.

————. 2007. Older people and political engagement: From avid voters to "cooled out marks." *Generations* 30 (4): 24–31.

Campbell, A. L. 2003. *How Policies Make Citizens: Senior Political Activism and the American Welfare State.* Princeton, N.J.: Princeton University Press.

Cauchon, D. 2007. Generation gap? About $200,000. *USA Today* (May 20), 1.

CNN. 2008. CNN exit polls. www.cnn.com/ELECTION/2008/results/ polls/.

Cohen, A. 2003. Too old to work? *New York Times Magazine* (March 1), 54.

————. 2009. New ways to reach boomers. Presented at Boomer Business Summit preview (Mar. 18), American Society on Aging/National Conference on Aging 2009 Aging in America Conference, March 15–19, Las Vegas, Nev.

Corporation for National Community Service. 2007. *Keeping Baby Boomers Volunteering: A Research Brief on Volunteer Retention and Turnover.* Washington, D.C.: Corporation for National Community Service.

Cost, J. 2008. Review of Obama's voting coalition, parts I–IV (May 27).

www.realclearpolitics.com/horseraceblog/2008/05/a_review_of_obamas_voting_coalition_1.html.

Dennis, H., and K. Thomas. 2007. Ageism in the workplace. *Generations* 31 (1): 84–90.

Dychtwald, K. 1999. *Age Power: How the 21st Century Will Be Ruled by the New Old*. New York: Tarcher-Putnam.

Economic Mobility Project. 2007. *Economic Mobility: Is the American Dream Alive and Well?* Washington, D.C.: Pew Charitable Trusts.

Employee Benefit Research Institute. 2007. Employment status of workers ages 55 and older, and assets in qualified retirement plans, 1985–2005: Updated. *Notes* 28 (8): 2–7.

Ernst and Young. 2008. *Retirement Vulnerability of New Retirees: The Likelihood of Outliving Their Assets* (July). Washington, D.C.: Ernst and Young, LLP, for Americans for Secure Retirement.

Fidelity Research Institute. 2007. *The Fidelity Research Institute Retirement Index*. Research Insights Brief. Boston: Fidelity Research Institute.

Focalyst/AARP. 2006. *The Focalyst View*. Washington, D.C. and New York: AARP and the Kantor Group.

Frey, W. H. 2006. *America's Regional Demographics in the '00s Decade: The Role of Seniors, Boomers, and New Minorities*. New York: Research Institute for Housing America.

———. 2008. America's regional demographics in the early 21st century: The role of seniors, boomers, and new minorities. *Public Policy and Aging Report* 18 (1): 1–31.

Galston, W. A., and M. H. Lopez. 2006. Civic engagement in the United States. Pp. 3–20 in L. B. Wilson and S. P. Simpson (eds.), *Civic Engagement and the Baby Boomers*. New York: Russell Sage Foundation.

Galston, W. A., and P. S. Nivola. 2008. Vote like thy neighbor. *New York Times Magazine* (May 11).

Garner, R. 1996. *Contemporary Movements and Ideologies*. New York: McGraw-Hill.

Gillon, S. 2004. *Boomer Nation*. New York: Free Press.

Gist, J., and K. Wu. 2004. *The Inequality of Financial Wealth among Boomers*. Washington, D.C.: AARP Public Policy Institute.

Greenberg, Quinlin, Rosner Research. 2005. *2005 Likely Voter Survey*. Washington, D.C.: Greenberg, Quinlin, Rosner Research, Inc.

Gross, M. 2000. *My Generation*. New York: Cliff Street Books.

Hacker, J. 2006. *The Great Risk Shift: The Assault on American Jobs, Families, Health Care, and Retirement—and How You Can Fight Back*. New York: Oxford University Press.

Hayes-Bautista, D. E. 2004. *La Nueva California: Latinos and California Society, 1940–2040*. Berkeley: University of California Press.

Helman, R., M. Greenwald, and J. VanDerhei. 2008. *The 2008 Retirement Confidence Survey.* Issue Brief No. 316. Washington, D.C.: Employee Benefit Research Institute/Mathew Greenwald Associates.

Helman, R., J. VanDerhei., and C. Copeland. 2007. *The Retirement System in Transition: The 2007 Retirement Confidence Survey.* Issue Brief No. 304. Washington, D.C.: Employee Benefit Research Institute/Mathew Greenwald and Associates.

Howe, N., and W. Strauss. 2007. The next 20 years: How customer and workforce attitudes will evolve. *Harvard Business Review* 85 (July/Aug.): 41–53.

Hughes, M. E., and A. M. O'Rand. 2004. *The Lives and Times of the Baby Boomers.* New York: Russell Sage Foundation.

Jones, L. Y. 1980. *Great Expectations.* New York: Ballantine.

Keating, P. 2004. Wake-up call. *AARP Magazine* (Sept./Oct.): 48.

Kotlikoff, L. J., and S. Burns. 2004. *The Coming Generational Storm.* Cambridge, Mass.: MIT Press.

Lang, M.-E. 2007. Not a "baby," never "boomed." CBC News and Viewpoint (May 31). www.cbc.ca/news/viewpoint/vp_lang/20070531.html [retrieved June 2, 2007].

Levitz, J., and P. Shishkin. 2009. More workers cite age bias after layoffs. *Wall Street Journal* (Mar. 10), A1.

Light, P. C. 1988 [1999]. *Baby Boomers.* New York: Replica Books.

Lusardi, A., and O. S. Mitchell. 2006. Baby boomer retirement security: The roles of planning, financial literacy, and housing wealth. Working Paper 2006-114, University of Michigan Retirement Research Center.

Macunovich, D. 2002. *Birth Quake.* Chicago: University of Chicago Press.

Mannheim, K. 1952. The problem of generations. Pp. 276–321 in K. Mannheim, *Essays in the Sociology of Knowledge.* New York: Oxford University Press.

Marx, G. T., and D. McAdam. 1994. *Collective Behavior and Social Movements: Process and Structure.* Englewood Cliffs, N.J.: Prentice-Hall.

McManus, S. A. 1996. *Young v. Old: Generational Combat in the Twenty-First Century.* Boulder, Colo.: Westview Press.

Merrill Lynch. 2005. *The New Retirement Survey.* New York: Merrill Lynch & Co., Inc.

Metlife Mature Market Institute. 2004. *Demographic Profile: American Baby Boomers.* New York: Metropolitan Life Insurance.

———. 2009. *Boomer Bookends: Insights into the Oldest and Youngest Boomers.* Westport, Conn.: Metlife Mature Market Institute.

Munnell, A. H. 2009. Retirement dreams face new reality. National Public Radio *Marketplace* (May 15).

Munnell, A. H., M. Soto, A. Webb, F. Golub-Sass, and D. Muldoon. 2008. *Health Care Costs Drive Up the National Retirement Index.* Chestnut Hill, Mass.: Center for Retirement Research, Boston College.

Munnell, A. H., A. Webb, and L. Delorme. 2006. *A New National Retirement Risk Index.* Issue in Brief No. 48. Chestnut Hill, Mass.: Center for Retirement Research, Boston College.

Myers, D. 2007. *Immigrants and Boomers: Forging a New Social Contract for the Future of America.* New York: Russell Sage Foundation.

———. 2009. Aging baby boomers and the effect of immigration: Rediscovering the intergenerational social contract. *Generations* 32 (4): 18–23.

Okrent, D. 2000. Twilight of the boomers. *Time Magazine* (June 12): 68–74.

Peterson, P. G. 1999. *Gray Dawn: How the Coming Age Wave Will Transform America—and the World.* New York: New York Times Books.

———. 2004. *Running on Empty: How the Democratic and Republican Parties Are Bankrupting Our Future and What Americans Can Do about It.* New York: Farrar, Strauss, & Giroux.

Petrumo, T. 2008. The case for a new national frugality. *Los Angeles Times* (Aug. 9), C1.

Pew Research Center. 2007. *Trends in Political Values and Core Attitudes, 1987–2007.* Washington, D.C.: Pew Research Center.

Political Wire. 2008. Baby boomers could be key swing vote. http://politicalwire.com/archives/2008/06/20/baby_boomers_could_be_key_swing_vote.html (June 20) [no longer available].

Putnam, R. D. 2000. *Bowling Alone: The Collapse and Revival of American Community.* New York: Simon & Schuster.

Reich, R. 2007. *Supercapitalism: The Transformation of Business, Democracy, and Everyday Life.* New York: Knopf.

Rivlin, A. M., and I. V. Sawhill. 2007. *Restoring Fiscal Sanity: Meeting the Long-Run Challenge.* Washington, D.C.: Brookings Institution.

Rix, S. 2004. *Aging and Work: A View from the United States.* Washington, D.C.: AARP Public Policy Institute.

———. 2006. *Update on the Aged 55+ Worker.* Washington, D.C.: AARP Public Policy Institute.

Roberts, S. 2007. New demographic racial gap emerges. *New York Times* (May 17), A1.

Rotenberg, J. 2006. The retirement challenge: Expectations v. reality. Presentation at the EBRI/AARP Pension Conference, May 15, Washington, D.C.

Samuelson, R. J. 2007. Making the think tanks think. *Washington Post* (Aug. 1), A17.

Schmich, M. 2007. Basic premise for a column boomerangs. *Chicago Tribune* (Aug. 15), A14.

Schrag, P. 2006. *California: America's High Stakes Experiment.* Berkeley and Los Angeles: University of California Press.

Schulz, J. H., and R. H. Binstock. 2006. *Aging Nation: The Economics and Politics of Growing Older in America.* New York: Praeger Books.

Seelye, K. 2008. In Clinton v. Obama, age is one of the greatest predictors. *New York Times* (Apr. 22), A1.

Smelser, N. J. 1962. *Theory of Collective Behavior.* New York: Free Press.

Smolka, G., L. Purvis, and C. Figueiredo. 2007. *Health Coverage among 50-to-64-Year-Olds.* Washington, D.C.: AARP Public Policy Institute.

Stein, R. 2007. Baby boomers appear to be less healthy than parents. *Washington Post* (Apr. 20), A1.

Steinhorn, L. 2006. *The Greater Generation.* New York: St. Martin's Press.

Stewart, A., and C. Torges. 2007. Social, historical, and developmental influence on the psychology of the baby boom at midlife. Pp. 23–43 in S. K. Whitbourne and S. L. Willis (eds.), *The Baby Boomers Grow Up: Contemporary Perspectives on Midlife.* Mahwah, N.J.: Lawrence Erlbaum Associates.

Strauss, W., and N. Howe. 1991. *Generations.* New York: William Morrow.

Teixeira, R. 2009. *New Progressive America.* Washington, D.C.: Center for American Progress.

Turner, R. H., and L. M. Killian. 1987. *Collective Behavior,* 3rd ed. Englewood Cliffs, N.J.: Prentice-Hall.

U.S. Bureau of the Census. 2007. Minority population tops 100 million. *U.S. Census Bureau News* (May 17). Washington, D.C.: U.S. Department of Commerce, U.S. Bureau of the Census.

VanDerhei, J. 2009. *The Impact of the Recent Financial Crisis on 401(k) Account Balances.* Issue Brief No. 326. Washington, D.C.: Employee Benefit Research Institute.

Verma, S. K. 2006. *Retirement Plan Coverage of Boomers: Analysis of 2003 SIPP Data.* Washington, D.C.: AARP Public Policy Institute.

Williamson, J. B. 1998. Political activism and the aging of the baby boom. *Generations* 22 (1): 55–59.

Wolfe, T. 1980. The "Me" decade and the third great awakening. *New York Magazine* (August 23). http://nymag.com/news/features/45938/.

6. Theoretical Approaches to the Development of Aging Policy in the United States

Robert B. Hudson, Ph.D.

There can be little doubt that older people have today assumed a special place in the U.S. social policy and political landscape. They constitute a large and growing population, they are increasingly well organized, and they are the recipients of public benefits that are the envy of every other social policy constituency in the nation.

This chapter reviews and assesses different theoretical approaches that may help account—in full or in part—for these fairly recent and remarkable developments. While there is some variety in how welfare state analysts have organized and distinguished between these approaches (Skocpol, 1991; Pampel and Williamson, 1992; Myles and Quadagno, 2002), each has identified a fairly common set of alternatives. The organization here centers on seven separate (though potentially reinforcing) possibilities. These, in turn, can be clustered into two economic, three society-centered, and two state-centered approaches.

The two economic theories—the logic of industrialization and neo-Marxist concepts—represent contrasting functionalist representations of how emerging industrial economies conditioned welfare state development. Both approaches are centered on the unrelenting economic forces of the industrial age, the former emphasizing the massive increase in economic resources and its subsequent social dislocations, the latter focusing on the inevitable consequences of wealth being concentrated in fewer and fewer hands. The aged, understood as an increasingly notable demographic presence, play an important role in each of these understandings.

The society-centered approaches bring into play the values, behaviors, and actions of individuals and groups that inform and structure the demands made of government that are tied to individual and social well-being. The first of these, based on cultural norms, is usually discussed under the rubric of national values. This lens has often been focused on U.S. social policy developments because of the country's *exceptionalist* political culture. However, as this culture allegedly impedes broad-based welfare state developments as seen in Europe, the aged emerge as a unique beneficiary group, being indulged where others are denied. A second society-centered approach finds mobilization of the working class to be central to welfare state developments: workers come to influence or even organize political parties, using their strength in numbers to press for benefits they are unable to gain from owners in the money-dominated economic realm. The aged are found to gain (or lose) relative advantage depending on the success of these forays into politics by labor.

The third society-centered approach looks to the participation of individual and organized interests manifested as groups or as constituencies, rather than as classes. Groups organize around various identities individuals may have, and in modern society these may be more particularistic than class goals. In a nation such as the United States, where working-class cohesion was never firmly established, multiple demands emerge, organized along these lines of identity. By the 1980s, the aged in the United States could be easily seen as one such interest.

The third theoretical clustering is state-centered, directing attention to the autonomy and cohesion of public and quasi-public institutions. These institutional elements include formal constitutional conditions, such as federalism and governmental structure; quasi-public entities, such as political parties; and, importantly, the product of those structures (i.e., *public* policy). It is worth distinguishing between two variants of state-centered theory, one focused on the state itself and the second on policy outcomes. How the state is structured and, in particular, how much autonomy its incumbents—both political and administrative—enjoy is critical to the first of these. The second understands that the policies generated by the state have crucial effects in shaping and constraining subsequent political activity. Put differently, policy is understood here as an independent rather than as a dependent variable in explaining welfare state developments. A substantial body of publications focusing on age-related policy has, in recent years, come to serve virtually as exhibit 1 in pushing this perspective to the theoretical fore.

The following pages review these seven theoretical understandings. Each discussion frames the particular approach, places it in both U.S.

and comparative contexts, and finds the place of the aged in these understandings. As will be seen, there exists a rich literature on the first two of these three elements; the principal value-added aspect of this chapter is in the aging-related material. The old—until recently—have often been treated more in passing than as central players in social policy development.

The Logic of Industrialization

The birth of the modern welfare state in Western nations occurred in the wake of the processes of industrialization and urbanization in the nineteenth century. Analysts vary on how dominant the role of industrialization was by itself, but none question its essential contribution. The aged—through both their emerging plight and their growing numbers—provide a key link between the forces of industrialization and early welfare state development.

At the most basic level, industrialization enabled an accumulation of resources that was not possible in preindustrial society. Industrial organization and technological advances grew symbiotically and made investment, not just consumption, possible. By so doing, surpluses could accumulate, allowing for social welfare expenditures, among other uses. It is over the use of these surpluses that capitalist and anticapitalist ideologues have struggled since the dawning of industrialization.

These twin processes of industrialization and urbanization disrupt traditional economic, social, familial, and geographic relationships. The status that older people enjoyed in agricultural economies, where farmers have considerable control over their own employment and where "landed property is power" (Gratton, 1986), waned with the onset of industrialization. Over time, workers become disabled or exhausted, and owners demanded ever-higher levels of productivity, especially during the industrial efficiency movements of the late nineteenth and early twentieth centuries. For their part, families found that the economic utility of children lessened in urban settings, abetted by small and squalid living arrangements. "At this point, all of the things that happen to old people become much more tragic" (Wilensky and Lebeaux, 1958, p. 77). In this *resources-plus-needs* formulation, the old come to hold a relatively unique, if unfortunate, place. Their family supports have been undermined (fewer children, higher divorce rates, disabled kin), and their economic value has been diminished (physically weak, technologically backward).

It is here that the state steps in, performing something of a regulatory function by instituting programs to provide for those necessarily (and appropriately) forced from the productive sector of the economy. The proximate factors that might create this—sympathy, assuring work for the young, responding to pressures from adult children—are not specified by this approach; however, cross-national analyses covering welfare state expansion from its inception through the 1970s find the aged to be a strong correlate, if not an established engine, of public social-expenditure growth. In Wilensky's (1975, p. 27) words, "as economic level climbs, the percentage of aged climbs, which shapes spending directly; with economic growth the percentage of aged goes up, which makes for an early start and swift spread of social security programs."

At one level (what Myles and Quadagno [2002] refer to as the weaker version), this approach is hard to fault; it would be difficult to account for welfare state growth absent the effects of economic growth and population aging. Importantly, these forces are as much at work today as they were formerly. Numerous analysts have posited economic growth as the absolutely essential (if not sole) factor behind the explosion in post–World War II social welfare expenditures (Cameron, 1978). Indeed, the potentially dominant role of economic growth (today associated more with technology than industrialization)—played down in the 1980s and 1990s by those emphasizing political factors in accounting for welfare state expansion—has received renewed attention in explaining assaults on the welfare state since the mid-1970s. That is, if economic growth fuels expansion, why would economic stagnation not contribute to program contraction? Yet while welfare state cutbacks have been observed in numerous national settings over the period (Huber, Stephens, and Ray, 1999), disagreement remains about whether the economics and politics of austerity are the mirror image of the economics and politics of expansion (Pierson, 1994).

A second, stronger version of the economic development approach is more contested. Cross-nationally, there is great variation between levels of economic growth, on the one hand, and the growth and size of welfare states, on the other—a divergence that strongly suggests that forces other than narrowly economic ones must be at work. Perhaps the U.S. is the most notable instance where industrial growth was early and fierce yet where social welfare spending has long lagged behind (Skocpol, 1991). A critique of this approach holds that it does not account for the proximate activities that generate change. For example, it does not take a terribly advanced understanding of human behavior to intuit that it is relatively easy to raise public revenue when gross domestic product (GDP) is expanding, but countries have nonetheless done so at far different rates.

These larger debates about welfare state growth aside, the place of the aged is notable in the industrialism approach. In a historical context, population aging appears to be a driver of pension and (later) health care spending, and today analysts on both sides of "the coming crisis in age-related spending" debate employ a GDP/aging-expenditure ratio to make their points—based on very different assumptions (Teles, 2007; Gist, 2008). There is some irony in this concern being spurred on by *population aging* (a.k.a. the aging of the baby boomers), in that the causal arrows are again up for grabs: whereas population aging presumably helped drive welfare state development one hundred years ago, it is also true that the enormity of today's welfare state expenditures has centrally contributed to the imposing presence represented by the current generation of seniors. If this is at least partially the case, the role of industrialization and economic growth must be augmented by other theoretical considerations that will be enumerated below.

Neo-Marxist Theory

A second deterministic economic approach borrows from and modifies Marxist arguments about the logic of capitalism and its relentless imperative toward the concentration of wealth into fewer and fewer hands. More than the original, contemporary Marxist theory finds in the welfare state an expanded, if limited, role for the state itself. Beyond being a handmaiden to capitalism in abetting capital accumulation (via infrastructure, education, and security), the state takes on the burden of caring for those who cannot meet the demands of labor imposed by organized capital. At the very time the state is doing capitalists' bidding by preparing workers with the skills needed to assume new occupations, the state also plays a legitimating role by enacting programs to prevent widespread suffering for those who cannot measure up. As Piven and Cloward (1971, p. 7) put it, "without work, people cannot conform to familial and communal roles; and if the dislocation is widespread, the legitimacy of the social order itself may come to be questioned."

In this understanding, the welfare state leads vulnerable populations to believe that the overall system can be reasonably supportive of them even if they have been cast out of the labor market. In something of an updated version of the original Marxian false-consciousness formulation, the populace sees beneficence, rather than control, in these interventions. This is accomplished through a pervasive yet subtle power mechanism whereby one party succeeds in "influencing, shaping, or determining [a second party's] very wants" (Lukes, 1974, p. 34). In so doing, the welfare state performs what Edelman (1964) terms a *quiescent function*.

Before the rise of a critical gerontology literature in the 1990s, the aged had not been centrally featured in these discussions, although they had been implicitly addressed in many (O'Conner, 1973; Gough, 1979). In borrowing from neo-Marxist literature, *critical gerontology* "differs from other gerontological perspectives by viewing the situation of the aged as the product of social structural forces rather than natural or inevitable individual and psychological processes" (Estes, 1991, p. 21). Thus income-maintenance policy for the old should not be understood merely as offsetting physical declines in late life but, rather, as a means to remove older workers from the industrial labor force (Graebner, 1974) in the name of promoting economic efficiency. Modern health care interventions for the old are less about addressing their indisputable needs than about siphoning public monies into the largely private hospital, nursing home, and mental health industries (Estes and Binney, 1991). The success of these efforts can be partially understood as the result of the overt power of dominant private sector actors, but a more adequate explanation is again found in the false-consciousness idea, here applied to the old, wherein "people accept as legitimate the conditions that lead to their own exploitation" (Hendricks and Leedham, 1991, p. 55).

The most interesting case for testing neo-Marxist and critical gerontology tenets on older people in the United States is found in the Townsend Movement of the 1930s. As elders suffered perhaps more than any other population, Francis Townsend proposed that each of them receive $200 per month on the conditions that they spend it immediately (in order to stimulate the economy) and agree not to work (to free up jobs for younger workers). The movement caught fire and, at its height during the Depression, there were hundreds of Townsend chapters with tens of thousands of adherents. How much pressure it generated on the Roosevelt administration as it designed its Social Security legislation is a matter of scholarly debate (Orloff, 1988; Amenta, 2006), but Franklin Roosevelt's Committee on Economic Security was keenly aware of its presence (Witte, 1963). The neo-Marxist interpretation holds that Old Age Insurance is best understood as a means of appeasing older people and, in so doing, defanging the Townsend Movement. In lieu of the Townsend Plan, "what the old folks got instead—if it did not entirely placate them, it placated their public supporters—was the Social Security legislation." Ultimately, this "meager concession spelled the demise of the movement" (Piven and Cloward, 1971, p. 101).

Critical gerontology's placating hypothesis is one of several that can tie the Townsend Movement and the Social Security Act to one another. Not to be lost in this theoretical discussion, however, is the fact that the most notable social movement that came out of the Depression is by and about old people. Nowhere else have older people ever been organized to such a degree. Moreover, this was no radical movement; it was carried on by "solid folk" (Piven and Cloward, 1971) and was overtly intended to restore, not to overthrow, the prevailing system. While the logic of the neo-Marxist approach can hold—Social Security did hasten the Townsend Movement's demise—the need to calm conservative old people rather than radical workers says a good deal about the U.S. political culture, to which I turn next.

Political Culture and Values

An exceptionalist and reinforcing set of national values served as the predominant theme in post–World War II writings about the unique place the United States appeared to occupy in comparative welfare state development (Orloff, 1988). Americans' historical attachments to individualism, self-reliance, voluntarism, free markets, and a Protestant-based moralism were seen as instrumental both in understanding the etiology of poverty and ill health and in limiting the role government should play in their amelioration (Rimlinger, 1971). Poverty and ill health were attributed largely to individual failings and immoral behavior, a diagnosis which left little room or justification for government involvement (Rosenberg, 1962). In early New England, the "old and the disabled were proper objects of relief, but not the able-bodied poor, who received harsher treatment" (Quadagno, 1988, p. 25). During this period, Americans warmed to Herbert Spencer's juxtaposing Charles Darwin and Protestantism, "a philosophy of liberation from the trammels of government" (Fleming, 1963, p. 127).

This value set poses a direct challenge to the logic of industrialization approach, because the country underwent massive economic dislocations in the almost complete absence of public intervention on behalf of those who were dislocated. While other countries were instituting unemployment, health care, and pension policies, social policy efforts in the United States were largely limited to the regulatory and "good government" initiatives of the Progressives. And even these followed the more substantive European developments by more than a decade. Skocpol's (1992) work highlighting early Civil War pensions and state-level mothers' pensions has served as a partial correction to these earlier understandings of how delayed U.S. developments were and, as such, adds a cautionary note about the national values argument. Nonetheless, these Civil War benefits being confined to veterans, women, and children was in sharp contrast to the European experience, where the needs, grievances, and demands of the working class were the essential ingredient.

Differences in national value structures also inform conceptual understandings of different welfare regimes. Under one formulation, the exceptionalism of the United States takes on particular salience. In a series of lectures delivered at Oxford University in 1949, British sociologist T. H. Marshall (1964) delineated three types of citizenship—*civil, political,* and *social*—that have marked the evolution of modern societies and contrasted their pattern of development cross-nationally. Civil citizenship encompassed a basic set of rights necessary to freedom in the modern world: the right to liberty, the right to property, and the right to the even-handed administration of justice. A second set of rights were political ones: the rights to vote, to organize, and to hold office. The third stage involved social rights, referring to economic security and the right to enjoy a reasonable level of well-being, understood not only in terms of absolute well-being but also in relationship to one's fellow citizens.

Writing at a time when the postwar Labour government was building the British welfare state, Marshall guardedly forecast that the historical victories involving civil and political citizenships would be joined by the social set of rights. Not only was it happening in Britain, but it had already happened to a significant degree in continental Europe and the Scandinavian nations. Indeed, in Germany social citizenship preceded the civil and political stages, leading to a highly paternalistic state—one, tragically, open to demagoguery, given the relative absence of the vital free and participatory spheres.

As for the United States, it clearly and famously succeeded at the civil and political stages, both sets of rights being firmly established before anywhere else, including Britain. The Bill of Rights, early white manhood suffrage, and expansions of organizing rights set the United States apart for many years, although with the notable omission of women and African Americans (Fraser and Gordon, 1992). Yet the third stage has never developed as fully as elsewhere. The right to health care, decent housing, employment, and a reasonable standard of living has never been codified here in a manner seriously approaching most other nations. There may be more than one way to account for this relative failing, but an entrenched set of deeply rooted exceptional values is certainly high on the list.

Value salience can also help account for the rationales associated with U.S. social policy interventions when they did ultimately occur. Franklin Roosevelt and his advisors were nearly obsessed with the work disincentives that might be associated with New Deal initiatives. Writing of that and subsequent periods, long-time Social Security Commissioner Robert Ball (2000, p. 43) repeatedly emphasized how important the idea of work was to all discussions: "Private pensions, group insurance, and social insurance all belong, along with wages and salaries, to the group of work-connected payments, and it is this work connection, the fact that it is earned, which gives social insurance its basic character." Indeed, the controversy that sprung up in 1939 about extending Old Age Insurance to cover survivors centered on the absence of any work history among those individuals.

The values perspective can also help account for what many observers see as major gaps in U.S. social policy. Most notable is the absence of any kind of family allowance policy acknowledging the costs and contributions of child-rearing in the modern world. U.S. policy toward young families, especially low-income young families, has been marked by exclusionary (Ryan, 1971), residual (Wilensky and Lebeaux, 1958), and behaviorist (Marmor, Mashaw, and Harvey,

1990) policies, most recently associated with welfare reform and the Temporary Assistance to Needy Families program. Mead's (1998, p. 109) writings on the need for a new paternalism to guide the unworthy poor ("Individuals need self-restraint . . . Those who would be free must first be bound") rival the writings of William Graham Sumner a century earlier ("The ill-endowed are also made radically unfree by yielding up their claim to fend for themselves" [quoted in Fleming, 1963, p. 129]).

Finally, focusing on the aged, the national values perspective has much to offer theoretically. Indeed, both sympathy for the aged and antipathy for much of the remaining population is a suggestive framework. Firsts for the aged in the United States include Civil War pensions for Northern veterans in 1862, Old Age Assistance and Old Age Insurance in 1935, Disability Insurance in 1956 (initially only for those over age 50), Medicare in 1965 (for the old alone until 1972), and Supplemental Security Income in 1972 (for the poor old, blind, and disabled). Because the old were assumed to be poor and frail, they alone could pass the American values litmus test around work and self-sufficiency. This also made the aged a favored group among social policy reformers who wished to institute benefits that would ultimately extend beyond the aged to other population groups.

Mobilization of the Working Class

This approach to understanding welfare state development has the organized presence of industrial workers at center stage. Not to be confused with neo-Marxist theories, analysts here see workers as having agency and as actively challenging the presumed imperatives of monopoly capital. Because the presence of workers and their economic and political organizations—unions and parties—are readily measured, assessing the utility of the working-class-struggle approach is more straightforward than addressing the imperatives and values addressed above.

In this model, politics matters, in that industrial workers use their numbers and organizations to affect the political system. If the strike is the workers' economic weapon, the vote is the workers' political one. And, because workers will always outnumber owners in free-market economies, the political realm is fertile, especially when parties organize to mobilize and channel workers' concerns. The organizational element is critical: the extension of political democracy absent effective organization is not sufficient to generate needed pressures on the existing system. Early on in the European experience, expansion of the franchise—largely through the efforts of left-wing parties (and by conservative parties trying to co-opt workers)—created political opportunities propitious for welfare state development.

There is a well-established empirical literature supporting the positive relationship between left-wing legislative presence and welfare state growth (Cameron, 1978; Esping-Andersen, 1985). The logic of the theory is, obviously enough, that social democratic parties will prevail, form governments, and enact expansive programs. That, of course, happened, but one also finds that the approach can be operative even when rightist parties are in power. This occurred most famously in the case of Bismarck's creation of the German welfare state in the 1880s. Antecedent to this, but related, would be Conservative Prime Minister Benjamin Disraeli extending the franchise to workers in 1860s Britain. In both cases, a co-optation hypothesis prevails— the paternalistic privilege of the Right indulges the emerging working class and forestalls the further organization of the Left.

Not surprisingly, little is said of the U.S. experience in these discussions. As has been well documented, in comparative perspective the United States failed to generate permanent, sizeable, or cohesive left-wing political (or economic) movements. On the economic side, there were periodic appearances—the Industrial Workers of the World, the Knights of Labor—but these were mercurial and fleeting. When mainstream labor did organize, it was the more-skilled craft unions that first emerged, ultimately forming the American Federation of Labor (AFL). Far from an orthodox leftist union leader, the AFL's founder, Samuel Gompers, opposed federal unemployment insurance well into the early years of the Depression. In the political domain, an American Socialist Party emerged around the turn of the century—Eugene Debs won nearly 7 percent of the vote in the 1912 election—but the Democratic Party has served as the closest approximation of a leftist party in the United States for more than a century.

A vast literature exists on why socialism failed in America (Greenstone, 1969; Lipset and Marks, 2001). Most obviously at work are the exceptionalist values discussed earlier. Geography and the frontier have long been argued to have played a role in dispersing the disgruntled and in defusing tensions. Much has been laid at the door of race and ethnic animosities, whereby "blood being thicker than class" vitiates attempts to bring workers of different backgrounds together. And, of course, employers vehemently opposed organizing efforts on behalf of workers and attacked those workers and their leaders who attempted organization. As a result of these various factors, it is widely agreed that the United States failed to generate a viable and cohesive working-class-based political movement.

There are interesting ramifications of this failure for the emerging older population. On the one hand, an effective working-class movement would appear to benefit the aged, if only because current workers would become old, and pension benefits have almost always been included as one of a package of worker demands. Indeed, pensions can be seen as a way for workers to press for (future) benefits in a manner that is less threatening to employers than demands for improvements in current wages and working conditions. As Myles (1984) argues, pensions are a form of deferred wage and, because most jobs are onerous but necessary, the promise of future leisure time through the pension mechanism is appealing. That U.S. workers pressed for and received some private (and, later, public) pension coverage is consistent with the working-class-struggle approach. In fact, invoking Marshall's terminology, Myles sees these pensions as "a citizen's wage." Because public pensions have come to constitute a comparatively enormous portion of U.S. welfare state expenditures, and because pension and health benefits form the lion's share of fringe benefits negotiated for by workers, the aged in the United States can be seen as both conceptually and economically advantaged through leftist (or at least progressive) efforts at benefit expansion. The passage of Medicare in the 1960s serves as further evidence of this advantage. Its passage has been partially attributed to organized labor trying to push union-funded retiree health care costs—another form of deferred income—off onto the public sector so that those energies and resources could be channeled into efforts on behalf of current workers (Quadagno, 2005).

On the other hand, as Pampel and Williamson (1992) observe, the workings of this theory could be seen as inimical to the concerns of the aged. To the extent that the theory postulates and behaviors might follow, organized labor's political action efforts might work to exclude other groups. In addition to the aged, these might include women and populations of color, who might or might not be workers. Certainly the segregationist impulses of mainstream American labor would serve to substantiate such a concern.

As for current workers, there is no reason to believe that pensions would be their primary bargaining item unless circumstances forced some other, more immediate concerns of workers off the table; unemployment and workers' compensation benefits certainly might be seen as more central. And, moving to a more contemporary concern, Pampel and Williamson (1992) note that intergenerational tension might emerge for unions (and, conceivably, the Democratic Party) in a situation where there was a call for higher dues (or taxes) be imposed to support pension benefits for current retirees. Despite these theoretical possibilities, the dangers of such a split are reduced in the U.S. case by, once again, the limited impact of purely working-class political movements. The recent erosion of union membership, to say nothing of an influx of hard-to-unionize, low-wage immigrant workers, makes this potential working-class "threat" to the old a marginal possibility at best.

Democratic and Group Participation

Perhaps the most commonly presented construct of how a (social policy) bill becomes a law in the United States centers on how interests are articulated, aggregated, and realized. In the classic democratic participation model, citizens express their views through voting, letter-writing, campaigning, and contributing; interest groups are organized around clusters of citizen concerns, and these concerns are then carried by them to political parties and directly into the halls of government; and political parties merge separate demands into coherent platforms as a means of structuring political debate (Easton, 1957).

This model, associated very much with pluralist theories of the political system (Polsby, 1963), has both empirical and normative dimensions. Mainstream political scientists saw these pluralistic impulses as marking how the U.S. government worked from World War II through the 1960s, but it was widely held that the pluralists often conflated depictions of how the system worked with how they preferred it to work. Subscribing to an "order paradigm" (Horton, 1966), the pluralists saw individual and group competition taking place within a larger world of shared values and common assumptions. Voter, group, and party competition functioned not unlike the workings of the free economic market, with myriad demands being muted and compromises being forged. In all of this, the government served as something of a referee, ratifying the winners and losers and lending formal recognition to the balance of political powers at any given point in time. A growing tide of criticism (Lowi, 1967; Parenti, 1970) and events of the 1960s and 1970s led to the model's fall from grace. Nonetheless, the pluralists' desire to document and defend democratically stable political systems in light of the widespread failure of democratic governments earlier in the century was more than understandable.

There can be no question that the basic ingredients of the model were (and are) much in evidence in the United States. Long seen as a nation of joiners, the United States has more interest groups, many of them highly particularistic, than found elsewhere. Whereas political parties in other nations do, in fact, perform critical aggregating functions around candidate selection and policy formulation, in the United States it is said to be on K Street in Washington—home to hundreds of special interest groups, many of them generously funded—where a disproportionate influence on these key functions is effectively exercised. The logical basis for this reality derives in part from what the United States does not possess. Lacking strong working-class structures or consciousness and marked by a highly fragmented Constitutional structure, the policy process itself in the United States becomes balkanized. Put differently, of the two *demand theories* presented here, the unit of analysis in the pluralistic model is groups; in the social democratic model, it is classes.

If the democratic participation model worked as advertised, it would represent a highly reasoned if comparatively underorganized political system. Over time, however, observers found many elements to fault in both its workings and its outcomes. As most famously argued by Lowi (1967), referring to the model as "interest group liberalism," the group process does not yield bargaining and negotiated outcomes. Many unfiltered demands, indulging numerous program constituencies, sail through a fragmented committee structure in Congress and through a maze of subcabinet agencies in the executive branch. Beyond the excessive noise created by such a system, there are also negative distributional consequences, with the "have" groups being better able to organize, generate resources, and press their demands, creating, in Lowi's words, "a system of privilege." Yet other theorists see no checks at work offsetting the relentless series of demands those in search of governmental largesse make, potentially resulting in "an overload of democracy" (Buchanan and Tullock, 1962; Niskanen, 1971) and impeding governance itself.

The aged present a fascinating case study of the potential validity of the interest group model and its limitations, both empirical and normative. They are a large and growing population, they are active politically, they are extremely well organized, they have particularistic policy concerns, and roughly one-third of the federal budget is devoted to their interests. As they say, that is a potent political cocktail. However, correlation is not causation, and, as we will see subsequently, exactly how the cocktail is mixed may make all the difference.

First, it is important to note that the aged's organized presence in Washington is reinforced by its imposing electoral standing. No longer just a large population, seniors now have higher voting-participation rates than any other age group (U.S. Bureau of the Census, 2004). In off-year and primary elections, that disproportionate presence is even more pronounced. Yet it is equally important to observe that older people vote much like younger ones in general elections (Binstock, 2000), suggesting that their particularistic interests do not necessarily determine their voting decisions. Of course, because no candidate campaigns on an antiaging platform, this nonevent becomes a potent illustration of how elders exercise a "second face of power" (Bachrach and Baratz, 1962), namely, keeping unwanted alternatives off the political agenda altogether. There is little evidence that the voting patterns of older people directly shape aging-related policy results, but a fair summation of the older voters' place in the policy process may simply be that "they are there, and they are aware."

Seniors' interest-group presence in Washington is formidable, and it is here that the potential exercise of the first face of power is in full view. Organizations ranging from AARP (with 34 million members) to smaller ones such as the National Academy of Elder Care Attorneys and the American Society of Consulting Pharmacists are among the 54 organizations that constitute the Leadership Council of Aging Organizations (i.e., an organization of aging organizations). A few of the members, such as AARP, are mass-membership organizations, but the majority represent professionals and other providers that serve older Americans, all of whom have interests in Washington.

While these organizations' significant presence is beyond dispute, their exact role in securing the enormous benefits today's elders enjoy is a matter of some controversy. Certainly, there has been much commentary in both popular (Peterson, 1999; Samuelson, 2005) and scholarly circles (Pratt, 1976; Price, 1997) pointing—usually with alarm—to the influence the organized aged have in Washington. AARP has been portrayed as the capital's most powerful group, and its support of President Bush's Medicare Part D prescription drug program is widely believed to have been crucial to its passage (Iglehart, 2004).

In many other legislative episodes, however, it has been difficult to isolate a determinative role that these senior interest groups have played. Because the groups themselves have been organized only recently—AARP and the National Council of Senior Citizens (NCSC) were the first, both dating back only to the late 1950s—they played no role in the formative years of aging policy. And accounts of particular legislative episodes also report mixed results. In each of the following cases, the organized aged and their allies were engaged, but evidence of their role in determining the ultimate policy outcomes is varied: Social Security (Derthick, 1979b; Campbell, 2003); Medicare (Marmor, 1970); the Age Discrimination in Employment Act, or ADEA (Pratt, 1993); Supplemental Security Income, or SSI (Burke and Burke, 1974); repeal of the Medicare Catastrophic Coverage Act (Himelfarb, 1995); and private pension benefit protection (Madland, 2007).

These cautionary comments do not ignore the reality that the aged and their organized representatives have assumed a major place in U.S. political life. It is no longer possible, as it was 50 years ago, for politicians to ignore older people as they went about their business. The question of concern here, however, is, How do different theoretical approaches understand and account for what has now become that imposing presence? In the democratic and group participation model, the literal presence of the aged is less mediated than in any of the competing approaches. Nonetheless, as imposing as seniors' political presence may now be, it does not necessarily account for aging-based welfare state development, appealing as that direct linkage may appear.

The Role of the State: Structure

Having reviewed two functionalist theories and three society-centered ones, I now turn to the role of the state in aging-related welfare state developments. In a literal sense, it is, of course, the state that formally enacts and funds policies of all sorts. Yet, in the approaches reviewed thus far, the role of the state is remarkably marginal. Industrialization theory sees it as responding in some quasi-automatic and unspecified way to an emerging combination of technological innovation and human suffering; neo-Marxists see it as abetting organized capital in a wholly subordinated manner; the working-class approach sees the state as the prize that one or the other of two class-based interests will control; and the pluralism inherent in the democratic organized-interest model finds state actions to be largely a ratification of the balance of organized group influence within the polity.

The 1980s saw the reemergence of the state as a central analytical ingredient in accounting for welfare state developments. The center of attention in political science's very early years—Woodrow Wilson wrote famously about it while at Princeton (Robertson, 1993)—the role of the state lost standing to the alternative approaches above, especially in the post–World War II years. Two scholars in particular are associated with this reemergence of interest in the state. Theodore Lowi (1964) suggested that what the state does critically affects the subsequent political process, not simply the reverse, as is suggested by social democratic and democratic-process approaches. At the 1981 American Political Science Association's annual meeting, Lowi and his cochair, Sydney Tarrow, argued: "We do not reject the perspective that focuses on the political process, or on political behavior—even when it is *mass* behavior—but we argue that processes and behavior can best be studied within the context of institutions" (quoted in Robertson, 1993, p. 20, italics in the original).

Theda Skocpol and her colleagues have produced a significant body of literature over the past twenty years under the rubric of "bringing the state back in," the essential argument being that "states conceived as organizations claiming control over territories and people may formulate and pursue goals that are not simply reflective of the demands or interests of social groups, classes, or society" (Skocpol, 1985, p. 9).

The crux of the argument is that state structures play an independent role in shaping political activity and political outcomes. These structures include all significant elements of the state—formal constitutional structures and quasi-public institutions such as political parties. Robertson (1993) sees measures of both *political capacity* and *political coherence* as being critical elements in any state-centered analysis.

Three key measures of capacity are the boundaries of legitimate governmental intervention, fiscal capacity, and the expertise of legislators and administrators. Coherence involves two dimensions: the extent to which authority within a level of government is unified or fragmented, and the autonomy possessed by different levels of government.

If not once again exceptional, the U.S. experience is at least notable if we briefly examine it against these five items. In comparative perspective, the boundaries of legitimate governmental action in the social policy realm are noticeably narrow. The exceptionalism of the national values perspective weighs in heavily here, as does Marshall's (1964) formulation noting how far social citizenship trails behind the civic and the political in the United States. A famous passage from Thomas Paine captures Americans' historical disdain for the state: "The more perfect civilization is, the less occasion it has for government, because the more does it regulate its own affairs and govern itself."

The fiscal capacity of the U.S. national government has been historically weak, one of many examples being that the budget of the State Department was drawn exclusively from consular fees until just before World War I. While decreasing the gap modestly, the United States continues to spend considerably less on social welfare functions than do other advanced nations (table 6.1).

The United States also trails other nations in critical aspects of administrative expertise. For myriad reasons, the civil service in the United States has never enjoyed the autonomy and prestige of its counterparts in other nations. In France, for example, a majority of senior civil servants and a significant number of senior politicians are graduates of L'École Nationale d'Administration, the training academy of France's political elites. The traditions surrounding the administrative sphere of government differ sharply on either side of the Atlantic. In Europe, the autonomy of the state is long established and taken as an institutional reality across a range of critical social activities (Nettl, 1968). This is in direct contrast to the U.S. experience, in which "the civil administration of the early twentieth-century U.S. state was weak, given the lack of an established state bureaucracy and the dispersion of authority inherent in U.S. federalism and the division of powers" (Orloff, 1988, p. 59).

The lack of cohesiveness of U.S. political structures is known, if not fully appreciated, by generations of students. Cohesion was intention-

Table 6.1 Gross Public Social Expenditure,
2003

Country	% of GDP
Sweden	37.1
France	33.1
Denmark	32.2
Belgium	30.0
Norway	28.2
United Kingdom	23.7
Germany	21.7
Australia	20.3
Canada	19.6
United States	17.4

Source: Data from Organisation for Economic Cooperation and Development, Social Expenditure
Database for 2003 (www.oecd.org/els/social/ex
penditure/).

ally attenuated from the beginning: a federal structure with divided areas of sovereignty, separated branches of government, checks and balances, a bicameral legislature (with the Senate embodying overt state-level representation), and staggered elections within and between the legislative and executive branches. Samuel Huntington (1966, p. 392) argues that U.S. governmental institutions are more incoherent than even the textbook version of checks and balances would suggest: "sovereignty was divided, power was separated, and functions were combined in many different institutions." In Huntington's analysis, it is America's consensual society that makes this institutional chaos possible: "In America, the ease of modernization within society precluded the modernization of the political system. The United States thus combines the world's most modern society with the world's most antique politics" (p. 406).

It is not hard to deduce why this state of institutional events would impede social policy development. In the bastardized words of a popular advertisement: "You expect less of the U.S. government, and you get it." Limited capacity and coherence—especially when intended— does not bode well for the reformers' agenda. That, in the nineteenth century, all levels of U.S. government were also marked by high levels of patronage and cronyism adds fuel to the fire. In short, in the eyes of the theory's proponents, weak political institutions can go a long way toward explaining America's peculiar social policy posture.

For our purposes, it also can be used to account for how the aged have fared in the United States. The most interesting application comes in Theda Skocpol's widely heralded rethinking of when the U.S. version of the welfare state actually began. For decades, scholars have pointed to the New Deal period as the time when the United States entered the welfare policy game, occasionally with the grudging acknowledgment that the Progressives at the turn of the century made tentative moves in that direction. Yet in her work highlighting the importance of Civil War pensions and mothers' pensions, Skocpol (1992) argues that, however selectively, the United States preceded what famously occurred elsewhere. By the late nineteenth century, these payments were roughly equal to any expenditure category in the federal budget, and in 1910 about 28 percent of men over age 65—more than one-half million—were receiving these benefits.

More interesting than their size, however, is their theoretical relevance: these pensions were awarded in great numbers to farmers and townspeople who were not central to industrialization, and they were not demanded by industrial workers or principally extended to them. Instead, pension expenditures expanded greatly until the end of the century, caught up in a uniquely American political process whereby they moved from "relatively straightforward compensation for wartime disabilities into fuel for patronage politics" (p. 120). Of course, coterminous with the growth of these politics was the aging of the veterans themselves; the combination of the "distributive politics" (Lowi, 1964), associated with politicians' ability to dispense benefits freely, and beneficent attitudes toward the old proved a powerful policy combination. In Skocpol's words, the Civil War pension "evolved from a generous partially utilized program of compensation for combat injuries and deaths into an even more generous system of disability and old age benefits which were taken up by 90 percent of the Union veterans surviving in 1910" (pp. 109–10). In short, political incoherence and limited fiscal capacity did not impede the ability of elected representatives to inaugurate social welfare benefits for the old.

A second and final application of this perspective to old age policy in the United States revolves around on the role of governmental civil servants in the welfare state enterprise. That such individuals were central to European developments has been well established (Beer, 1966; Heclo, 1974). In perhaps the first of the state-centered monographs, Heclo (1974, p. 156) reviews and downplays the roles of industrialization, elections, political parties, and interest groups: "At no time did organizations of the aged or pensioners themselves play any prominent part." Rather, he concludes that "the bureaucracies of Britain and Sweden loom predominant in the policies studied" (p. 301).

Despite the shortcomings of capacity and coherence in the United States (or perhaps because of them), there are important instances of policy elites making a crucial difference in social policy developments. And many of these involved the aged. Most notable in this regard is Franklin Roosevelt's Committee on Economic Security, which fashioned the original Social Security Act. As Ikenberry and Skocpol (1987, p. 405) bluntly conclude: "The policy process through which Social Security was planned and drafted in the mid-1930s was strikingly closed." Martha Derthick (1979b) famously chronicled how closed Social Security policy making was from its beginnings through the mid-1970s. Two commissioners, Arthur Altmeyer and Robert Ball, held the job for two-thirds of that period, and longer if one realizes Ball's influence in the years both preceding and following his official term in this post. As to their relationship to the elected officials with whom they interacted, Derthick concluded: "Program specialists in executive bureaus are one of the principal sources of supply for politicians who are looking for ideas for things to do. In the case of Social Security, for several decades they were almost the only source of supply" (p. 210).

Policy elites inside government were essential to later social policy successes, again disproportionately involving the aged. Wilbur Cohen, Oscar Ewing, and two key Congressional figures—Senator Patrick McNamara of Michigan and Representative Aime Forand of Rhode Island—centrally fashioned Medicare strategy from the mid-1950s until its enactment in 1965 (Marmor, 1970). John Veneman, undersecretary of the Department of Health, Education, and Welfare, was the central actor in the phoenixlike transformation of President Nixon's failed Family Assistance Plan for Aid to Families with Dependent Children into the Supplemental Security Income program, providing a modest guaranteed income for the poor old, the blind, and the disabled in 1973 (Burke and Burke, 1974).

In the U.S. situation, the working of policy elites was far less institutionalized than in the European case. But these key actors, operating in an admittedly semi-coherent political system, grasped critical opportunities and were able to strike when the policy moment was hot. And, in these efforts, they often seized on the plight of the aged and the sympathy they engendered in the U.S. context. In this manner, the aged served as something of an ideological loss-leader for these reformers, eager not only to help aged people but also to use them in advancing policy agendas to other groups (Hudson, 1978).

The Role of the State: Policy

In various ways, each of the perspectives above addresses factors and actors who may be seen as responsible for the timing and shape of welfare state policies. This last perspective reverses the causal arrows by asking, instead, To what degree do the policies shape subsequent political activity? Here, policy becomes an independent variable affecting politics and, in turn, future policy. This hypothesis derives directly from the state-centered perspective in that policies, being the formal product of states, both contribute to and derive from the state's autonomy and capacity.

Schattschneider (1935) was the first to identify and examine the phenomenon of how policy causes politics in his early discussion of tariff policy. Later investigations of policy types (Lowi, 1964; Wilson, 1973) demonstrated how the scope and distributive consequences of various enactments shaped subsequent activity. More recently, Schneider and Ingram (1993) added yet another key dimension, inquiring how the power and political construction of particular target populations can create arenas generating very different political processes. In particular, different policies can draw individuals into the political system, alienate them from it, or leave them indifferent. Policies are a powerful mechanism in attaching citizens to the political world; they can see what government can do for them or what it may do to them. Because levels of political participation have been declining and U.S. civic engagement has been called into question (Putnam, 1995), the role of public policy in fostering citizen involvement has normative as well as empirical ramifications.

Contemporary scholars have shown the impact that governmental policy can have. Skocpol's (1992) treatment of Civil War pensions reveals how patronage politics developed out of what was initially a reasonably constricted set of benefits, but the policy later created political opportunities. Mettler (2007, p. 196) shows how the enactment of the G. I. Bill following World War II both contributed to broad-based economic gains and "also prompted higher levels of subsequent involvement in civic and political activities." Given the extraordinary growth in social welfare expenditures after 1960, the argument can be made more broadly: government spending on behalf of individual citizens created widespread interest in and commitment to the broader civic enterprise. During this period, the New Deal programs grew dramatically (after little growth in their early years) and the Great Society programs of the Kennedy/Johnson years were enacted as well. By the mid-1970s, as Mettler notes, one sees "the expansion of the American welfare state, the growth of the middle class and the reduction of economic inequality, and high levels of positive attitudes and civic involvement among citizens" (p. 196).

Within this policy-causes-politics template, the place of older people has a stunning presence. In part it is because the programs—Social Security, Medicare, a large part of Medicaid, and numerous lesser ones—dominate the federal domestic spending landscape. But the connection and timing between the growth in policies and the subsequent actions of older citizens and their interest groups is yet more remarkable. Looking at the role of aging-related interest groups, a simple chronology hints at this possibility, as notable policy enactments and expansions appear to have preceded rather than followed interest group developments. Thus, AARP (formerly known as the American Association of Retired Persons) had virtually no policy presence until the 1970s and, even then, one of its first political positions was to oppose, as inflationary, a 1972 Democratic proposal to raise Social Security benefits by 20 percent (Pratt, 1976). Somewhat later, Walker (1983) determined that more than one-half of the 43 aging-related interest groups in his study came into being after 1965, the breakthrough year that saw the enactment of Medicare, Medicaid, and the Older Americans Act. In Walker's words, "in all of these cases, the formation of new groups was one of the *consequences* of major new legislation, not one of the *causes* of its passage. A pressure model of the policymaking process in which an essentially passive legislature responds to petitions from groups of citizens who have spontaneously organized because of common social or economic concerns must yield to a model in which influences for change come as much from inside the government as from beyond its institutional boundaries" (p. 403, italics in the original).

Actions subsequent to the passage of the Older Americans Act—a program funding an array of social and in-home services to people aged 60 or older—provide a concrete example of this process at work. The state agencies charged with administering the program formalized their trade association, the National Association of State Units on Aging, in the years after 1965; the substate agencies, brought into existence through amendments in 1972, created their trade association, the National Association of Area Agencies on Aging, in the wake of that authorization (Hudson, 1994). Groups of nutrition, transportation, and legal service providers were also formed subsequent to these amendments.

Yet more compelling evidence of the policy-generating politics chain is seen in the creation of seniors themselves as a self-identified political constituency. In her pathbreaking book, Campbell (2003) documents how the growing presence of older Americans in the political process owes much of its existence to the expansion of Social Security. In carefully crafted research juxtaposing public opinion and voting data with Social Security program expansion, Campbell shows how levels of political consciousness, participation, and salience followed in the wake of Social Security's growth. Seniors are the only group whose electoral participation in presidential elections over the past 40 years has increased, while the participation rates of voters aged 18–24, 25–44, and 45–64 have declined. In relative terms, a higher proportion of seniors now vote than does any other age group; in 1964, they exceeded only the youngest age group. Campbell shows, as well, that the participation rates of seniors in other forms of political activity— letter-writing, campaigning, and contributing—have also increased in both relative and absolute terms.

In assessing these findings, Campbell concludes that Social Security, by dramatically improving the economic well-being of older people, created both time and interest—what Pierson (2007) calls material and cognitive incentives—for seniors to involve themselves in political matters more heavily than had ever been the case. "Senior mass membership groups did not create Social Security policy. Rather, the policy helped create the groups. Social Security's effects on individuals—the increases in income, free time due to retirement, and political interest—enhance the likelihood of group membership. Social Security created a constituency for interest group entrepreneurs to organize, just as it defined a group for political parties to mobilize" (Campbell, 2003, p. 77).

While the causal role of policy is the principal contribution of this analysis, the secondary effects of policy's role is equally important. Thus, at *time* 1, public policy may have been critical in the creation and institutionalization of the organized aging, but at *time 2* the groups become crucial in efforts to expand or—more recently— to defend the policies against outside encroachment. Put differently, the Walker/Campbell argument does not dismiss the role of interest groups; rather, it helps explain both their origins and the dynamic (i.e., benefit protection) that keeps formal members or informal adherents tuned in to their messages. In short, while AARP may be the biggest lobby in Washington, it would not be where it is if (1) Social Security had not helped galvanize the elderly and if (2) Social Security and other programs were not there as a policy fulcrum around which AARP could rally its membership.

Conclusion

This chapter reviewed seven approaches that may help to account for the prominent place of the aged in America's truncated welfare state. That aged people have fared better than other groups in the United States is beyond dispute, although it is worth noting that in European welfare states, where working-age and younger populations have been much more generously provided for than in the United States, the aged are still relatively better off than those in the United States (table 6.2). Smeeding (2006), using standardized poverty-rate data from the Luxembourg Income Study, finds the United States with the highest rate of poverty of eleven rich nations and the second highest rate of poverty among elderly people (after Ireland) of those nations.

It is neither necessary nor possible to find any one of these approaches accounting for the entirety of aging-related policy events. Some may be more attuned to particular time periods of particular episodes, but even then, no single perspective can be expected to explain the totality of events.

That said, some theoretical speculations are in order to conclude this voyage through U.S. old age policy. First, it seems fair to conclude that the aged have been transformed from being a group overwhelm-

Table 6.2 Relative Poverty Rates (Percentage below 50 Percent Median Adjusted Income), both Overall and for Elders

Nation	Overall (rank)	Elders (rank)
United States	17.0 (1)	28.4 (2)
Ireland	16.5 (2)	48.3 (1)
Italy	12.7 (3)	14.4 (6)
United Kingdom	12.4 (4)	23.9 (3)
Canada	11.4 (5)	6.5 (10)
Germany	8.3 (6)	11.2 (7)
Belgium	8.0 (7)	17.2 (5)
Austria	7.7 (8)	17.4 (4)
Netherlands	7.3 (9)	2.0 (11)
Sweden	6.5 (10)	8.3 (9)
Finland	5.4 (11)	10.3 (8)
Overall Average	10.3	17.0

Source: Data from Smeeding, 2006.

ing defined by need into a fully institutionalized population capable of articulating its own interests. The elites and reformers that have historically made the policy case on behalf of older people have no contemporary equals. The likes of Arthur Altmeyer, Robert Ball, Arthur Flemming, and Claude Pepper are nowhere to be found around aging policy today (Browdie, 2004). But, more importantly, the landscape has changed; aging policy has become institutionalized and routinized.

Second, in Schattschneider's (1960) famous words, "the scope of conflict has expanded." Derthick (1979a), in her article "How easy votes on Social Security came to an end," was among the first to observe that the closed decision-making circle she described in *Policymaking for Social Security* (1979b) has ceased to exist. Whether generationally or ideologically motivated (Hudson, 1999; Williamson and Watts-Roy, 2009), organized resistance has brought to an end Social Security's long existence in splendid isolation. Indeed, these twin factors—the new institutional presence of the aged (in both politics and policy) and the ideological and fiscal pressures bearing down on this presence—have created something of a perfect political storm.

Third, and last, if this loggerhead is to be broken as baby boomers enter old age, it may be the result of a reassessment of what old age is and who, in fact, the old are. People aged 65 or older enjoy an aggregate level of well-being that is stunning in comparison with the situation 50 years ago (e.g., poverty levels are down by a factor of four, health insurance coverage has risen from less than half to virtually the entire older population). Having celebrated those developments in the face of looming fiscal pressures, the question then emerges, Should benefits be cut either through increasing the age of eligibility or through some other mechanism? To further raise the age of eligibility for full Social Security benefits would, in policy terms (if not beyond), have old age begin at, say, age 75. Doing so would certainly save enormous sums and would probably arguably improve the program's target efficiency. Yet to do so might well have the ethically charged consequence of reresidualizing the aged, literally re-creating them as the singularly vulnerable group of a century ago.

Despite aging populations, globalization, and other contemporary pressures, it is not at all clear that the welfare state in general, or America's "old age welfare state" in particular, will be retrenched. It is clear, however, that the aged's new policy and political presence will represent an impressive counterweight against those who would pare away existing benefits.

References

Amenta, E. 2006. *When Movements Matter: The Townsend Plan and the Rise of Social Security*. Princeton, N.J.: Princeton University Press.

Bachrach, P., and M. Baratz. 1962. The two faces of power. *American Political Science Review* 56 (4): 947–52.

Ball, R. 2000. *Insuring the Essentials: Bob Ball on Social Security*. New York: Century Foundation Press.

Beer, S. H. 1966. *British Politics in the Collectivist Age*. New York: Alfred A. Knopf.

Binstock, R. H. 2000. Older people and voting participation: Past and future. *Gerontologist* 40 (1): 18–31.

Browdie, R. (ed.). 2004. Advocacy and aging. *Generations* 28 (1).

Buchanan, J., and G. Tullock. 1962. *The Calculus of Consent: Logical Foundations of Constitutional Democracy*. Ann Arbor: University of Michigan Press.

Burke, V. J., and V. Burke. 1974. *Nixon's Good Deed: Welfare Reform*. New York: Columbia University Press.

Cameron, D. R. 1978. The expansion of the public economy: A comparative analysis. *American Political Science Review* 72 (Dec.): 1243–61.

Campbell, A. L. 2003. *How Policies Make Citizens: Senior Political Activism and the American Welfare State.* Princeton, N.J.: Princeton University Press.

Derthick, M. 1979a. How easy votes on Social Security came to an end. *Public Interest* 54 (Winter): 94–105.

———. 1979b. *Policymaking for Social Security.* Washington, D.C.: Brookings Institution.

Easton, D. 1957. An approach to the analysis of political systems. *World Politics* 9 (3): 383–400.

Edelman, M. 1964. *The Symbolic Uses of Politics.* Urbana: University of Illinois Press.

Esping-Andersen, G. 1985. *Politics against Markets: The Social Democratic Road to Power.* Princeton, N.J.: Princeton University Press.

Estes, C. 1991. The new political economy of aging: An introduction and critique. Pp. 19–36 in M. Minkler and C. Estes (eds.), *Critical Perspectives on Aging.* Amityville, N.Y.: Baywood.

Estes, C., and E. A. Binney. 1991. The biomedicalization of aging: Dangers and dilemmas. Pp. 117–34 in M. Minkler and C. Estes (eds.), *Critical Perspectives on Aging.* Amityville, N.Y.: Baywood.

Fleming, D. 1963. Social Darwinism. Pp. 123–46 in A. Schlesinger (ed.), *Paths of American Thought.* New York: Houghton-Mifflin.

Fraser, N., and L. Gordon. 1992. Contract versus charity: Why is there no social citizenship in the United States? *Socialist Review* 22 (3): 45–67.

Gist, J. 2009. Population aging, entitlement growth, and the aging. Pp. 173–96 in R. B. Hudson (ed.), *Boomer Bust? Economic and Political Issues of the Graying Society.* Westport, Conn.: Praeger.

Gough, I. 1979. *The Political Economy of the Welfare State.* London: Macmillan.

Graebner, W. 1974. *A History of Retirement.* New Haven, Conn.: Yale University Press.

Gratton, B. 1986. The new history of the aged: A critique. Pp. 3–29 in D. Van Tassel and P. Stearns (eds.), *Old Age in a Bureaucratic Society.* Westport, Conn.: Greenwood.

Greenstone, J. D. 1969. *Labor in American Politics.* New York: Vintage.

Heclo, H. 1974. *Modern Social Politics in Britain and Sweden: From Relief to Income Maintenance.* New Haven, Conn.: Yale University Press.

Hendricks, J., and C. Leedham. 1991. Dependency or empowerment: Toward a moral and political economy of aging. Pp. 51–66 in M. Minkler and C. Estes (eds.), *Critical Perspectives on Aging.* Amityville, N.Y.: Baywood.

Himelfarb, R. 1995. *Catastrophic Politics: The Rise and Fall of the Medicare Catastrophic Coverage Act of 1988.* University Park: Pennsylvania State University Press.

Horton, J. 1966. Order and conflict theories of social problems as competing ideologies. *American Journal of Sociology* 71 (6): 701–13.

Huber, E., J. Stephens, and D. Ray. 1999. The welfare state in hard times. Pp. 164–93 in H. Kitschelt, P. Lange, G. Marks, and J. Stephens (eds.), *Continuity and Change in Contemporary Capitalism.* Cambridge: Cambridge University Press.

Hudson, R. B. 1978. The "graying" of the federal budget and its consequences for old-age policy. *Gerontologist* 18 (5, part 1): 428–40.

———. 1994. The Older Americans Act and the defederalization of community-based care. Pp. 45–75 in P. Kim (ed.), *Services to the Aged: Public Policies and Programs.* New York: Garland.

———. 1999. Conflict in today's aging politics: New population encounters old ideology. *Social Service Review* 73 (3): 358–79.

Huntington, S. 1966. Political modernization: America vs. Europe. *World Politics* 18 (3): 378–414.

Iglehart, J. 2004. The new Medicare prescription drug benefit: A pure power play. *New England Journal of Medicine* 350 (8): 826–33.

Ikenberry, G. J., and T. Skocpol. 1987. Expanding social benefits: The role of Social Security. *Political Science Quarterly* 102 (3): 389–416.

Lipset, S. M., and G. Marks. 2001. *It Didn't Happen Here: Why Socialism Failed in the United States.* New York: W.W. Norton.

Lowi, T. J. 1964. American business, public policy, case-studies, and political theory. *World Politics* 16 (4): 677–715.

———. 1967. The public philosophy: Interest group liberalism. *American Political Science Review* 61 (1): 5–24.

Lukes, S. 1974. *Power: A Radical View.* London: Macmillan.

Madland, D. 2007. The politics of pension cuts. Pp. 187–214 in T. Ghilarducci and C. E. Weller (eds.), *Employee Pensions: Policies, Problems, and Possibilities.* Champaign, Ill.: Labor and Employment Relations Association.

Marmor, T. R. 1970. *The Politics of Medicare.* Chicago: Aldine.

Marmor, T. R., J. L. Mashaw, and P. L. Harvey. 1990. *America's Misunderstood Welfare State.* New York: Basic Books.

Marshall, T. H. 1964. *Class, Citizenship, and Social Development.* Garden City, N.Y.: Doubleday.

Mead, L. 1998. Telling the poor what to do. *Public Interest* 132 (Summer): 97–112.

Mettler, S. 2007. The transformed welfare state and the redistribution of voice. Pp. 191–222 in P. Pierson and T. Skocpol (eds.), *The Transformation of American Politics*. Princeton, N.J.: Princeton University Press.

Myles, J. 1984. *Old Age in the Welfare State*. Boston: Little Brown.

Myles, J., and J. Quadagno. 2002. Political theories of the welfare state. *Social Service Review* 76 (1): 34–57.

Nettl, J. P. 1968. The state as a conceptual variable. *World Politics* 20 (4): 559–92.

Niskanen, W. 1971. *Bureaucracy and Representative Government*. Chicago: Aldine.

O'Conner, J. 1973. *The Fiscal Crisis of the State*. New York: St. Martin's.

Orloff, A. S. 1988. The political origins of America's belated welfare state. Pp. 37–80 in M. Weir, A. S. Orloff, and T. Skocpol (eds.), *The Politics of Social Policy in the United States*. Princeton, N.J.: Princeton University Press.

Pampel, F., and J. Williamson. 1992. *Age, Class, Politics, and the Welfare State*. New York: Cambridge University Press.

Parenti, M. 1970. Power and pluralism: A view from the bottom. *Journal of Politics* 32 (3): 501–30.

Peterson, P. G. 1999. *Gray Dawn: How the Coming Age Wave Will Transform America—and the World*. New York: New York Times Books.

Pierson, P. 1994. *Dismantling the Welfare State? Reagan, Thatcher, and the Politics of Retrenchment*. New York: Cambridge University Press.

———. 2007. The rise and reconfiguration of activist government. Pp. 19–38 in P. Pierson and T. Skocpol (eds.), *The Transformation of American Politics*. Princeton, N.J.: Princeton University Press.

Piven, F. F., and R. Cloward. 1971. *Regulating the Poor: The Functions of Public Welfare*. New York: Vintage.

Polsby, N. 1963. *Community Power and Political Theory*. New Haven, Conn.: Yale University Press.

Pratt, H. J. 1976. *The Gray Lobby*. Chicago: University of Chicago Press.

———. 1993. *Gray Agendas*. Ann Arbor: University of Michigan Press.

Price, M. C. 1997. *Justice between Generations: The Growing Power of the Elderly in America*. Westport, Conn.: Greenwood.

Putnam, R. D. 1995. Bowling alone: America's declining social capital. *Journal of Democracy* 6 (1): 65–78.

Quadagno, J. 1988. *The Transformation of Old Age Security*. Chicago: University of Chicago Press.

———. 2005. *One Nation, Uninsured: Why the U.S. Has No National Health Insurance*. New York: Oxford University Press.

Rimlinger, G. 1971. *Welfare Policy and Industrialization in Europe, America, and Russia*. New York: Wiley.

Robertson, D. B. 1993. The return to history and the new institutionalism in American political science. *Social Science History* 17 (1): 1–36.

Rosenberg, C. 1962. *The Cholera Years.* Chicago: University of Chicago Press.

Ryan, W. 1971. *Blaming the Victim.* New York: Knopf.

Samuelson, R. J. 2005. AARP's America is a mirage. *Washington Post* (Nov. 16), A19.

Schattschneider, E. E. 1935. *Politics, Pressures, and the Tariff.* New York: Prentice-Hall.

———. 1960. *The Semi-Sovereign People.* New York: Wiley.

Schneider, A. L., and H. Ingram. 1993. Social construction of target populations. *American Political Science Review* 87 (2): 253–77.

Skocpol, T. 1985. Bringing the state back in: Strategies of analysis and current research. Pp. 3–43 in P. Evans, D. Rueschemeyer, and T. Skocpol (eds.), *Bringing the State Back In.* New York: Cambridge University Press.

———. 1991. State formation and social policy in the United States. *American Behavioral Scientist* 34 (4/5): 559–84.

———. 1992. *Protecting Soldiers and Mothers.* Cambridge, Mass.: Belknap Press.

Smeeding, T. 2006. Poor people in rich nations. *Journal of Economic Perspectives* 20 (1): 69–90.

Teles, S. 2007. Conservative mobilization against entrenched liberalism. Pp. 160–88 in P. Pierson and T. Skocpol (eds.), *The Transformation of American Politics.* Princeton, N.J.: Princeton University Press.

U.S. Bureau of the Census. 2004. *Current Population Survey* (Nov., and earlier reports). Washington, D.C.: U.S. Department of Commerce, U.S. Bureau of the Census.

Walker, J. 1983. The origins and maintenance of interest groups in America. *American Political Science Review* 77 (2): 390–406.

Wilensky, H. 1975. *The Welfare State and Equality.* Berkeley: University of California Press.

Wilensky, H., and C. Lebeaux. 1958. *Industrial Society and Social Welfare.* New York: Free Press.

Williamson, J. B., and D. Watts-Roy. 2009. Aging boomers, generational equity, and the framing of the debate over Social Security. Pp. 153–72 in R. B. Hudson (ed.), *Boomer Bust?: Economic and Political Issues of the Graying Society.* Westport, Conn.: Praeger.

Wilson, J. Q. 1973. *Political Organizations.* New York: Basic Books.

Witte, E. E. 1963. *The Development of the Social Security Act.* Madison: University of Wisconsin Press.

II. The Populations of Aging Policy

7. On Time and Ties
Why the Life Course Matters for Old Age Policies

Richard A. Settersten, Jr., Ph.D., and
Molly E. Trauten, M.G.S.

The emergence and maturation of the life-course perspective is one of the most significant social science developments of the last half-century. This chapter explores how some of the key emphases of a life-course perspective might yield new insights for old age policies. These emphases include the need to describe the experiences of individuals and groups over long stretches of time and to explain the short- and long-ranging causes and consequences of these patterns. They also include the need to understand how these experiences are shaped by the many social settings in which people grow up and age. A life-course perspective also emphasizes how the lives of individuals are intimately affected by the circumstances and choices of other people. For these and other reasons, there is a natural, mutual attraction between scholarship on the life course and scholarship on aging (for an overview, see Settersten, 2006a; see also Elder and Johnson, 2003).

Sociological research on the life course has especially pointed to the macro, or *distal*, social forces that guide and govern how life unfolds for individuals and groups—historical events and periods of social change, population processes, the economy and the labor market, and the like (Mayer, 2004; Settersten, 2005, 2009). The government, with its corresponding welfare state, is chief among these forces. Social policies at federal, state, and local levels powerfully determine opportunities and outcomes in every realm of life—education, employment, finances, family, health, leisure, and more. The reach of policies is far, their hold is strong, and their legacies are made even more powerful by the fact that, as individuals, we are often not even conscious of their presence. The policies and programs of a welfare state are also based on, and reinforce, core cultural ideas about how the life course is (or is supposed to be) organized and what people do (or should be doing) in different periods of life. Policies are even used to define particular periods of life or to regulate when people leave one period and enter the next.

In this chapter, we illustrate some of the ways that the life course matters for old age policies, especially during the *young-old*, or early postretirement, years—what James and Wink (2006) call the *crown of life*. We point especially to dynamics related to two key themes: time and age, and social ties.

On Time and Age

A Slice of Life

The programs and policies of most welfare states are likely to address particular periods of life, or particular kinds of experiences regardless of when they happen in life, rather than the whole of life. The U.S. welfare state extends its greatest support to individuals at the two ends of life—children and old people—because both groups are assumed to be especially vulnerable and dependent or, in the case of older people, to be at risk of becoming dependent or to be deserving of support because of their prior contributions to society (see also Skocpol, 2000).

For adults who are not yet old, minimal and temporary spot coverage is to be found around specific events or periods of risk, especially those that interfere or intersect with paid work, such as spells of unemployment, poverty, disability, or family leave. Programs kick in to keep some semblance of equilibrium, attempting either to restore these individuals or groups to a prior state or to provide a small boost in resources while they encounter especially difficult times, often with the aim of reducing the degree to which individuals are dependent on others. Policies that provide money or in-kind assistance to those without jobs, health insurance, food, or housing are good examples. These policies carry assumptions about the individuals and groups that are neediest and most deserving of help, as well as what kinds of resources they should get and how long they should get them.

These approaches reflect the premium that the U.S. welfare state places on personal responsibility and self-reliance (Hacker, 2006). That is, for working age adults who are not yet eligible for old age policies, the message sent by the welfare state is that individuals are largely on their own to cope with problems using the safety nets, resources, and skills they have or those they can garner through others.

This is consistent with the emergent philosophy of many modern welfare states, which, even when they extend support, prefer strategies that *equip* individuals and families with skills to actively manage their lives through their own actions rather than strategies that simply *protect* them from changes and risks (Esping-Andersen, 2002).

As welfare states around the world grew in the second half of the twentieth century, social policies established and reinforced markers for some of life's stages. This is particularly true in defining both the beginning of adulthood and the beginning of old age. In the latter case, old age has traditionally been signaled by retirement—or, more specifically, the age of eligibility for Social Security or pension benefits. In the United States this has historically been at age 65, even though many people over 65 today would not declare themselves to be "old." This threshold has been incrementally increased for later birth cohorts. Retirement patterns have, however, undergone significant changes in recent decades. Whether out of choice or necessity, older workers have increasingly found alternatives to moving directly into full-time retirement, such as bridge jobs, part-time work, and limited-time returns to work during retirement (e.g., Cahill, Giandrea, and Quinn, 2006). An abrupt transition from work to nonwork is no longer the norm. These changes may eventually prompt new markers of old age that are not as bound to work (for illustrations, see Settersten and Trauten, 2009).

Old age is also now life's longest period, extending three or more decades and comprised of early and late phases that are often extremely different from each other (see also chapter 9). Gerontologists have responded by splitting old age, or the population of older people, into categories such as the *young old*, *old old*, and *oldest old*, or the *third* and *fourth ages*, in an effort to create a more nuanced view of life's final decades and the people in them. For example, in the young-old, or third-age, years, individuals are free of responsibilities in work and child care and are in good health, have adequate resources and time left to live, and can realize new forms or a greater degree of self-fulfillment (Gilleard et al., 2005). While the third age and other periods are often defined in chronological terms, they are not bound to age as much as to physical health, attitudes, and lifestyle.

Policy makers, like scholars, develop extensive portfolios of initiatives around the particular circumstances and needs of individuals in different periods of life or around particular transitions. To some degree, it is necessary and effective to slice up life into manageable units. In doing so, however, we create a vast and fragmented array of policies and we lose sight of the life course as a whole.

The Accumulation of Experience and Inequality

Old age policies are based on an assumption that once people reach their mid- to late 60s, they have a common set of needs or are at risk by virtue of their age. Policies use age or age groups as a basis for providing opportunities and allocating resources. Yet people of every age exhibit significant variability in their physical, psychological, and social statuses. This is particularly true of old age. In part this is the result of the accumulation of individual experiences over many decades that creates life courses as unique as fingerprints. But the differences among old people are also generated by processes related to social inequality, such that those who are more advantaged at the beginning of life accumulate greater resources and opportunities throughout their lives relative to those who start life in more disadvantaged positions. These processes increase the disparities among people by the time they are old (Dannefer, 2003).

As the variability among old people grows, it is unclear what they have in common or what makes old age different from any other period of life. One of the primary ways in which old age does seem distinct from other periods is that life's later years have a highly contingent quality. Old age is embodied with so much possibility, as individuals can count on a long and largely healthy old age. Revolutionary declines in mortality and morbidity in the last century have made a vibrant third age possible. But the potentials of these years, if they are to be realized, hinge on having health, resources, and relationships—all of which can suddenly, unexpectedly, and permanently change in late life with the onset of illness, the illness or loss of a spouse, the inability to live independently, the limited capacity of children to help, the instability of markets, and the like. As these contingencies come undone, so do futures that have been counted on or taken for granted. They quickly make the maintenance of the third age difficult. These contingencies, and the ability of individuals and families to manage them, are also exacerbated by the inequalities described earlier and the fact that there is relatively less time to recover when things go awry.

Old age policies are particularly important in ensuring stability, or at least minimizing some of the fallout, when these changes occur. Some changes associated with aging may also be postponed but rarely escaped, such as normative declines in physical health or cognitive abilities. Still, those with greater resources of many kinds are better positioned to manage or compensate for those universal declines. Most aspects of aging can be expected to be shaped by social class: life expectancy, physical and psychological health, family structure and relationships, social integration and engagement, personal resources, and so forth. In the future, social class seems likely to become an even more powerful factor in determining patterns of aging and in creating serious cleavages within societies (Furstenberg, 2003; Kohli, 2007). Old age policies must therefore be more sensitive to how social class produces different worlds of old age, especially in combination with race, ethnicity, and immigration status, which are radically altering the composition of the U.S. population. Given the variability among old people, it seems likely that subgroups of people *within* the aged population have greater competing needs—especially in terms of wealth and health—than ever before, which also fractures the political solidarity they may have as a group (Binstock, 2004). These inequalities are likely to make aging and the life course even greater sources of political regulation and conflict, and potentially leave old age policies highly contested.

Looking Back to Look Ahead

A life-course perspective emphasizes the need to understand human lives *prospectively* (forward in time) and *retrospectively* (backward in time). Some old age policies have both prospective and retrospective aspects of time at their core. Social Security and pension plans are good examples. These policies are future oriented because they are ultimately aimed at providing or improving income security throughout late life. This is done under the assumption that old age is or should be a period of retirement or leisure, whether because health challenges may make it difficult to continue working or because elders should be rewarded for their prior contributions to society and should therefore be able to more freely enjoy their final years.

These policies, however, are also bound to the past, as benefit levels in old age are tightly tied to an individual's work history. For example, in defined-benefit plans, pension levels are generally a function of the duration of employment and the last few years of earnings. Vesting rules may bring about a complete loss of benefits if an employee leaves the position before the vestment period has passed or may penalize workers who leave before official retirement ages. In defined-contribution plans, by contrast, an employer makes annual investments based on a percentage of an employee's annual income. These plans generally have much shorter vesting periods and are often portable. Defined-contribution plans therefore do not penalize individuals with fragmented work histories (e.g., those who alternate between full- and part-time status, take leaves, change jobs) to the same degree as defined-benefit plans. The shift toward contingent models of work, to be discussed shortly, has been accompanied by a shift toward defined-contribution plans and an increase in the proportion of workers who are without pensions and, in some cases, without benefits of any kind.

Whether individuals are entitled to Social Security benefits, and how much they receive, also depends on a number of factors. These include the year a person was born, his or her age at retirement, his or her average career earnings in employment covered by Social Security, and, most importantly, a relatively constant work history, one with relatively few zeros in the formula used to calculate retirement benefits. These formulas disadvantage workers who have discontinuous employment histories due to family responsibilities, limited skills or low-wage work, discrimination in the workplace, involuntary job separation, periods of joblessness, physical or mental health conditions, and other factors. Because less-stable employment is typical of women, racial and ethnic minorities, and those in more vulnerable sectors of the labor market, these benefit formulas exacerbate economic inequality among old people (Flippen and Tienda, 2000).

In understanding the welfare of old people, it is therefore important to know about the many decades they have already lived, especially where earlier pathways may have resulted in or increased risks for problematic outcomes in old age. But in some ways it is the limited time left that constrains the abilities of either individuals or policies to make up for past inadequacies. This contrasts with policies created for children, adolescents, and young adults, who have much of their lives in front of them and for whom current investments are presumed to yield future payoffs in well-being both for the individuals themselves and for society at large. For these reasons, policies for the young are more often construed as preventative, even if they are ultimately ameliorative (e.g., Head Start, foster care). Because children have many decades of life in front of them, attempts to improve their circumstances will (potentially) have positive effects that accumulate throughout their lives—or at least suppress or minimize overtly negative effects later on. Policies for the old, in contrast, are framed more as being ameliorative and designed with a shorter time horizon in mind. One could argue that Social Security is the biggest ameliorative policy related to income, and Medicare for health, in providing basic income security to most old people and health coverage to all old people.

Anticipating the Future of Old Age

Virtually everything known about aging is based on cohorts born early in the first few decades of the twentieth century. The last century was punctuated by remarkable events and changes related to war, economic hardship and prosperity, health epidemics, civil rights, and shifts in medicine, communication, and transportation. The Great Depression and military service during World War II, in particular, heavily marked the lives of men and women who are now old (Settersten, 2006b). These historical events and changes may lurk beneath much of the scientific knowledge base in gerontology. In terms of policies, these cohorts are also unique. Their early lives saw and benefited significantly from the inception of the New Deal and its programs in the early 1930s; their military service, too, brought educational, housing, and other benefits related to the G. I. Bill after World War II; and they later saw and benefited from the programs of the Great Society of the mid-1960s.

This means that we do not know how much of our current knowledge base about aging will apply to future cohorts whose historical experiences have been very different from those who are currently old. Later cohorts have also grown up and older with different resources, expectations, and needs, and they have been subject to different constellations of government programs and policies, with different types and levels of support.

We do not need to wait to see how they are different. The future of aging is already here. It can be understood by getting more intimately acquainted with cohorts who are *not yet old*. Understanding cohorts now in middle age is particularly important, for they are next in the queue. For example, doom-and-gloom public discourse surrounding the baby boom generation has focused on how its size has strained the social institutions through which its members have moved during early and middle adulthood (Schulz and Binstock, 2007). There is little doubt such challenges will continue to affect members of the baby boom as its individuals move through old age. But it is important to remember that the physical, psychological, and social statuses of the boomers are rather favorable relative to cohorts past. One could argue, in fact, that in the future there may not be another group of people who enter old age as *uniformly* well positioned and with as much potential as the older boomers, in particular. The recent surge of interest in the civic engagement of the young old seems symbolic of the new potentials inherent in the boomers (Morrow-Howell and Freedman, 2006–7). Important insights for policy making will be found by probing the implications of their better positions for all aspects of aging, as well as in examining their aspirations and expectations for old age.

We should also become intimately acquainted with cohorts currently in early adulthood. For example, members of these cohorts are experiencing a significantly prolonged transition to adulthood, with substantial delays accompanying many specific transitions, including leaving home, finishing school, starting work, being married or partnered, and having children (Settersten, 2007a). The routes they are taking toward adult roles and responsibilities are also more circuitous and do not match the linear models of life that underlie many contemporary policies related to education, work, and family. These mismatches will play out in ways never before seen. Relative to other cohorts, younger generations are in some ways better off (e.g., men, women, and members of racial and ethnic minority groups have had greater access to higher education and unparalleled educational attainment), and in some ways worse off (e.g., their housing and educational debts are greater, and they have encountered new vulnerabilities as the service and knowledge sectors of the economy have grown; see Danziger and Rouse, 2008). Their world views are also clearly different from previous cohorts (e.g., they are more liberal on a wide range of social and political measures, but they have much lower social engagement; see Smith, 2005). As these young adults grow older, they, like the boomers, will further challenge much of what we now take for granted about aging.

These shifts—from the boomers, to current young adults, and further down—serve as reminders that lives and times seem always to be in flux, and that change is the rule rather than the exception. As change occurs, we cannot treat new conditions as if they have become permanent, for these conditions, too, will eventually be displaced by others. The constant presence of change is what makes updating policies both so important and so difficult.

Breakups in the Lock-Step Life

Human lives can change dramatically, but social policies and institutions lag behind the times, resist change, and become stagnant. Policy makers must be sensitive to these dynamics, not only because it is important to tune them up or make them over, but also because *not* doing so creates serious risks for people whose lives do not or *cannot* meet the expectations in those policies and institutions, given the realities of the world today.

A good example is that work has traditionally been the central force in organizing the life course in Western societies into three successive "boxes": education, work, and retirement. This three-box structure has characterized the lives of men, and increasingly of women as the latter's educational attainment and labor force participation have grown. Recent decades, however, have brought not only important changes to the boundaries that demarcate these three boxes, but also challenges to the viability of the model itself (Settersten, 2003).

The early part of adult life, for example, has seen major extensions in education. Entry into full-time work has been delayed because young people often pursue education and work simultaneously or alternate between spells of school and work. These changes mean that individuals from recent cohorts have gotten a late start in building private and public pension funds. This will potentially reduce their resources in old age, a problem made worse by the fact that gains in longevity have also extended the retirement period.

In the middle part of life, modernization and rapid technological change have similarly made it necessary for working adults to return to school or seek training that will allow them to update their skills and knowledge to remain competitive in new markets. Yet most scholarships, federal grants, work-study funds, and low-interest loans are generally awarded only to full-time, degree-seeking students, which most adults cannot be. As a result, expenses for educational activity must be paid out of pocket, making a return to school unaffordable or impossible for many adults, especially if it also means losing their health insurance. These constraints make it difficult for adults to improve their economic standing in the job market.

The need to remain competitive in new markets has especially grown as *lifetime models of work*—in which employers and employees invest in a long-term partnership, and the longer an employee spends with the firm, the better his or her wages, job security, job mobility, and pension—have eroded. Stable work has itself become uncertain, and many jobs no longer come with health insurance or benefits or, if they do, the jobs come with much lower levels of protection than they did in the past. Additionally, while growing numbers of middle-aged individuals must reduce their work commitments to care for elderly parents, growing numbers of middle-aged parents are also extending significant support to adult children in their 20s and 30s (e.g., Schoeni and Ross, 2005). The provision of support to old parents or young-adult children may bring financial and other kinds of strain or alter plans for retirement.

We noted earlier that in late life, a wider array of routes into retirement is now more common. For some time, there was also a surprising trend toward early retirement. Coupled with delays in full-time work at the start of adult life, the trend toward early retirement meant that the period of gainful work became shorter. There is now evidence, however, that the trend toward early retirement is reversing and will eventually jump ahead by at least a few years. This is partly produced by incremental changes in eligibility ages for Social Security and partly by the need for individuals to remain employed longer in order to support themselves and their family members. For many, the need to remain employed may now have grown in the face of the current economic recession, prompted by the subprime mortgage crisis, which has significantly reduced the resources at their disposal. Changes such as these would seem to undermine the future of the third age, described earlier, which is predicated on traditional retirement.

Despite these and other changes, the three-box structure is created and reinforced by policies that regulate education, work, and retirement. This means that when the lives of individuals depart from this three-box structure, whether by choice or out of need, they are penalized for it. A simple example of such a penalty is health insurance. In the United States, having health insurance hinges on the good fortune of either having full-time employment and employer-provided health insurance benefits, or of being legally attached (as a spouse or dependent) to someone who does. If one makes choices or finds oneself in a position that strays from these conditions, there are no protections. Having to live without basic health insurance is a scary thing. It is therefore hard to break free from this three-box structure, especially intentionally, when some of life's basic protections—for oneself and for one's family—are bound to it.

Another brief example concerns the replacement of lifetime models of work, described earlier, by *contingent models of work*. These models are characterized by time-bound contracts with no promise of work beyond those parameters—and even no contracts at all. Movement toward contingent models of work has been driven by technological change, foreign competition, concerns about the cost of labor, the decline of manufacturing, and the growth of service-sector positions, which offer few benefits, low wages, and are generally not unionized. The result is that employers keep fewer employees in their lifetime pools and more employees in their contingent pools. This shift carries significant implications for social policies and for the security of individuals and families. For example, such a shift means that health care coverage, pension plans, and Social Security benefit levels may be jeopardized or significantly lowered. Because careers have become more disjointed, it may also mean that individuals need unemployment insurance more often and for longer periods of time. Changes such as these affect the well-being not only of employees, but also of the spouses and children attached to them as dependents and beneficiaries.

On Social Ties

The Interdependence of Lives

A life-course perspective emphasizes the linked or *interdependent* nature of human lives. Quite simply, this principle states that the lives of individuals are intimately affected by, and themselves affect, the circumstances and choices of others. Family relationships are, of course, a prime example of this. Despite the easy recognition that individual lives cannot be understood in isolation from others, *individuals* are almost always the targets of policies and, rather ironically, policies are often intended to decrease the dependence of individuals on others (Mayer and Schöpflin, 1989; Leisering, 2003).

To compensate for life's new risks and for the often limited resources of families and welfare states, an effective strategy for success in every period of life is to build stronger and wider webs of relationships with others who can provide guidance and support. Of course, this is the default solution in a welfare state such as the United States, which emphasizes individual responsibility and limited government support. If this is to be the solution, the irony is that those who have the greatest personal resources thrive and those who are most disadvantaged remain that way because they have few resources themselves and are not part of extensive, resource-rich networks that can be mobilized for support.

For example, as old age has become longer and more individualized, the family is the primary institution that is called on to absorb the costs of new vulnerabilities and risks. The ability of families to manage this long and complex period varies extensively, according to the resources they possess or those they can access through formal and informal ties. Experiences in old age can therefore be drastically different, depending on personal and family resources and connections. Old people in relatively privileged families may have the luxury of using the later years for purposes of exploration—to return to school, to switch careers or work as desired, to volunteer, to pursue activities aimed at personal growth and development, and the like. In contrast, for old people in less-privileged families, these possibilities seem more tenuous and even out of reach, as they may be required to work beyond retirement age; their lives must be managed with limited means or poorer health, as their own family members also struggle to stay afloat and cannot readily provide or buy support.

Family relationships extend across the life course, but the nature of family relationships changes as members grow older and as the structure of the family, and the place of individuals in it, changes over time. Many policies target special family circumstances that emerge at particular points in life. For example, policies are often targeted at periods when families are being formed (e.g., maternity or paternity leave), children are young (e.g., child care, child abuse, child support, custody, or parental leave), children are adolescents and young adults (e.g., school vouchers, college financial aid), or parents are old (e.g., elder care). In most of these cases, dependent children are targeted through their parents. In the case of elder care, middle-aged children are targeted because of their increased responsibility for their parents.

Women, Men, and Social Relationships

To date, women's family relationships and friendships have been more active, positive, and have offered greater protection than those of men (Settersten, 2007b). But as women's educational attainment surpasses that of men, and as their work patterns more closely approximate those of men, one begins to wonder whether these commitments will also take a toll on women's social relationships. The long-term legacies of divorce and remarriage on social relationships in old age are also unknown. Still, the greater human capital of women suggests that they will have new resources and choices as they move into old age in the future. Women's lifelong commitments to more diverse and multiple roles may also make it easier for them to adjust to change and manage hardships when they are old.

Men's family relationships are especially important to watch in the future, particularly the connections between men and children (for further discussion, see Settersten, 2007b). Surprisingly, a range of social indicators reveal that men are, as a group, becoming less—not more—intensely involved with and committed to children (Eggebeen, 2002). The widespread prevalence of divorce is particularly important, because divorce generally leads to a loss or a restriction of fathers' ties to their children.

What will these trends mean for men's future experiences in old age? The picture is bleak if men's social relationships in late life become even more tenuous than they are today. Yet it is also possible that subgroups of fathers who clearly *are* making bigger investments in children when they are little will end up with more protective relationships with those children when they are grown. Cohorts of young men currently entering adulthood also have more fluid attitudes about masculinity and manhood, which may open up men's experiences in family relationships and friendships and result in deeper and more resourceful ties when they are old (Cohler and Smith, 2006). The growing instability of work for men, and its corresponding losses in income and benefits, will also reduce the resources that men can build for themselves and provide to others, undermine their role in families, and make their need to invest in relationships even stronger.

Relationships as Risks in Policies

We cannot assume that our ties to other people are merely sources of help and protection. They can also bring hardship, limit opportunities, and create risk. This is true in the policy context, as it is in everyday life. As an example, consider the spousal benefits for Social Security. These benefits are tied to not only the work history of the spouse, but also to the marital history of the couple. This has especially important implications for women's lives. Social Security rules are based on a model of marriage in which men are the sole wage-earners within marriages that start early and last long. These rules protected current and past cohorts of older women because most of these women did not have either earnings histories of their own or histories that matched eligibility expectations. What these women did have were long-lasting marriages to men who met eligibility criteria; they could count on benefits through their husbands. Even so, these spousal benefits devalue women's contributions because they are generally equivalent to about half of what their husbands received.

Against contemporary divorce and remarriage patterns, however, women have become even more vulnerable. A little-known Social Security regulation is that divorced women can draw on spousal benefits only if their marriages last a minimum of 10 years. While women from recent cohorts have longer work histories than their predecessors, they nonetheless continue to cycle in and out of the labor force, or between part- and full-time work statuses, in response to family demands, leaving their work histories more sporadic than men's. The work histories of many women will not be enough to meet basic eligibility requirements related to work duration, though their levels of support are affected by work patterns and positions, since benefit values increase with longer, more continuous employment.

But what many women no longer have are long-lived marriages, and this may place future cohorts of women at greater risk than their predecessors in old age. These risks also are heightened by the fact that divorced men are more likely to remarry than divorced women, which may leave men less likely to deliver on alimony or other forms of support and leave women with fewer resources of their own. It is also prudent to remember that divorce comes not only to young marriages, but also increasingly to marriages of people in the second half of life, making the experience of divorce inherently different for them and bringing more immediate consequences for their situations in late life because they have less time to rebound or recover from any hardships.

The combination of higher rates of remarriage for men, the trend for men to marry women who are younger, and the sex differential in life expectancy mean that the majority of men spend most of their adult lives with a spouse and that they are much more likely to have wives living when they face illness, serious impairment, and death. In contrast, women are likely to spend several, if not many, years alone after the death of their husbands and, consequently, be more dependent on care from others, especially their children.

There are many such examples of the explicit and implicit assumptions in social policies about the presence and nature of relationships, many of which are no longer warranted in light of dramatic changes in marriage, divorce, and remarriage, as well as in light of the new diversity of family forms, such as single-parent households, cohabitating couples, gay and lesbian couples, interracial or multiethnic families, and individuals and couples who are intentionally single and childless. This diversity seems likely to increase in the future (Bianchi, Robinson, and Milkie, 2006). Some of these diverse families, such as gay and lesbian families, are socially and politically contested and their ties to one another are neither recognized nor permitted in the eyes of the law. Legal definitions of family reward some kinds of relationships and penalize others, spilling over onto every policy that rests on those definitions. They alter, often in life-changing ways, the options that individuals and their families face. For example, according to Lambda Legal (www.lambdalegal.org), marriage brings as many as 1,400 legal rights at the federal and state levels. When gay and lesbian families are not permitted to marry, or when long-term heterosexual couples do not marry, these protections and benefits are not extended to them—including joint parental rights for their children, joint adoption, next-of-kin status for hospital visitation and medical decisions, Social Security survivor benefits, and bereavement or sick leave for a partner or child. Similar problems exist for immigrants and other types of families whose relationships are uncertain or excluded in the eyes of the law.

The new diversity of families has changed the look and feel of the extended families in which elders now exist, and it will change the look and feel of old age when members of younger cohorts, whose family patterns have been so different, reach later life. It will also eventually require that legal definitions of "the family" be enlarged, even if this continues to come with some resistance.

Conclusion

Great shake-ups are afoot in every period of life, including old age. Too exclusive a focus on any particular period of life compromises what is most important about a life-course perspective: a dynamic and process-based approach to understanding the transitions and trajectories of individuals and cohorts as they grow older. Gerontologists and policy makers must actively take into account matters of time; the phenomena we study or seek to affect demand it. Even if our primary concerns ultimately relate to old age, there are six or more decades of life that precede and profoundly shape it. Old age itself also spans three or more decades, which requires us to understand how experiences in it are both highly variable and susceptible to change.

The need to take a long view of life, whether in looking back or looking forward, is at odds with key emphases of the U.S. welfare state, which provides temporary spot coverage for unusual events or periods of significant transition or risk, and which clings heavily to age as a simple administrative tool for allocating entitlements and benefits, regardless of individuals' capacities or resources. The state's emphasis on individuals as targets of activity is also at odds with a fundamental fact of human life: that the circumstances, options, and resources of individuals are intimately bound to other people. Almost everything that happens in our lives—the good, the bad, and the ugly—is connected to other people. The people to whom we are connected also change as we grow older, shifting in response to our personal circumstances and the everyday settings in which we exist.

A life-course perspective emphasizes the importance of updating or remaking social policies to better keep up with the times. It begs us to better anticipate the future: not only to pursue immediate answers to current problems by focusing on individuals who are already old, but also to ready ourselves for future needs by focusing of those who are not yet old. In addition, it underscores the need to understand and respond to the sources and consequences of social inequalities. A more *anticipatory gerontology*, to use Cain's (2003) term, will enrich the field by fostering the perspective of jurisprudence, not just politics, in confronting issues of equitability within and across age groups. These prospects will not only promote more effective social planning and policy making, but ultimately bring about important opportunities and obligations to foster greater compassion and concern for people of all ages.

The welfare state touches the lives of everyone and has profound and sometimes unintended bearings on the whole life course. While most U.S. policies *affect* the life course, however, they are not *life-course policies* designed with the whole of life in mind and intended to integrate multiple life periods (Leisering, 2003). Policies and programs for particular life periods cannot be designed in isolation from other periods, for the changes occurring in one period have repercussions for others. A key challenge is to figure out how to articulate a more coherent, coordinated, and comprehensive set of policies and programs for the entire life course. Movement in these directions is essential for ensuring the well-being of societies and their citizens now and in the future, at home and around the world.

References

Bianchi, S. M., J. P. Robinson, and M. A. Milkie. 2006. *Changing Rhythms of American Family Life*. New York: Russell Sage Foundation.

Binstock, R. H. 2004. The prolonged old, the long-lived society, and the politics of age. Pp. 362–86 in S. G. Post and R. H. Binstock (eds.), *The Fountain of Youth*. New York: Oxford University Press.

Cahill, K. E., M. D. Giandrea, and J. F. Quinn. 2006. Retirement patterns from career employment. *Gerontologist* 46 (4): 514–23.

Cain, L. 2003. Age-related phenomena: The interplay of the ameliorative and the scientific. Pp. 295–325 in R. A. Settersten, Jr. (ed.), *Invitation to the Life Course: Toward New Understandings of Later Life*. Amityville, N.Y.: Baywood.

Cohler, B. J., and G. D. Smith. 2006. The dilemma of masculinity and culture. Pp. 3–26 in V. H. Bedford and B. F. Turner (eds.), *Men in Relationships: A New Look from a Life-Course Perspective*. New York: Springer.

Dannefer, D. 2003. Cumulative advantage/disadvantage and the life course: Cross-fertilizing age and social science theory. *Journals of Gerontology, Series B: Social Sciences* 58 (6): S327–37.

Danziger, S., and C. Rouse (eds.). 2007. *The Price of Independence: The Economics of Early Adulthood*. New York: Russell Sage Foundation.

Eggebeen, D. J. 2002. The changing course of fatherhood: Men's experiences with children in demographic perspective. *Journal of Family Issues* 23 (4): 486–506.

Elder, G. H., Jr., and M. K. Johnson. 2003. The life course and aging: Challenges, lessons, and new directions. Pp. 49–81 in R. A. Settersten, Jr. (ed.), *Invitation to the Life Course: Toward New Understandings of Later Life*. Amityville, N.Y.: Baywood.

Esping-Andersen, G. 2002. Towards the good society, once again? Pp. 1–25 in G. Esping-Andersen, D. Gallie, A. Hemerijck, and J. Myles (eds.), *Why We Need a New Welfare State*. Oxford: Oxford University Press.

Flippen, C., and M. E. Tienda. 2000. Pathways to retirement: Patterns of labor force participation and labor market exit among the pre-retirement population by race, Hispanic origin, and sex. *Journals of Gerontology, Series B: Social Sciences* 55 (1): S14–27.

Furstenberg, F. F., Jr. 2003. Reflections on the future of the life course. Pp. 661–70 in J. T. Mortimer and M. J. Shanahan (eds.), *Handbook of the Life Course*. New York: Kluwer Academic/Plenum.

Gilleard, C., P. Higgs, M. Hyde, R. Wiggins, and D. Blake. 2005. Class, cohort, and consumption: The British experience of the third age. *Journals of Gerontology, Series B: Social Sciences* 60 (6): S305–10.

Hacker, J. 2006. *The Great Risk Shift: The Assault on American Jobs, Families, Health Care, and Retirement—and How You Can Fight Back*. New York: Oxford University Press.

James, J., and P. Wink (eds.). 2006. *Crown of Life: Dynamics of the Early Post-Retirement Period*. Annual Review of Gerontology and Geriatrics, Vol. 27. New York: Springer.

Kohli, M. 2007. The institutionalization of the life course: Looking back to look ahead. *Research in Human Development* 4 (3–4): 253–71.

Leisering, L. 2003. Government and the life course. Pp. 205–25 in J. T. Mortimer and M. J. Shanahan (eds.), *Handbook of the Life Course*. New York: Kluwer Academic/Plenum.

Mayer, K. U. 2004. Whose lives? How history, societies, and institutions define and shape life courses. *Research in Human Development* 1 (3): 161–87.

Mayer, K. U., and U. Schöpflin. 1989. The state and the life course. *Annual Review of Sociology* 15: 187–209.

Morrow-Howell, N., and M. Freedman (eds.). 2006–7. Civic engagement in later life. *Generations* 30 (4).

Schoeni, R. F., and K. E. Ross. 2005. Material assistance from families during the transition to adulthood. Pp. 396–416 in R. A. Settersten, Jr., F. F. Furstenberg, Jr., and R. G. Rumbaut (eds.), *On the Frontier of Adulthood: Theory, Research, and Public Policy*. Chicago: University of Chicago Press.

Schulz, J., and R. Binstock. 2007. *Aging Nation: The Economics and Politics of Growing Old in America.* Baltimore: Johns Hopkins University Press.

Settersten, R. A., Jr. 2003. Rethinking social policy: Lessons of a life-course perspective. Pp. 191–224 in R. A. Settersten, Jr. (ed.), *Invitation to the Life Course: Toward New Understandings of Later Life.* Amityville, N.Y.: Baywood.

———. 2005. Toward a stronger partnership between life-course sociology and life-span psychology. *Research in Human Development* 2 (1–2): 25–41.

———. 2006a. Aging and the life course. Pp. 3–20 in R. Binstock and L. George (eds.), *Handbook of Aging and the Social Sciences,* 6th ed. Boston: Academic Press.

———. 2006b. When nations call: How wartime military service matters for the life course and aging. *Research on Aging* 28 (1): 12–36.

———. 2007a. Passages to adulthood: Linking demographic change and human development. *European Journal of Population* 23 (3–4): 251–72.

———. 2007b. Social relationships in the new demographic regime: Potentials and risks, reconsidered. *Advances in Life Course Research* 12: 3–28.

———. 2009. It takes two to tango: The (un)easy dance between life-course sociology and life-span psychology. *Advances in Life Course Research* 14: 74–81.

Settersten, R. A., Jr., and M. E. Trauten. 2009. The new terrain of old age: Hallmarks, freedoms, and risks. Pp. 455–69 in V. Bengtson, M. Silverstein, D. Putney, and S. Gans (eds.), *Handbook of Theories of Aging,* 2nd ed. New York: Springer.

Skocpol, T. 2000. *The Missing Middle: Working Families and the Future of American Social Policy.* New York: Norton.

Smith, T. W. 2005. Generation gaps in attitudes and values from the 1970s to the 1990s. Pp. 177–221 in R. A. Settersten, Jr., F. F. Furstenberg, Jr., and R. G. Rumbaut (eds.), *On the Frontier of Adulthood: Theory, Research, and Public Policy.* Chicago: University of Chicago Press.

8. Public Policies and Older Populations of Color

Jeffrey A. Burr, Ph.D., Jan E. Mutchler, Ph.D., and Kerstin Gerst, Ph.D.

Regardless of race or ethnic background, the lives of older persons have been dramatically improved during the last 70 years, due largely to the implementation of Social Security, Medicare, Medicaid, and the Older Americans Act, among other federal and state programs (Hungerford et al., 2002). These programs provide income security and health insurance, as well as a wide range of social services. Nevertheless, many groups—including older women, poor people, low-income elderly people, older members of some minority racial and ethnic groups, the oldest old, and elderly immigrants—continue to lag behind the older white population in terms of their quality of life and overall well-being (Hudson, 1996).

This chapter provides an overview of some of the policy issues that differentially affect the well-being of several major racial and ethnic groups in the United States. These groups include, where data permit, blacks, Hispanics, Asians, and non-Hispanic whites. We begin by providing a brief demographic profile of America's diverse elderly population. Next, we discuss some of the intersecting themes that condition our understanding of the adequacy of old age policy for different racial and ethnic groups. We then address three broad policy areas—income security, health insurance and health care barriers, and formal and informal long-term care—showing how these intersect with the well-being of the white, black, Hispanic, and Asian elderly populations. Finally, we discuss policy modifications that may alleviate some of the inequities found among elderly members of these different racial and ethnic groups.

Much of old age public policy is based on a homogeneous view of the elderly population, an approach that does not reflect the myriad realities of a heterogeneous population (Wallace and Villa, 2003). As the United States becomes both older *and* more diverse (Torres-Gil and Moga, 2001), policy makers, service providers, and relatives of older persons face many challenges when it comes to supporting vulnerable older persons of color. These challenges include shifting value systems that define who is deserving of public support, balancing the needs of younger and older persons, accounting for the unique situations of new immigrants, and constructing fair and adequate support programs in the context of economic constraints (Ozawa, 1999).

Even the definition of old age is in flux (Gonyea, 2005), a development that may have unanticipated consequences for black, Hispanic, and Asian seniors, whose health and economic profiles are often uneven. Some of the most important programs supporting the elderly population employ age thresholds to define eligibility. Policy makers and academics are engaged in an active discourse over whether age is an appropriate marker for program eligibility. The principal policy option this discussion raises is whether thresholds for income security and health insurance programs should be increased as a result of increasing life expectancy and added years of disability-free life. However, groups that do not share equally in these advances may be negatively affected by an extension of age thresholds. Importantly, however, it might be the case that if old age and, in turn, eligibility for old age programs were to be defined by health and functional status rather than by age (Takamura, 2002), the impact would be less severe among minority population groups, which continue to lag behind the majority population in terms of their relative physical and mental health.

Cross-Cutting Themes

Several themes provide context for examining the impact of public policy on the well-being of older members of America's largest racial and ethnic groups. These include (1) the gradual ideological shifts and budgetary constraints that have emerged over the last few decades on social insurance, welfare, and collective responsibility for vulnerable populations; (2) the increasing racial and ethnic diversity of the elderly population, including cultural diversity; and (3) the recent high levels of immigration from Latin America and Asia.

Public discourse about the deservedness of older persons' receipt of public benefits has shifted substantially over the years (Takamura, 2002; Binstock, 2005b), resulting in a growing emphasis to place more responsibility for well-being on the shoulders of vulnerable individuals and their families and, in turn, diminishing the role of government and the private sector (Hacker, 2006). The national political climate and tight budgets have politicians and other officials looking, in Binstock's words (2005a), for scapegoats in making zero-sum or negative-sum spending decisions.

Added to this picture is the robust growth of younger age groups among minority populations, especially Asians and Hispanics. This development is occurring in conjunction with the rapid growth of the elderly population, especially elderly whites (Hayes-Bautista et al., 2002). As a result, the potential for intergenerational and interethnic conflict may be substantial (Hayes-Bautista, Schink, and Chapa, 1988; Torres-Gil and Moga, 2001), particularly in localities and states that have relatively high proportions of persons from Latin America, whether U.S.- or foreign-born (e.g., California, Texas, Florida). Some observers argue that in a number of such states, there will be pressure to shift public resources from support for children, who are disproportionately Hispanic, toward older populations, who are disproportionately white (Hayes-Bautista, Schink and Chapa, 1988). These observers even point to the possibility of tax revolts if younger Hispanic populations are unwilling or unable to pay the taxes that support programs for seniors.

The different racial and ethnic groups in the United States contain an array of values, shared beliefs, customs, and histories of discrimination and adaptation. Broad labels such as "Asian" and "Hispanic" mask the rich cultural variability and experiences that exist across these groups. The Hispanic population, for example, includes persons whose heritage may be Cuban, Puerto Rican, Mexican, South American, or Central American. The diversity of experiences and needs is substantial across these peoples. Yet there is even greater heterogeneity within each of these groups (R. Angel and J. Angel, 1997). For example, the potential income and health needs, including long-term care, of a Mexican American elder whose family has been in the United States for six generations is likely to be very different from a Mexican American elder who migrated to the United States three years ago.

A key indicator of well-being in later life is located in the complex web of family relationships, which are in part culturally defined. Hispanic and Asian cultures are argued to have strong value systems and norms regarding attachments to and manifestations of familialism, including variable patterns of expectations of support for elderly persons and levels of reverence for elders (R. Angel and J. Angel, 1997). Because families provide the vast majority of support for older persons, it is assumed that elders from these groups benefit from their unique cultural systems. Increasingly, however, this assumption does not represent current realities, due to increases in marital disruption, labor force participation among women, and growth in the numbers of children living with one parent. Clearly, issues of family connectedness and a sense of mutual responsibility should play into policy considerations. This is especially true for the provision of informal and formal long-term care, where public policy is problematic.

Immigrants, particularly those from Latin America and Asia, represent a special case when it comes to public policy geared toward supporting older persons. Crucial to generating effective immigration *and* old age policies is an understanding of the different life chances associated with the age at which a person immigrates, the duration of his or her residence in the United States, and his or her immigration status (refugee, economic, or family reunification). Those who immigrate as children or younger adults have time to adapt to American culture—including learning the language and earning work credits to become eligible for Social Security benefits—along with developing their social, financial, human, and cultural capital. Older, recent immigrants are much less likely to generate and possess these advantages and are thus at a distinct disadvantage with respect to achieving an acceptable quality of life in old age (R. Angel and J. Angel, 1997).

Demographic Profile of a Diverse Aging Population

The U.S. Census Bureau estimates the median age for (non-Hispanic) whites in 2010 to be 41.3 years; for blacks, 31.7; for Asians, 36.0; and for Hispanics, 27.5 (table 8.1). Projections for the year 2050 show white median age at 44.6 years, blacks at 38.9, Asians at 43.4, and Hispanics at 31.2 (U.S. Bureau of the Census, 2008b). The gap in median age between blacks, Asians, and whites will decrease substantially over the next 40 years, but the gap between Hispanics and whites will narrow only slightly, due to the projected higher fertility and immigration patterns of Hispanics. Thus Hispanics will remain a relatively young population compared with the other groups.

The Census Bureau estimates also show that 80.1 percent of per-

Table 8.1 Age Characteristics (in Percentages), by Race and Hispanic Origin Group

Race/ethnic group	Median age		Among ages 65 or older	
	2010	2050	2010	2050
White alone (non-Hispanic)	41.3	44.6	80.1	58.5
Black alone	31.7	38.9	8.5	11.9
Asian alone	36.0	43.4	3.3	8.5
Hispanic origin (of any race)	27.5	31.2	7.1	19.8

Source: Data from the U.S. Bureau of the Census, 2008b.
Note: In the 2000 Census, respondents were asked to self-identify their race and Hispanic ethnicity. Respondents were permitted to choose more than one race. In this table, white (non-Hispanic), black, and Asian figures are reported for persons who selected only one of the race categories.

sons aged 65 or older in 2010 are non-Hispanic white, 8.5 percent are black, 3.3 percent are Asian, and 7.1 percent are of Hispanic origin (of any race; see table 8.1). By 2050, the proportion of the population that is non-Hispanic white will decline substantially, falling to 58.5 percent of the elderly population, with blacks rising to 11.9 percent, Asians to 8.5 percent, and Hispanic-origin persons to 19.8 percent (U.S. Bureau of the Census, 2008b). The proportion of Hispanic and Asian elders in the older population will nearly triple over the next 40 years. This development will likely have wide-ranging impacts on federal and state budgets and on the political discourse surrounding the balance between public and private support for the elderly.

Immigration trends represent a key component of the growing diversity of the U.S. population, including among elderly people. Elderly immigrants represented about 10 percent of the overall elderly population in 2005; by 2050, that figure is projected to increase to 20 percent (Passel and Cohn, 2008). Most of this increase in the immigrant elderly population will be the result of younger adult immigrants aging into the later stages of the life course rather than from a significant increase in the number of persons who immigrate after age 65 (Passel and Cohn, 2008). Nevertheless, many immigrants who migrate to the United States in later life have unique issues that intersect with old age policy, including limited or no public or private pension resources and immigration status that could impinge upon program eligibility, such as for Supplemental Security Income or Medicaid (R. Angel and J. Angel, 1997).

Income Security

We now turn to three major policies that can directly affect well-being in later life among populations of color. We begin by describing the economic situation of the different racial and ethnic groups. In 2006, the overall poverty rate for persons aged 65 or older was 9.4 percent; however, vast differences in poverty exist among specific racial and ethnic groups. For elderly non-Hispanic whites, the poverty rate was 7.0 percent; for blacks, 22.8 percent; for Asians, 12.0 percent; and for Hispanics, 19.4 percent (Federal Interagency Forum on Aging-Related Statistics, 2008). Poverty among America's elderly black and Hispanic persons remains distinctly high, despite the overall positive effect associated with the implementation of old age policies during the twentieth century.

A similar pattern of disadvantage in later life is reflected in income differences across racial and ethnic groups. The median household income in 2007 for elderly non-Hispanic whites was $29,617; for blacks, $19,450; for Asians, $33,263; and for Hispanics (of any race), $21,860 (U.S. Bureau of the Census, 2009).

Income Support

Most observers consider that postretirement income should rest on the three legs of Social Security, private pensions, and individual savings. Earnings from employment may also be important sources for many persons in later life. Table 8.2 shows the percentage of individuals aged 65 and above receiving any income from different sources in 2006, separated by racial and ethnic groups. The data indicate that a higher percentage of elderly whites receive income from earnings, Social Security, private pensions, and assets (including savings) than do elderly blacks, Asians, or Hispanics. Thus white elders, on average, have more sources of income on which to draw for a comfortable retirement compared with older persons of color.

Social Security has been central to the reduction in poverty among the old (Ozawa and Yoon, 2002). In addition, for some older persons, especially those who have experienced a lifetime of income insecurity, Social Security also stabilizes their income flow (Hendley and Bilimoria, 1999; Martin, 2007). However, having to rely largely on Social Security benefits, a common reality among elderly blacks and Hispan-

Table 8.2 Income Sources (in Percentages) for Persons Aged 65 or Older, by Race and Hispanic Origin, 2006

	White alone	Black alone	Asian alone	Hispanic origin
Earnings	25.2	20.1	23.5	22.5
Social Security	90.0	82.1	68.2	74.5
Private pensions or annuities	30.9	18.4	14.3	12.9
Income from assets	58.9	25.6	40.2	22.6
Supplemental Security Income	2.6	9.3	10.7	10.1

Source: Data from the U.S. Social Security Administration, 2009.

ics, leaves these persons at a greater risk of poverty (R. Angel and J. Angel, 2006; Favreault and Mermin, 2008). Social Security constitutes nearly 90 percent of the income for persons 65 or older located in the bottom 20 percent of the income distribution curve, and it constitutes roughly 50 percent of the retirement income for Hispanics and blacks. This compares with Social Security representing only about one-third of whites' retirement income (Favreault and Mermin, 2008).

The benefit and financing elements of Social Security have a mixed effect on older populations of color. While the Social Security payroll tax is regressive because of the cap on taxable earnings and a flat tax rate, the benefit structure is progressive, because the income replacement ratios are higher for persons with lower lifetime earnings. However, when taking into consideration racial differences in longevity (black life expectancy after age 65 is lower than that of other groups) and marital history (black spouses receive fewer survivor benefits because the differences in their lifetime earnings profiles are narrower than whites), the progressive nature of Social Security is seriously compromised (Ozawa and Kim, 2001; Steuerle et al., 2004).

Poor and low-income persons, including a disproportionate number of older persons of color, are much less likely to have private pensions or substantial savings. While 30.9 percent of white elders received private pension income in 2006, only 18.4 percent of black, 14.3 percent of Asian, and 12.9 percent of Hispanic elders received such benefits (table 8.2). Reasons for the low rates of private pension receipt among some racial and ethnic groups include employment in jobs that do not offer pensions and a lack of knowledge about pension availability and investment strategies. In addition, it is unlikely that poor or near-poor persons of color would be able to save substantial portions of their income for retirement, given their need to pay for everyday sustenance and a lack of discretionary funds. The importance of Social Security for vulnerable groups is underscored in light of their lower levels of access to private pensions, federal and state retirement systems, and low rates of saving (Morgan and Eckert, 2004).

One means for making Social Security more equitable across groups would be to provide caregiver credits, which would benefit women in general, and black and Hispanic women in particular (Favreault and Mermin, 2008). Another suggestion for reducing poverty among those persons who are eligible for Social Security benefits would be to provide a minimum benefit tied to the poverty cutoff line (Favreault et al., 2007), so that no individual would find him- or herself receiving Social Security and yet still be living in poverty. However, in the current political and economic environment, the likelihood of such initiatives coming into effect is remote.

Supplemental Security Income (SSI), a means-tested program, provides income to disabled persons of any age and to persons aged 65 or older based on financial eligibility (Martin, 2007), with most states supplementing the federal payment. The percentage of elderly blacks, Asians, and Hispanics receiving SSI is more than 4 times as high as that for elderly whites (table 8.2). However, the program provides only a modest amount of support, which is generally not adequate as a sole source of support. SSI is also underused, due to a lack of knowledge about the program, the stigmatization associated with accepting welfare, perceived hassles of working with large agencies that control the distribution of the funds, and the chilling effect brought on by welfare reform (see below).

Immigrants and Income Security

It is instructive to compare the U.S.-born elderly population's economic situation with that of the Hispanic and Asian immigrant elderly population. In 2005–6, the median household income for U.S.-born elderly persons was $33,718; for Hispanic elder immigrants, $30,469; and for Asian elder immigrants, $52,689 (Burr et al., 2008). Household and family income differences for older Asian and white immigrants show a large gap, one that is influenced in part by group variability in living arrangement patterns (e.g., on average, older Asians live in households with more persons participating in the labor market, increasing the median household income).

The poverty rate is 22.7 percent for older Hispanic immigrants and 15.0 percent for older Asian immigrants, while the rate for U.S.-born elders is 10.8 percent (Burr et al., forthcoming). Thus Hispanic (at 16.1%) and Asian (at 12.5%) immigrant elders are more dependent on SSI than are U.S.-born elders (at 3.4%). Yet the passage of the Personal Responsibility and Work Opportunity Reconciliation Act (PRWORA) in 1996 has negatively affected the financial safety net for older immigrants. The PRWORA reduced or eliminated public support for many immigrant elders, depending on when they arrived relative to the date of the legislation and whether they had become naturalized citizens (J. Angel, 2003; Gerst and Burr, 2009). Research also shows that there may have been a *chilling effect* associated with this legislation, that is, welfare uptake rates, especially under SSI, have been reduced among eligible native-born and foreign-born elders, possibly because of confusion over the new welfare eligibility rules and fear of deportation (Van Hook, 2000, 2003; Gerst, forthcoming). Further, the variability in the level of state generosity toward immigrants with respect to public support is substantial, meaning that geography also plays a role in this form of the safety net for older immigrants (Gerst and Burr, 2009).

Health Insurance and Barriers to Health Care

Racial and ethnic health disparities in the United States currently occupy a central position in the nation's public health agenda (National Institutes of Health, 2002; Hummer, Benjamins, and Rogers, 2004). Life expectancy at birth shows a clear disadvantage for blacks compared with non-Hispanic whites, Asians, and Hispanics (U.S. Bureau of the Census, 2008a). In 2010, life expectancy is projected to be 78.9 years for whites, 78.8 for Asians, 81.1 for Hispanics, and 73.8 for blacks. By the year 2050, these racial and ethnic group gaps are projected to narrow. Further, among those persons who reach age 65, differences in mortality risk among the groups narrow significantly, in some cases showing a well-known, if suspect, mortality crossover effect (Hummer, Benjamins, and Rogers, 2004).

Ethnic disparities are also found when considering disability rates.

Elderly non-Hispanic black males have higher rates of disability than elderly non-Hispanic white males, but Hispanic and Asian males have lower disability rates later in life than both blacks and whites. A similar pattern holds for females, except that Hispanic females and white females have about the same rates of disability (Hummer, Benjamins, and Rogers, 2004). Once health and socioeconomic status are taken into account, differences in the prevalence of disabilities are reduced but are not erased (Dunlop et al., 2007).

Elderly non-Hispanic white males and females generally report lower rates of poor or fair health, and they report fewer activity limitations than elders from all other major racial and ethnic groups except for Asians (Hummer, Benjamins, and Rogers, 2004). Research also demonstrates that elderly blacks and Hispanics have higher prevalence and incidence rates of dementia than do elderly whites (Manly and Mayeux, 2004). These racial and Hispanic-origin group health and mortality differences are believed to be related to a complex mixture of genetic makeup, cultural background, social characteristics, economic stratification, and access to health care, including differential access to adequate health insurance.

Health in later life is a consequence of cumulative (dis)advantages and increased disease risk over the life course—both at the group and individual levels (O'Rand, 2006). The primary reason for a lack of access to health care among all age groups is a lack of health insurance. Among other factors, a lack of health insurance among vulnerable populations earlier in life contributes to reduced well-being later (Fitzpatrick et al., 2004). Thus a lack of health insurance coverage among some of America's largest non-white racial and Hispanic-origin groups puts them at a significant disadvantage (R. Angel and J. Angel, 1997). In 2007, 10.4 percent of non-Hispanic whites, 19.5 percent of blacks, 16.8 percent of Asians, and 32 percent of Hispanics were without either government or private health insurance (DeNavas, Proctor, and Smith, 2008). Health insurance coverage also varies dramatically by one's state of residence, further demonstrating the role geography plays in the quality of later life (Williams, Neighbors, and Jackman, 2003).

Medicare and Medicaid

The Medicare program provides nearly universal health insurance coverage for the elderly population. However, gaps in coverage and cost-sharing requirements (principally copayments, deductibles, and premiums) leave poor and near-poor elderly persons (including women, the oldest old, and older blacks and Hispanics) with inadequate access to health care (Rowland and Lyons, 1996). The poor and low-income elderly also are more likely to have health problems that require attention, making this an even more untenable situation. While only 12 percent of elderly whites receiving Medicare in 2002 had incomes below the poverty line, 37 percent of black elderly persons and 36 percent of Hispanic elderly persons receiving Medicare lived in poverty (Kaiser Family Foundation, 2009). However, for some poor elders, Medicaid fills some of the gaps in Medicare coverage by paying premiums and various other out-of-pocket costs.

Despite the availability of Medicaid to cover costs associated with limitations in the Medicare program, a substantial fraction of elderly poor and low-income persons do not take advantage of Medicaid (Rowland and Lyons, 1996; Pezzin and Kasper, 2002). Some estimates show that as many as two-thirds of those who are eligible do not participate in the program (Harrington Meyer, 2001). Reasons for underuse include the perceived stigmatization associated with Medicaid use, a lack of knowledge about the program, and a fear of consequences for immigrant groups who may see interacting with representatives of local, state, and federal governments as risky to their status. This pattern is especially troubling because the poor, including older black and Hispanic persons, pay a much higher proportion of their incomes toward health care through out-of-pocket expenses than do elderly middle- and upper-class persons (Rowland and Lyons, 1996).

Other developments in health care do not bode well for minority elders. In firms with 200 or more employees, the availability of retiree health insurance fell by more than half between 1998 and 2008 (Munnell, Muldoon, and Saas, 2009). It is reasonable to expect that in the current economic climate, more companies will be dropping this type of coverage or will make it more expensive, further reducing the insurance coverage rates of older non-Hispanic whites disproportionately, given that they are more likely than Hispanics and blacks to work for firms that provide access to such benefits.

Medicare cost-containment efforts may also negatively effect Hispanic and black elders (Johnson, 2005). One strategy would be to raise the age limit of eligibility for Medicare benefits to 67 years old and allow near-elderly persons to buy into the program between the ages of 62 and 66 (Johnson, 2005). This approach acknowledges that for the population as a whole, age 65 may no longer be a reasonable threshold for the definition of old age. Moreover, delaying receipt of Medicare benefits would be an inducement to remain in the labor force longer. Yet many elders, disproportionately Hispanic and black ones, may be either unable to find employment or unable to work due to various levels of disability. Johnson (2005) shows that there would be cost savings for the Medicare program if these policy changes were made. However, without a heavy subsidization of premiums for poor persons, including poor persons of color, many of these persons would have no coverage in the near-elderly years.

Variability in the rates of use of health services among elderly members of different racial and ethnic groups is well documented (Gornick et al., 1996; Dunlop et al., 2002, 2007). For example, some, but not all, studies show that elderly blacks and Hispanics are more likely than elderly whites to make use of physician visits (Lum, Chang, and Ozawa, 1999), although they see relatively little difference between the groups in terms of hospital stays and home health care services. Others find that the overall number of health care services used is larger for elderly whites than for elderly blacks (Escarce et al., 1993), including certain types of cancer screening, eye examinations, and routine follow-up examinations for mental illness after hospital discharge (Schneider, Zaslavsky, and Epstein, 2002).

Across the life course, barriers to medical and dental care are more likely to be reported by blacks, Hispanics, and some Asians. Wallace and Villa (2003) group these barriers into three categories: acceptability (e.g., lack of cultural competence on the part of providers), accessibility (e.g., cost of care), and availability (e.g., location of medical facilities). Dissatisfaction with care, lack of any usual source of care, lack of trust in the medical establishment, and difficulties experienced in obtaining care (language, transportation difficulties), including delays in seeking care due to cost and long waiting lines, are more prevalent among blacks and Hispanics of all age groups, including elders, than among whites (Rowland and Lyons, 1996; Jackson and George, 1998; Hunt, Gaba, and Lavizzo-Mourey, 2005; Armstrong et al., 2007).

Immigrants and Health Care

Immigrants are often regarded as self-selected for migration, based on their better health status compared with their country-of-origin peers (Jasso et al., 2004); however, the effect of health is not always supported in research literature (Mutchler, Prakash, and Burr, 2007; Rubalcava et al., 2008). Many of today's immigrants come from countries with health care systems that are considered less effective than the U.S. system (including some Latin American and Asian countries); thus they are likely to be in poorer health than U.S.-born persons, especially if the former immigrated later in life (Jasso et al., 2004; R. Angel and J. Angel, 2006). Further, low pay, hazardous occupations, limited or no access to employer-sponsored health insurance, and dependence on nontraditional medicine, along with avoidance of the health care system in the United States, all leave many elderly immigrants in poorer health than their counterparts born in the United States.

Health insurance coverage among immigrants of all age groups is low, whereas differences between native-born persons and immigrants are affected primarily by citizenship status and whether a person works for a company that provides health insurance (Buckmueller et al., 2007). Recent legislation further widens this gap, with some research (Kaushal and Kaestner, 2005) finding that the PRWORA increased the likelihood that immigrant families headed by women with low levels of education would not have health insurance. Other research shows that the PRWORA has reduced Medicaid enrollment among eligible prereform immigrants, which provides further, indirect evidence for the chilling effect discussed earlier (Kandula et al., 2004). As a result, the outlook for elderly immigrants' health care is not favorable, especially among recent older immigrants who are not U.S. citizens.

Long-Term Care

The provision of long-term care comes from two sources: informal and formal. Both forms of care are often used in combination to support elders in need (Litwak, 1985). The vast majority of long-term care is performed by family members, usually a spouse or adult daughter or daughter-in-law (Bowles and Kington, 1998). Estimates based on mid-1990s data indicate that unpaid help (personal assistance services) given by family members to older persons with disabilities amounted to approximately $24 billion annually, based on a reasonable market wage applied to the number of hours of help provided (LaPlante, Harrington, and Kang, 2002).

Long-Term Care Coverage by Race and Ethnicity

To demonstrate relative group differences in potential informal long-term care support among older persons, we generated caregiver-care recipient dependency ratios—defined as the number of persons aged 45–54 divided by the number of persons aged 75 or older within each racial and ethnic category—based on U.S. Census data for the year 2000. This measure represents a crude (and conservative) indicator of potential support, especially because elderly blacks and Hispanics typically rely more heavily on grandchildren and fictive kin for informal support than do elderly whites (R. Angel and J. Angel, 1997). For every non-Hispanic white person aged 75 or older, there are 2.0 non-Hispanic whites in typical caregiving ages (aged 45–54); for elderly blacks, the ratio is 3.4:1; for elderly Asians, 4.5:1; and for elderly Hispanics, 4.8:1 (U.S. Bureau of the Census, 2009). The differences between whites and blacks are due to historically higher black fertility; the relatively high values for Asians are due to immigration patterns, and the high values for Hispanics are due to a combination of high fertility and high immigration. Whether the greater potential for these racial and ethnic group families to provide informal care might translate into less demand for formal caregiving alternatives will be a major issue in the years ahead.

Concerning formal care, table 8.3 shows the distribution of nursing home residence by race and Hispanic origin for different age groups. In 2004, older blacks exceeded the other three groups in terms of this cross-sectional picture of nursing home use, having a utilization rate of 47.7 per 1,000 population, compared with 36.2 for elderly whites, 20.3 for elderly Hispanics, and 15.6 for other races combined (Centers for Disease Control and Prevention, 2009). Until recently, older whites were more likely than older blacks to use a nursing home for long-term care. The data indicate this pattern has changed, which may be due in part to whites employing a wider range of alternative long-term care resources (such as assisted living and home health care) based on their ability to pay privately, and in part to blacks reducing their resistance to institutional care. However, it is worth noting that

Table 8.3 Nursing Home Utilization Rates (per 1,000 Persons), by Age, for Racial and Ethnic Groups, 2004

	White	Black	Other races	Hispanic	Non-Hispanic
65 or older	36.2	47.7	15.6	20.3	37.1
65–74	8.5	20.2	6.2	8.9	9.4
75–84	35.2	55.5	17.8	27.4	36.4
85+	139.4	160.7	65.3	66.5	141.3

Source: Data from the Centers for Disease Control and Prevention, 2009.

in the face of declining health, elderly blacks postpone home care and nursing home admission longer than elderly whites, which means that elderly blacks are less likely to leave a nursing home after entering it (Cagney and Agree, 1999).

Harrington Meyer (2001) finds that because the nursing home industry generally prefers private-pay patients, access to nursing homes among older blacks and Hispanics is restricted, due to their disproportionate reliance on Medicaid as a source of payment. The consequences include an added burden on the families of the poor—among which blacks, Hispanics, and some Asians are overrepresented—and delay in access to needed care. Assuring higher Medicaid reimbursement rates, or adding a comprehensive long-term care benefit to Medicare, would certainly alleviate this situation, but neither seems politically feasible in the current environment.

Through the Older Americans Act (OAA), the Administration on Aging (AoA) supports many social service programs that help elderly persons to live independently in their communities, although the demand for services greatly exceeds their supply. The best-known services include nutrition, long-term care ombudspersons, and transportation programs (Takamura, 1999). The OAA is specifically designed to provide services to disadvantaged elderly populations, and older persons from some racial and ethnic groups do receive a disproportionate amount of benefits. Native American, Alaskan, and Hawaiian elders are especially targeted for service provision by the OAA. Some research shows that social services tend to be underused by eligible blacks, Asians, and Hispanics, despite the fact that many elders from these groups report that their adult children have less time to devote to helping them with daily tasks (Torrez, 1998).

Immigrants and Long-Term Care

Older immigrants who do not qualify for Supplemental Security Income, especially those who immigrated recently, also do not qualify for Medicaid. These elders may have fewer public sources of funds to pay for long-term care than do their U.S.-born counterparts. Most recent arrivals do not typically have the wherewithal to purchase private long-term care insurance and do not have the resources to pay for nursing home care out of pocket. Unqualified (undocumented) elderly immigrants may be in the most serious straits, given that eligibility is now based on citizenship status. Naturalization, which is necessary for some elderly immigrants to qualify for Medicaid and requires a five-year waiting period, is a more difficult process for elderly immigrants entering the country in later life, due to language difficulties, a lack of knowledge, and confusion surrounding administrative requirements (J. Angel, 2003).

Conclusion

This chapter was written in the midst of an economic crisis that extends across the globe, the likes of which have not been experienced in more than three generations. The Congressional Budget Office (2009) projects a $1.2 trillion deficit in 2009, the largest in U.S. history. With federal outlays for programs supporting the elderly population comprising ever-larger shares of the total federal budget, pressure to control costs will likely be felt in many areas of both federal and state budgets, including programs that support elders and their families. When this happens, it will no doubt take its most substantial toll on vulnerable groups—such as poor people and low-income elders, members of vulnerable racial and ethnic groups, women, and the oldest old. Much of the discussion in this chapter must be considered in light of the uncertainties that these economic forces imply.

Research indicates that many black, Hispanic, and Asian elders lag behind their white counterparts in several areas that are addressed by welfare and entitlement policy. As we approach the second decade of the twenty-first century, a number of questions need to be addressed. Will various racial and ethnic group advocacy organizations combine efforts to press for a multicultural, multigenerational approach to old age policy, or will they fragment and support policies that best suit the most pressing of their core identity-group needs (Torres-Gil and Moga, 2001)? What will it take to raise public consciousness about the needs of vulnerable black, Hispanic, and Asian elders, including making politicians aware of their unique issues? Will plans to increase scientific research in the area of health disparities yield positive outcomes for older members of diverse racial and ethnic groups (National Institutes of Health, 2002; Wallace and Villa, 2003)? Will elders from black, Hispanic, and Asian groups and their supporters have more political clout now that there is an African American president in the White House?

In debates about policy issues related to families, there is a tendency to focus on children or elderly people, instead of focusing on both age groups within the context of the full life course (Ozawa, 1999). Taking a life-course approach to policy formation is important for older blacks, Hispanics, and Asians, because they often do not have income security in later life, or health insurance, or the resources to pay for long-term care—thus they rely more on family. Yet families of all groups are stretched thin, making it more difficult for them to provide care and support. One of the long-term policy solutions for improving the well-being of older members of diverse racial and ethnic groups may be to improve the well-being of children and young families. Improving the minimum wage, enforcing civil rights legislation, improving public schools, establishing a universal health insurance program, and making more funds available for college students would be a helpful beginning (Torres-Gil and Moga, 2001).

Is there a reason to be optimistic about a narrowing of the gap in well-being in later life among the diverse U.S. racial and ethnic groups as the baby boomers enter this stage of the life course? Mutchler and Burr (2009) argue that many members of America's racial and Hispanic-origin groups will find themselves relatively less well off than their white and non-Hispanic peers, because they continue to have lower levels of education, are less likely to be employed in jobs with pensions and adequate health insurance, and have lifetime earnings and savings that are less than those of their white counterparts. On the other hand, the gaps in the factors that account for disparities in life chances (social, human, cultural, and financial capital) have been closing in recent years, so it is likely that the distance between the groups will be lessened for the boomer generation.

References

Angel, J. L. 2003. Devolution and the social welfare of elderly immigrants: Who will bear the burden? *Public Administration Review* 63 (1): 79–89.

Angel, R. J., and J. L. Angel. 1997. *Who Will Care for Us? Aging and Long Term Care in Multicultural America.* New York: New York University Press.

———. 2006. Minority group status and healthful aging: Social structure still matters. *American Journal of Public Health* 96 (7): 1152–59.

Armstrong, K., K. Ravenell, S. McMurphy, and M. Putt. 2007. Racial/ethnic differences in physician distrust in the United States. *American Journal of Public Health* 97 (7): 1283–89.

Binstock, R. H. 2005a. The contemporary politics of old age policies. Pp. 265–93 in R. B. Hudson (ed.), *The New Politics of Old Age Policy.* Baltimore: Johns Hopkins University Press.

———. 2005b. Old-age policies, politics, and ageism. *Generations* 29 (3): 73–78.

Bowles, J., and R. S. Kington. 1998. The impact of family function on health of African American elderly. *Journal of Comparative Family Studies* 29 (2): 337–47.

Buckmueller, T., A. LoSasso, I. Lurie, and S. Dolfin. 2007. Immigrants and employer-sponsored health insurance. *Health Services Research* 42 (1, part 1): 286–310.

Burr, J., K. Gerst, J. Mutchler, and N. Kwan. 2008. The economic well-being and welfare program participation among older immigrants in the US. *Generations* 32 (4): 53–60.

Cagney, K., and E. M. Agree. 1999. Racial differences in skilled nursing care and home health use: The mediating effects of family structure and social class. *Journals of Gerontology, Series B: Social Sciences* 54 (4): S223–36.

Centers for Disease Control and Prevention. 2007. *Health, United States, 2007: With Chartbook on Trends in the Health of Americans.* National Center for Health Statistics. www.cdc.gov/nchs/data/hus/hus07.pdf#027 [retrieved January 29, 2009].

———. 2009. Table 1. Number, percent distribution, and rate per 10,000 population of nursing home residents by selected resident characteristics and age at interview: United States, 2004. *National Nursing Home Survey, 2004.* www.cdc.gov/nchs/data/nnhsd/Estimates/nnhs/Estimates _Demographics_Tables.pdf [retrieved January 2009].

Congressional Budget Office. 2009. The budget and economic outlook: Fiscal years 2009 to 2019. www.cbo.gov/ftpdocs/99xx/doc9957/01-07 -Outlook.pdf [retrieved January 2009].

DeNavas, W. C., B. C. Proctor, and J. C. Smith. 2008. *Income, Poverty, and Health Insurance Coverage in the United States.* Current Population Reports P60-235. Washington, D.C.: U.S. Government Printing Office.

Dunlop, D. D., L. M. Manheim, J. Song, and R. W. Chang. 2002. Gender and ethnic/racial disparities in health care utilization among older adults. *Journals of Gerontology, Series B: Social Sciences* 57 (4): S221–34.

Dunlop, D. D., J. Song, L. M. Manheim, M. Daviglus, and R. W. Chang. 2007. Racial/ethnic differences in the development of disability among older adults. *American Journal of Public Health* 97 (12): 2209–15.

Escarce, J., K. Epstein, D. Colby, and J. Schwartz. 1993. Racial differences in the elderly's use of medical procedures and diagnostic tests. *American Journal of Public Health* 83 (7): 948–54.

Favreault, M., and G. Mermin. 2008. *Are There Opportunities to Increase Social Security Progressivity Despite Underfunding?* Washington, D.C.: Urban Institute.

Favreault, M., G. Mermin, C. E. Steuerle, and D. Murphy. 2007. *Minimum Benefits in Social Security Could Reduce Aged Poverty.* Washington, D.C.: Urban Institute.

Federal Interagency Forum on Aging-Related Statistics. 2008. *Older Americans, 2008: Key Indicators of Well-Being.* Washington, D.C.: U.S. Government Printing Office.

Fitzpatrick, A., N. Powe, L. Cooper, D. Ives, and J. Robbin. 2004. Barriers to health care access among the elderly and who perceives them. *American Journal of Public Health* 94 (10): 1788–94.

Gerst, K. Forthcoming. Supplemental Security Income among older immigrants from Central and South America: The impact of welfare reform. *Journal of Aging and Social Policy.*

Gerst, K., and J. Burr. 2009. Welfare use among older Latin American immigrants: The effects of federal and state policy. Working paper, Gerontology Department, University of Massachusetts–Boston.

Gonyea, J. G. 2005. The oldest old and a long-lived society: Challenges for public policy. Pp. 157–82 in R. B. Hudson (ed.), *The New Politics of Old Age Policy.* Baltimore: Johns Hopkins University Press.

Gornick, M., P. Eggers, T. Reilly, R. Mentnech, L. Fitterman, L. Kucken, and B. Vladeck. 1996. Effects of race and income on mortality and use of services among Medicare beneficiaries. *New England Journal of Medicine* 335 (11): 791–99.

Hacker, J. 2006. *The Great Risk Shift: The Assault on American Jobs, Families, Health Care, and Retirement—and How You Can Fight Back.* New York: Oxford University Press.

Harrington Meyer, M. 2001. Medicaid reimbursement rates and access to nursing homes. *Research on Aging* 23 (5): 532–51.

Hayes-Bautista, D. E., P. Hsu, A. Perez, and C. Gamboa. 2002. The "browning" of the graying of America: Diversity in the elderly population and policy implications. *Generations* 26 (3): 15–24.

Hayes-Bautista, D. E., W. Schink, and J. Chapa. 1988. *The Burden of Support: Young Latinos in an Aging Society*. Stanford, Calif.: Stanford University Press.

Hendley, A., and N. Bilimoria. 1999. Minorities and Social Security: An analysis of racial and ethnic differences in the current program. *Social Security Bulletin* 62 (2): 59–64.

Hudson, R. B. 1996. The changing face of aging politics. *Gerontologist* 36 (1): 33–35.

Hummer, R., M. Benjamins, and R. Rogers. 2004. Racial and ethnic disparities in health and mortality among the U.S. elderly population. Pp. 53–94 in N. Anderson, R. Bulatao, and B. Cohen (eds.), *Critical Perspectives on Racial and Ethnic Differences in Health in Later Life*. Washington, D.C.: National Academies Press.

Hungerford, T., M. Rassette, H. Iams, and M. Koenig. 2002. Trends in the economic status of the elderly, 1976–2000. *Social Security Bulletin* 64 (3): 12–23.

Hunt, K., A. Gaba, and R. Lavizzo-Mourey. 2005. Racial and ethnic disparities and perceptions of health care: Does health plan type matter? *Health Services Research* 40 (2): 551–76.

Jackson, P. B., and L. K. George. 1998. Racial differences in satisfaction with physicians: A study of older adults. *Research on Aging* 20 (3): 298–316.

Jasso, G., D. Massey, M. Rosenzweig, and J. Smith. 2004. Immigrant health: Selectivity and acculturation. Pp. 227–66 in N. Anderson, R. Bulatao, and B. Cohen (eds.), *Critical Perspectives on Racial and Ethnic Differences in Health in Later Life*. Washington, D.C.: National Academies Press.

Johnson, R. 2005. *Raising the Medicare Eligibility Age with a Buy-In Option: Can One Stone Kill Three Birds?* Washington, D.C.: Urban Institute.

Kaiser Family Foundation. 2009. *A Profile of African Americans, Latinos, and Whites with Medicare: Implications for Outreach Efforts for the New Drug Benefit*. www.kff.org/minorityhealth/7435.cfm [retrieved January 2009].

Kandula, N., C. Grogan, P. Rathouz, and D. Lauderdale. 2004. The unintended impact of welfare reform on the Medicaid enrollment of eligible immigrants. *Health Services Research* 39 (5): 1509–26.

Kaushal, N., and R. Kaestner. 2005. Welfare reform and health insurance of immigrants. *Health Services Research* 40 (3): 697–722.

LaPlante, M. P., C. Harrington, and T. Kang. 2002. Estimating paid and unpaid hours of personal assistance services in activities of daily living provided to adults living at home. *Health Services Research* 37 (2): 397–416.

Litwak, E. 1985. *Helping the Elderly: The Complementary Roles of Informal Networks and Formal Systems.* New York: Guilford Press.

Lum, Y., H. Chang, and M. N. Ozawa. 1999. The effects of race and ethnicity on use of health services by older Americans. *Journal of Social Service Research* 25 (4): 15–42.

Manly, J., and R. Mayeux. 2004. Ethnic differences in dementia and Alzheimer's disease. Pp. 95–141 in N. Anderson, R. Bulatao, and B. Cohen (eds.), *Critical Perspectives on Racial and Ethnic Differences in Health in Later Life.* Washington, D.C.: National Academies Press.

Martin, P. P. 2007. Hispanics, Social Security, and Supplemental Security Income. *Social Security Bulletin* 67 (2): 73–100.

Morgan, L. A., and J. K. Eckert. 2004. Retirement financial preparation. *Journal of Aging and Social Policy* 16 (2): 19–34.

Munnell, A. H., D. Muldoon, and S. Sass. 2009. *Recessions and Older Workers.* Chestnut Hill, Mass.: Center for Retirement Research, Boston College.

Mutchler, J., and J. Burr. 2009. Varieties of well-being: Race, class, gender, and age. Pp. 23–46 in R. B. Hudson (ed.), *Boomer Bust? The New Political Economy of Aging.* Westport, Conn.: Praeger.

Mutchler, J., A. Prakash, and J. Burr. 2007. The demography of disability and the effects of immigration history: Older Asians in the United States. *Demography* 44 (2): 251–63.

National Institutes of Health. 2002. *Strategic Research Plan and Budget to Reduce and Ultimately Eliminate Health Disparities,* Vol. 1. Washington, D.C.: U.S. Department of Health and Human Services. http://ncmhd.nih.gov/our_programs/strategic/pubs/VolumeI_031003EDrev.pdf [retrieved February 2009].

O'Rand, A. 2006. Stratification and the life course: Life-course capital, life-course risks, and social inequality. Pp. 146–65 in R. H. Binstock and L. K. George (eds.), *Handbook of Aging and the Social Sciences.* Amsterdam: Academic Press.

Ozawa, M. N. 1999. The economic well-being of elderly people and children in a changing society. *Social Work* 44 (1): 9–19.

Ozawa, M. N., and H. J. Kim. 2001. Money's worth in Social Security benefits: Black-white differences. *Social Work Research* 25 (1): 5–14.

Ozawa, M. N., and H. S. Yoon. 2002. Social Security and SSI as safety nets for the elderly poor. *Journal of Aging and Social Policy* 14 (2): 1–25.

Passel, J., and D. Cohn. 2008. *U.S. Population Projections, 2005–2050.* Washington, D.C.: Pew Research Center.

Pezzin, L., and L. Kasper. 2002. Medicaid enrollment among elderly Medicare beneficiaries: Individual determinants, effects of states, and impact on service use. *Health Services Research* 37 (4): 827–47.

Rowland, D., and B. Lyons. 1996. Medicare, Medicaid, and the elderly poor. *Health Care Financing Review* 18 (Winter): 61–85.

Rubalcava, L., G. Teruel, D. Thomas, and N. Goldman. 2008. The healthy migrant effect: New findings from the Mexican Family Life Survey. *American Journal of Public Health* 98 (1): 78–84.

Schneider, E., A. Zaslavsky, and A. Epstein. 2002. Racial disparities in the quality of care for enrollees in Medicare Managed Care. *JAMA: Journal of the American Medical Association* 287 (10): 1288–94.

Steuerle, E. C., A. Carasso, and L. Cohen. 2004. *How Progressive Is Social Security and Why?* Washington, D.C.: Urban Institute.

Takamura, J. 1999. Getting ready for the 21st century: The aging of America and the Older Americans Act. *Health and Social Work* 24 (3): 232–38.

———. 2002. Social policy issues and concerns in a diverse aging society: Implications of increasing diversity. *Generations* 26 (3): 33–38.

Torres-Gil, F., and K. B. Moga. 2001. Multiculturalism, social policy, and the new aging. *Journal of Gerontological Social Work* 36 (3–4): 13–32.

Torrez, D. J. 1998. Health and social service utilization patterns of Mexican American older adults. *Journal of Aging Studies* 12 (1): 83–99.

U.S. Bureau of the Census. 2008a. *Projected Life Expectancy at Birth by Sex, Race, and Hispanic Origin for the United States, 2010 to 2050.* Washington, D.C.: U.S. Department of Commerce, U.S. Bureau of the Census, Population Division.

———. 2008b. Summary tables (with projections of the population by race, ethnicity, age, and sex for the United States, 2010 to 2050). *2008 National Population Projections (Based on Census 2000).* Washington, D.C.: U.S. Department of Commerce, U.S. Bureau of the Census, Population Division. www.census.gov/population/www/projections/summary tables.html [retrieved February 16, 2009].

———. 2009. Historical poverty tables—people. *Current Population Survey, Annual Social and Economic Supplements.* www.census.gov/hhes/ www/poverty/histpov/perindex.html [retrieved January 2009].

U.S. Social Security Administration. 2009. Table 1.8: Percentage with income from specified source, by sex, race, Hispanic origin, and age, 2004. *Income of the Population 55 and Older, 2004.* www.ssa.gov/policy/docs/ statcomps/income_pop55/2004/sect01.html#table1.8 [retrieved January 2009].

Van Hook, J. W. 2000. SSI eligibility and participation among elderly naturalized citizens and non-citizens. *Social Science Research* 29 (1): 51–69.

———. 2003. Welfare reform's chilling effects on non-citizens: Changes in non-citizen welfare recipiency or shifts in citizenship status. *Social Science Quarterly* 84 (3): 613–31.

Wallace, S. P., and V. M. Villa. 2003. Equitable health systems: Cultural and structural issues for Latino elders. *American Journal of Law and Medicine* 29 (2–3): 247–67.

Williams, D. R., H. Neighbors, and J. J. Jackson. 2003. Racial/ethnic discrimination and health: Findings from community studies. *American Journal of Public Health* 93 (2): 200–208.

9. The Oldest Old and a Long-Lived Society

Challenges for Public Policy

Judith G. Gonyea, Ph.D.

The definition of old age as beginning at age 65 is a relatively recent phenomenon. It reflects the decision of European nations to establish this chronological age as determining eligibility in the formation of their old age social insurance programs around the turn of the twentieth century. With the passage of the 1935 Social Security Act, the United States also instituted 65 as the marker of normal retirement and the beginning of old age. Increasing life expectancies, however, are causing us to rethink what we mean by old. Today, it is possible to consider a healthy, vigorous, and socially engaged person in his or her 60s or 70s as not being elderly. Indeed, one-third of Americans in their 70s perceive of themselves as middle aged (National Council on Aging, 2000).

Yet, using the conventional old age benchmark of one's 60s as representing old age, today's older population can span as much as five decades. Individuals in their 60s, 70s, 80s, 90s, and 100s are all found among the ranks of the elderly. Gains in both life expectancy and elder well-being have led to a remarkable increase in the heterogeneity of America's older population in critical areas, including economic standing, health status, behavioral and lifestyle customs, and living and social arrangements.

This *democratization of aging*—that is, the new reality that the vast majority of Americans are attaining old age and even advanced old age—has led researchers, practitioners, and policy makers to differentiate between the young old and the oldest old (Neugarten, 1974; Harris et al., 1978; Treas and Bengtson, 1982). The term *oldest old* was coined by Matilda White Riley and Richard Suzman in a presentation at the 1984 American Association for the Advancement of Science meeting, in which they strove to draw the scientific community's attention to this emerging age population. As editors of a special issue of *Milbank Quarterly* devoted to the topic of the oldest old, Suzman and Riley (1985, p. 177) wrote that it was "so new a phenomenon that there is little in historical experience that can help in interpreting it." Yet they also went on to predict that, given their rising numbers, the oldest old would "no longer remain invisible" in the economy, the polity, and the health and social service systems. Reflecting the accuracy of their prophecy, the oldest old or very old age category is now often employed by demographers; economists; social, behavioral, and health researchers; and policy makers to both describe and predict trends in America's older population.

The significance of the growth and extension of the older population—now including active and vigorous elders, often in their 60s or 70s, and frail and vulnerable elders, usually in their 80s or older—has not been lost on the world of public policy. As a result of these developments, the older population today is subjected to two negative but nonetheless competing stereotypes: being both "greedy" and "needy." Thus, to a number of analysts, the policy outlook of an aging United States, particularly being a long-lived society, has become increasingly dire, referents moving from "the graying of the federal budget" (Hudson, 1978), to "a fiscal black hole" (Callahan, 1987), to nothing less than "apocalyptic demographic forecasts" (Robertson, 1991).

Yet, as the following discussion makes clear, the oldest old are diverse. While they are the least likely to fit the new stereotype of elderly people, described by Binstock (1994) as "prosperous, hedonistic, selfish, and politically powerful," neither are they inevitably poor, frail, and isolated. Still, advanced old age is associated with a greater risk of experiencing economic hardship and disabling health conditions. Two key policy questions are: First, what will be the impact of an increasing number of the oldest old on systems of health care delivery and financing, on informal caregiving support systems, and on public and private pensions? And second, How do we as a society respond to the challenges of an aging population to promote a secure, positive, and meaningful later-life experience for all of our very oldest citizens? In particular, how can public policy better target benefits to those elders with greatest needs? In so doing, to what degree should policy rely on chronological age as a proxy for such need? Or should age instead be used as an adjunct to functional status and income tests, which can apply to persons of all ages?

Population Trends

Over the past century, the number of Americans aged 65 or older has increased more than tenfold, to today's 35 million. One in every eight Americans is aged 65 or older, and by 2030 that proportion is estimated to increase to nearly one in five. And among older Americans, it is the oldest old whose numbers are growing the fastest. In 2000, approximately 1.5 percent of the U.S. population, or about 4 million Americans, were aged 85 or older; by 2050, the ranks of the oldest old is projected to increase to approximately 5 percent, to nearly 21 million individuals (figure 9.1). As for the very oldest old, the current number of 84,000 individuals at age 100 or older in the United States is projected to reach 580,000 persons by 2040 (U.S. Bureau of the Census, 2000). The dramatic changes in the older population that will occur during the next four to five decades will be due to the baby boom cohort's arrival at old age. Thus, as reflected in figure 9.1, the most rapid increase in the population 85 years or older will occur between 2030 and 2050 as the baby boom generation join the ranks of the very old. Based on increasing life expectancies, the Census Bureau's population projections suggest that by the middle of this century, more than 40 percent of adults aged 65 or older can expect to live to at least age 90 (U.S. Bureau of the Census, 2000).

Studies of the impacts of this dramatic demographic age transition have typically focused on changes in the population proportions of three age groups: young people, working-age adults, and elderly people. More recently, however, based on the projected steep increase in the oldest old age group, a growing number of demographers are arguing for the use of a four-age-group model: young people, working-age people, younger retired people, and oldest people. Extending this concept further, Robine, Michel, and Herrmann (2007) proposed the adoption of an "oldest old support ratio" based on two age groups: a 50- to 74-year-old age group, the pivotal generation in providing care to the second group, and an 85+ oldest old age group. Although acknowledging that the specific age ranges of the two categories are somewhat arbitrary, Robine and colleagues emphasize that these two age groups are most often defined as encompassing the delivery and receipt of elder care. Importantly, they suggest that use of an oldest old support ratio may offer governments a better indicator of "the implications of substantial intergenerational changes that are occur-

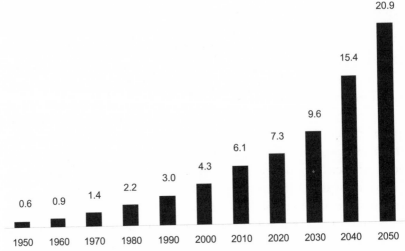

Figure 9.1. U.S. Population Aged 85 or Older, 1950 to 2050 (in Millions).
Source: Data from the Federal Interagency Forum on Aging-Related Statistics, 2006.

ring and aid policy makers to formulate appropriate social policies" (p. 571). Moreover, others argue that the four-age population model may offer a better mechanism for estimating the future long-term care needs of our oldest citizens.

The Social World of the Oldest Old

It is immediately striking that the oldest old are predominantly women, a phenomenon that has led some to refer to this age cohort as the "granny generation." At age 85 or older, the gender ratio in the United States is nearly 3 men for every 10 women, with women accounting for 68 percent—or 3.6 million individuals—of the 85+ population and men comprising 32 percent—or 1.7 million individuals (Federal Interagency Forum on Aging-Related Statistics, 2008). Yet in recent years, the sex ratio has narrowed a bit as the gap between male and female life expectancy has decreased, with the average life expectancy for women and men who survive to 85 years of age today being 7.2 years and 6.7 years, respectively (Federal Interagency Forum on Aging-Related Statistics, 2008). This narrowing of the gender gap in life expectancy is primarily due to declining male mortality rates in deaths due to heart disease (Federal Interagency Forum on Aging-Related Statistics, 2001). U.S. Census Bureau projections suggest that the sex ratio will continue to rise, leveling off by 2050 to about 6 men for every 10 women for those aged 85 or older (U.S. Bureau of the Census, 2000).

The nation's older population is also becoming more racially and ethnically diverse, although not as rapidly as the total U.S. population. Currently, the vast majority (87%) of Americans aged 85 or older identify themselves as non-Hispanic white; however, the percentages of elders of color and of Hispanic origin are projected to increase steadily throughout the coming decades. By 2050, the proportion of elderly blacks and Hispanics 85 years or older could increase to approximately one-third of the total 85+ population. Significant differences in life expectancies, however, do exist by race. Life expectancy at birth is lower for blacks than for whites; at most ages, the mortality rates of blacks are higher than for whites. In 2004 the life expectancy of white women at age 65 exceeded that of black women by about five years. However, this black-white life expectancy gap narrows, falls to zero, and leads to a *crossover* in the mortality rates for blacks and whites in advanced old age. After age 85, blacks have more years of additional life, at 7.1 years, than do whites, at 6.7 years (Federal Interagency Forum on Aging-Related Statistics, 2008). Debate exists regarding the meaning of the crossover phenomenon, with some suggesting it is an artifact of inaccurate birth dates (i.e., lack of birth records or overstatement of ages) and others offering sociobiological explanations of a select group surviving harsh conditions in early life (Elo and Preston, 1994; Johnson, 2000).

Given that women both live longer than men and also tend to marry men who are older than themselves, it is not surprising that women are less likely to share their later years of life with a spouse (figure 9.2). Whereas 60 percent of men aged 85 or older are married, only 15 percent of their female counterparts have husbands. Indeed, widowhood is normative for women late in life. More than three-quarters (76%) of women aged 85 or older are widows, compared with only 34 percent of men aged 85+. Although few of the current cohort of the oldest old women are either divorced (4%) or never married (4%), these percentages will undoubtedly rise as future generations enter the ranks of this age group (Federal Interagency Forum on Aging-Related Statistics, 2008). One-third of baby boomers are entering into old age as

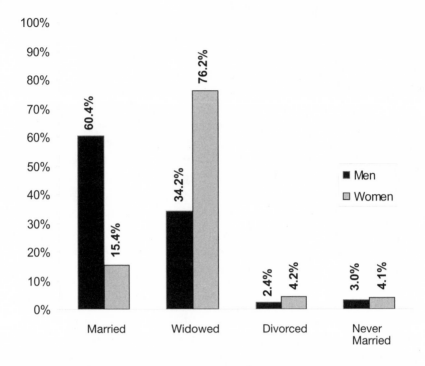

Figure 9.2. Marital Status of the U.S. Population Aged 85 or Older, by Gender, 2007. Source: Data from the Federal Interagency Forum on Aging-Related Statistics, 2008.

single persons, whether due to divorce, being widowed, or never marrying. These generational shifts in marital and divorce patterns may have a significant impact on the well-being of future cohorts of American elders. Marital status is correlated with a number of measures of economic, physical, and emotional well-being in later life. Older married individuals, on average, have higher household incomes, better physical health, lower rates of depression, and less risk of institutionalization than their unmarried counterparts. Importantly, spouses are the primary caregivers for their frail and disabled partners.

Not surprisingly, the gender gap in spouse survivorship affects living arrangements in later life. Older women are at least twice as likely as older men to live alone. By age 75, almost half (49%) of women live alone compared with less than one-quarter (22%) of men (Federal Interagency Forum on Aging-Related Statistics, 2008). Older persons typically enter nursing homes when physical disabilities and/or mental incapacity prevent them from living on their own or being cared for in other community settings. Although only a small percentage of the young old—approximately 1 percent of persons aged 65 to 74, and 4.7 percent of persons aged 75 to 84—resided in nursing homes in 2000, this figure rises dramatically to more than one in five (22.2%) for persons aged 85 or older (Centers for Disease Control and Prevention, 2002). Nursing homes are generally women's worlds. Not only do women have higher rates of nursing home residence than do men, but this gender difference also rises rapidly with age. Of the approximately 45 percent of elders residing in nursing homes who are 85 years of age or older, almost three-quarters are women, and nearly two-thirds are widowed (Gabrel, 2000).

Income, Wealth, and Expenditures of the Very Old

In recent decades, older Americans have experienced greater financial security as a result of a liberalization of Social Security benefits, the introduction of cost-of-living adjustments (COLAs) to Social Security, and the availability of health insurance through the Medicare and Medicaid programs. In 1959, 35 percent of persons aged 65 or older were living in poverty—a figure that exceeded the percentage of poor children or working-age adults. In 2006, only 8.6 percent of adults aged 65 to 74, 10 percent of adults aged 75 to 84, and 11.4 percent of those aged 85 or older were among the ranks of the poor—percentages that now fall below the poverty rates for both young children and adults (U.S. Bureau of Labor Statistics and U.S. Bureau of the Census, 2002; Federal Interagency Forum on Aging-Related Statistics, 2008).

Yet despite considerable economic gains, the oldest old, older women, and persons of color have a greater risk of facing poverty in late life. Among America's older population, total income declines with age. Median total income in 2006 was $20,518 for people aged 64 to 69, $16,447 for those aged 70 to 79, and $15,462 for people aged 80 or older. In fact, not only do slightly more than 1 in every 10 (11.4%) of America's oldest old currently live in poverty, but also an additional 3 out of the 10 have family incomes that are less than 150 percent of the poverty threshold in 2006.

Table 9.1 presents the percentages of the poor by age, gender, race, and Hispanic origin for the older population in 2006 (Federal Inter-

Table 9.1 Older Americans Living in Poverty (in Percentages), by Age, Gender, Race, and Hispanic Origin, 2006

	Total	White	Black	Asian	Hispanic origin[a]
Males					
65 to 74 years	6.9	4.5	17.8	11.6	18.1
75 or older	6.2	4.4	14.6	13.0	16.7
Females					
65 to 74 years	10.1	7.3	23.9	7.5	19.3
75 or older	12.9	10.5	30.2	17.0	23.1

Source: Data from the Federal Interagency Forum on Aging-Related Statistics, 2008.
[a] Hispanic can be of any race.

agency Forum on Aging-Related Statistics, 2008). The interactive effects of gender, race, and age on experiencing poverty are reflected in the fact that the poorest group of elderly people is comprised of black or African American women aged 75 or older, followed by Hispanic-origin women aged 85 or older. Indeed, in advanced old age, African American women are more than seven times as likely as white men to experience poverty, at 30 percent versus 4 percent. This gender-based economic disparity in old age has led some to comment that although older men experience a mortality disadvantage, they do have a quality-of-life advantage—particularly older white men (Longino, 1988; Barer, 1994). As Thompson (1994, p. 10) suggests, "death may come sooner, but later life for older men presents fewer problems." Four factors contribute to the risk of poverty for both men and women in older life: living longer, being widowed, living alone, and a lifetime of working in the secondary sector of the labor force. Yet each of these factors is more likely to occur in women's lives, especially for women of color.

Relative expenditures on food, housing, and health care are also an indicator of economic well-being. In 2005, the largest single component of expenditures for households headed by people aged 75 or older was for housing, which accounted for 36 percent of total spending; the federal government defines a "housing cost burden" as 30 percent or more of total household expenditures. Health care expenses, which include health insurance, medical services, and drugs and medical supplies, represented about 16 percent of all expenditures for seniors aged 75 or older. Finally, transportation expenses accounted for about 14 percent of their total spending, and food for an additional 13 percent (Federal Interagency Forum on Aging-Related Statistics, 2008).

There is a growing awareness of the circular relationship between income, housing, and health for older adults. As Lawler (2001, p. 1) notes: "When a living environment is affordable and appropriate, an aging individual is more likely to remain healthy and independent. When an individual maintains good health, he or she is more able to keep up with the maintenance of his or her living environment. As the population ages in an aging housing stock, it becomes difficult to distinguish a health concern from a housing concern." A fixed income or poor health may prevent an older adult from undertaking necessary home repairs, while substandard housing conditions may further compromise an individual's health.

Wealth, or *net worth*—the difference between assets and liabilities— can provide individuals with the resources to weather difficult life circumstances or transitions as they age. Net worth generally continues to rise throughout adulthood but begins to decline at age 75. Median net worth (excluding home equity) is an important indicator of well-being for elderly householders, as the vast majority of older Americans express a strong preference to *age in place* in their current dwelling. The concentration of wealth among a relatively few households and the extreme vulnerability of householders in the lowest income quintile is striking. In 2000, the 1.6 million elderly (aged 65 or older) householders in the highest (fifth) quintile of income distribution had a median net worth, excluding home equity, of $328,432, while the 7.9 million elderly householders in the lowest (first) quintile had a median net worth, again excluding home equity, of only $3,500. The bottom line is that America's oldest old, who find themselves in the lower income quintiles, have little or no cushion to meet any emergency—whether it be for clothing, food, medicine, and/or utilities (U.S. Bureau of the Census, 2003).

Health and the Oldest Old

Historically, the image of very old people has been one of frailty. Yet, as Camacho and colleagues (1993, p. 439) note, while "this is an accurate picture for some of the oldest old, we know that there are many

others who are able to maintain a high level of function at this age."
In fact, the oldest old's self-assessments of their health status suggest
that the majority view their health positively. Although self-assessed
health (rated as excellent, very good, good, fair, or poor) declines with
age, the majority of our oldest citizens perceive themselves as faring
well relative to their own age group; approximately 78 percent of the
young old (aged 65–74), 72 percent of the middle old (75–84) and 66
percent of the oldest old (85+) rated their health at least as "good" in
2006 (Federal Interagency Forum on Aging-Related Statistics, 2008).
This is a significant finding, as a self-rating of health as "good to excellent" is highly correlated with a lower risk of mortality (Centers
for Disease Control and Prevention, 2002). There are, however, significant racial and ethnic differences in health ratings. Among the 85+
population, only about half of blacks (54%) and Hispanics (47%)
offer a positive assessment of their own health, compared with approximately two-thirds (67%) of whites (Federal Interagency Forum
on Aging-Related Statistics, 2008). These discrepancies are seen as reflecting objective differences in health status and disability, as well as
cultural and class differences in health assessment.

Although noting that the chronological age of older adults is not
a good indicator of health status because interindividual variations
in health are greatest in later life, Santos-Eggimann (2002, p. 287)
emphasizes that "from a public health perspective, young and old
populations are undoubtedly different. With the emergence of large
cohorts of individuals reaching and dying at an advanced age, aging
countries are experiencing an epidemiological transition characterized
by changes in the main cause of death and morbidity profile." The
two current leading causes of death for persons aged 85 or older in
the United States are heart disease and cancer, followed by cerebro-
vascular diseases, Alzheimer's disease, and chronic obstructive lower
respiratory diseases (Federal Interagency Forum on Aging-Related
Statistics, 2008). These are diseases in which, as Santos-Eggimann
stresses, a prolonged period of functional decline, disability, and high
rates of health services use typically precede death. Although other
chronic diseases have lower fatality rates, they also can significantly
compromise older adults' quality of life (Santos-Eggimann, 2002).

According to the Federal Interagency Forum on Aging-Related Statistics (2008), the most common chronic health conditions reported by
the elderly are hypertension (53.3%), arthritis (49.5%), heart disease

(30.9%), any type of cancer (21.1%), and diabetes (18.0%). Again, the prevalence of certain chronic conditions varies by gender, race, and ethnicity. For example, among the elderly, Hispanic and non-Hispanic black women have diabetes prevalence rates that are twice as high as non-Hispanic white women. Finally, a significant proportion of the 85+ population have a number of sensory and oral health impairments; 62 percent report having trouble hearing, 27 percent report having trouble seeing, and 32 percent have no natural teeth.

Chronic health conditions often restrict elders' ability to perform the activities of daily living (ADLs)—such as dressing, bathing, and eating—and the instrumental activities of daily living (IADLs), such as meal preparation and housecleaning. Once again, the risk of functional limitations increases dramatically with age (Centers for Disease Control and Prevention, 2009). As table 9.2 reveals, compared to their younger counterparts, a greater percentage of the oldest old living in the community face difficulties performing the activities of daily living on their own and require assistance to bathe or shower (23%), dress (14%), eat (5%), get in and out of bed or chairs (20%), walk (43%), or use the toilet (10%). Similarly, a sizeable proportion of the oldest old living in the community report difficulties performing the instrumental activities of daily life and need help to use the telephone (17%), do light housework (24%), do heavy housework (52%), prepare meals (23%), shop (32%), and manage money (20%).

Cognitive impairments, particularly Alzheimer's disease and other dementias, also dramatically compromise the quality of life of both an affected elder and his or her family. Although only about 5 percent of adults aged 65 to 69 experience either moderate or severe memory loss, this figure climbs to almost one in five persons by ages 80 to 84, and it leaps dramatically to almost one-third of elders aged 85 or older (Federal Interagency Forum on Aging-Related Statistics, 2006). It is estimated that about half of the population aged 85 or older will have a major cognitive impairment or dementia as part of their final phase of life (Alzheimer's Association, 2008). Moreover, poor cognitive functioning is a significant risk factor for entering a nursing home. Higher rates of depressive symptoms—which are correlated with poorer physical health, greater functional limitation, and higher rates of health services use—are also found among the oldest old. While severe depressive symptoms are experienced by approximately 13 percent of adults aged 65 to 74, the incidence of severe symptoms of

Table 9.2 Noninstitutionalized Medicare Beneficiaries Age 65+ Who Have Difficulty Performing the ADLs and the IADLs (in Percentages), 2006

	Age		
	65–74	75–84	85+
Activities of daily living (ADLs)			
Bathing/showering	6.0	10.9	23.0
Dressing	4.9	6.8	13.5
Eating	1.7	2.4	4.5
Getting in/out of bed/chairs	8.8	13.5	20.3
Walking	17.7	25.9	42.7
Using the toilet	3.1	5.4	10.2
Instrumental activities of daily living (IADLs)			
Using the telephone	4.5	7.7	16.9
Doing light housework	8.0	12.6	24.2
Doing heavy housework	22.2	32.7	52.0
Preparing meals	5.5	10.1	22.6
Shopping	8.5	14.8	32.0
Managing money	3.6	7.1	20.3

Source: Data from the Centers for Disease Control and Prevention, 2009.

depression reaches 19 percent among those aged 85 or older (Federal Interagency Forum on Aging-Related Statistics, 2008). Interestingly, while in earlier life stages women are more likely to report depressive symptoms than men do, there is no gender difference among the oldest old. Older adults are disproportionately likely to die by suicide. While constituting just 12 percent of the total population, people aged 65 or older accounted for about 16 percent of all U.S. suicide deaths in 2004. Non-Hispanic white men aged 85 or older were most likely to die by suicide; they had a rate of 49.8 suicides per 100,000 persons in that age group (Centers for Disease Control and Prevention, 2008).

Age-Based Programs

Clearly, many of the economic, social, and health characteristics of the oldest old differ significantly from those of the young old. Because of these factors, the differential importance of public policy allocations for the oldest old is hard to overstate.

Receipt of Social Security has become almost universal among America's older citizens, and it constitutes the largest single source of their income. Remarkably, Social Security contributed 90 percent of the income for almost 4 out of every 10 seniors, and it was the only source of income for one-fourth of seniors (Purcell, 2007). Not surprisingly, retirement income sources (i.e., Social Security, pensions, savings, employment) differ greatly by income level. According to Purcell, older adults in the lowest quartile receive their largest share of income from Social Security benefits (83%); public assistance provides the second largest share (6%). In contrast, for those older adults in the highest income quartile, earnings represent the largest share of income (35%), followed in importance by pensions (23%), assets (20%), and Social Security (20%). As the oldest age group has the highest poverty rate, the relative importance of Social Security benefits for this age population is apparent. In fact, in 2006 the 80+ age group received $336 more in Social Security benefits than their younger-age counterparts. This higher dollar amount primarily reflects the fact that the Social Security benefit formula is progressive, meaning that Social Security replaces a greater proportion of past lower earners' income than it does of higher earners' income.

More than 96 percent of older Americans are covered by Medicare, which provides affordable coverage for most acute health care services. Medicare provides critical access to such health services as inpatient hospital care, physician care, outpatient care, home health care, and care at a skilled nursing facility; yet older Americans still face significant out-of-pocket costs to meet their health care needs. And, once again, these out-of-pocket expenses increase as older adults age. In 2005 the 65–74 age group paid, on average, $1,725 in health care costs out of pocket, and the 75–84 age group had average out-of-pocket costs of $2,628, but those 85 or older typically faced $5,287 in out-of-pocket expenses (Centers for Disease Control and Prevention, 2009).

Analysis of Medicare beneficiary data from the Centers for Disease Control and Prevention (2009) reveals significant differences in health care expenditures and types of services by different age groups within the older population. In 2005 the 85+ age group's $22,244 average annual expenditures for personal health care was more than twice the

65–74 age group's average expenditure of $10,259. For those entering old age—the 65–74 age group—the largest share of health care costs was for physician or supplier care (32%), followed by inpatient hospitalization (25%) and prescription drugs (18%). In contrast, for the oldest old—the 85+ age group—the largest share of health care costs was for nursing home or long-term care facilities (40%), followed by inpatient hospital care (22%) and physician/supplier care (17%).

Long-Term Care

The growing ranks of the oldest old have increasingly focused attention on the issue of long-term care, an area that includes an array of medical, social, personal care, and support services needed by people who have lost some capacity for self-care as a result of a chronic illness or disability. Because they are more likely to experience functional limitations, older adults are much more likely to require long-term care services than are younger adults. Individuals aged 65 or older currently account for almost three-quarters of all long-term care spending.

Long-term care services are provided through both family-centered informal arrangements and organizationally based formal care systems. It is beyond dispute that informal supports provided by families are the backbone for the provision of the nation's long-term care services. The findings of the 1989 National Long Term Care Survey—that families provide the vast majority of social, emotional, and physical care to frail and disabled older adults—have been replicated in virtually every subsequent state and national study, as has its finding that the majority of these caregivers are women, typically a spouse, daughter, or daughter-in-law (Gonyea, 2008). Among older adults living in the community and receiving long-term care, 66 percent rely on informal care only, 26 percent rely on informal and formal care, and 9 percent use formal care only. Families perform a wide range of services for their older relatives; they not only help with performing the activities of daily living, but they often also provide behavioral supervision of their loved one, pay attention to pain management, and manage interactions with health care organizations. As Bookman and Harrington (2007, p. 1005) emphasize, family caregivers represent a shadow workforce in geriatric health care, often acting as "geriatric case managers, medical record keepers, paramedics, and patient advocates to fill dangerous gaps in a system that is uncoordinated, fragmented, bureaucratic, and often depersonalizing."

In fact, studies estimating the value of informal home care have consistently found that it exceeds the costs of paid home care. Arno, Levine, and Memott (1999), using national data sets, estimated that 25.8 million caregivers provided a weekly average of 17.9 hours of help for a total of 24 billion hours of care in the United States in 1997. Using a midrange wage rate of $8.18 per hour, they calculated the national economic value of this informal care at $196 billion. This $196 billion, Arno and colleagues argued, dwarfed the $32 billion spent for formal home health care and the $83 billion cost of nursing home care in the same year. More recently, the AARP Public Policy Institute attempted to calculate the economic value of family caregiving in the United States in 2006 (Gibson and Houser, 2007). Based on their midrange estimate of 34 million caregivers providing 1,080 hours of assistance yearly (or 21 hours of care per week) at an hourly wage of $9.63, the national economic value of family caregiving in 2006 was $345 billion. They compared this $345 billion figure to the $342 billion spent on total expenditures for the Medicare program in 2005.

Clearly, the provision of informal care represents enormous cost-savings to the formal health care system and the billions of dollars in public expenditures which support it. Nonetheless, it is the rising cost of publicly supported, formal long-term care services that has captured national attention. As figure 9.3 reveals, the total amount spent on formal long-term care services in the United States in 2005 was $206.6 billion (U.S. Department of Health and Human Services, 2009). The biggest share—almost half—is paid for by Medicaid, followed by Medicare, which paid an additional 21 percent. Thus Medicare and Medicaid together accounted for approximately $142.6 billion (or 69%) of long-term care expenditures of older Americans in 2005. As this figure also shows, individuals pay 18 percent of the remaining costs out-of-pocket. Despite numerous efforts to expand its coverage in recent years, private insurance still pays for only about 7 percent of long-term care expenses.

The Congressional Budget Office (1999), estimated that total long-term care expenditures would increase at a rate of 2.6 percent a year above inflation over the following forty years, from $123 billion in 2000 to $346 billion by 2040 (in 2000 dollars). Although the Budget

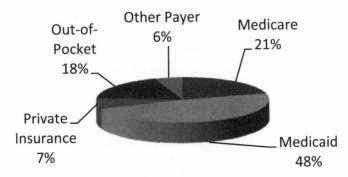

Figure 9.3. $206.6 Billion in Total Long-Term Care Expenditures in the United States, by Payer Source, 2005. Source: Data from the U.S. Department of Health and Human Services, 2009.

Office predicted some reduction in the age-specific prevalence of functional disability, this reduction was viewed as being offset by increasing demand as, by 2040, the baby boomer generation enters the ranks of the very old and the 85+ population grows to more than three times its current size.

The U.S. system of long-term care remains firmly planted in a residualist tradition, wherein the government provides benefits only when the individual's or their families' resources and market sources have failed. Indeed, Medicaid, the federal grant-in-aid program that helps states pay for medical assistance for individuals with a low income and few resources, has emerged as a key payer of long-term care expenditures, particularly institutional care. In 2001, 81 percent of Medicaid funds for long-term care for the elderly were directed toward nursing home services, and 2 percent went to care in intermediate care facilities for older persons with mental retardation. Only 17 percent was devoted to home and community-based services (O'Brien, 2005). The disproportionate amount of funding for institutional care has been strongly criticized by a number of advocates for older adults. These critics argue that Medicaid's heavy emphasis on nursing home care means that many frail elders in the community go without services that could better support their independence in their own homes (Kane, Kane, and Ladd, 1998). In many states, a large portion of Medicaid dollars support poor, elderly nursing home residents who had been middle class prior to their institutionalization. There is growing public sentiment that individuals and families should not be forced to spend down their assets and face impoverishment as a result of long-term care costs and that a financing mechanism that provides an alternative to means-tested Medicaid is needed.

Although Medicare pays primarily for acute medical services, beneficiaries may also receive long-term care coverage through the program's skilled nursing and home health care benefits. Medicare spent $32.8 billion on home health care and skilled nursing care facilities in 2005. Indeed, Medicare is the largest purchaser of home health care. However, the reality is that Medicare coverage of home care and nursing home care is very limited. Medicare pays for 100 days of nursing home care for individuals with a prior hospital stay who require skilled nursing care or rehabilitative therapy. Medicare pays for the first 20 days of a nursing home stay; after that, the older adult faces a substantial copayment. Similarly, Medicare covers home health care only for older adults with skilled care needs. The older adult must be homebound, require intermittent skilled nursing or therapy services, and be under the care of a physician who prescribes the plan of care.

Concerns about the rising costs of Medicare's home health benefit led to policy changes to eligibility criteria and payment methods in the Balanced Budget Act of 1997. The outcome was a dramatic decline in the number of beneficiaries using home health care for extended periods. The average number of Medicare home health visits per user has also declined, from 73 visits in 1996 to 27 visits in 2005 (Gibson and Houser, 2007). Some experts have sounded alarms that elder care responsibilities and costs are increasingly being shifted onto the informal care system. For example, at the same time that access to Medicare home services has become more restrictive, the average length of hospital stays for Medicare patients has declined from 11.7 days in 1973 to 5.5 days in 2005 (Gibson and Houser, 2007). Thus families are increasingly being asked to assume and perform complex and technical care responsibilities for their older relatives.

Since the mid-1980s, there has been considerable growth in the number of private insurance companies offering long-term care insurance. Yet from a public policy perspective, private insurance is unlikely to provide adequate funding for long-term care. For many Americans, the cost of purchasing long-term care insurance is prohibitive. Moreover, economic models suggest that even by the year 2030, only 10 percent of elderly persons will be able to purchase long-term care insurance at a cost of less than 5 percent of their total income (Zedlewski and McBride, 1992).

As an alternative to either public-assistance Medicaid or the private market, the United States could offer families more complete protection against the catastrophic costs of long-term care by adopting a public insurance model. Despite the nation's historic residualistic philosophy, social insurance models have been successfully implemented to avert two other potential economic catastrophes confronted by families. Social Security represents a social insurance approach to protect families from impoverishment caused by inadequate retirement income and savings. Similarly, Medicare protects individuals against poverty caused by a lack of acute medical care coverage in old age.

A clear advantage of a compulsory and universal public insurance model for protection against the cost of long-term care is that it allows the creation of large risk pools. By so doing, it avoids the adverse selection problem found in private-market insurance, which ultimately drives cost upward and makes policies unaffordable to most potential consumers. Mired in an economic recession and now facing the largest national debt ever incurred, the current economic climate would not appear to make such an initiative likely. However, recognizing that the U.S. health care system is broken, President Obama has identified fixing health care for our nation's families as one of his top priorities. If he is to design a health care system for the twenty-first century, addressing access, quality, and affordability of a continuum of long-term services must be part of this formulation. Most experts agree that the United States is in the midst of a growing elder care crisis. A significant number of frail older adults living in the community already go without the help they need, and this care gap can only widen as baby boomers join the ranks of America's older population.

Perhaps the best prospects for the challenges of developing and financing a public insurance model of long-term care which emphasizes community-based services lies in building coalitions of advocates for the aging and of advocates for children and younger adults with disabilities. Such a strategy suggests that this social insurance must be functionally based and not population centered. Although the presence of chronic illnesses and disabilities is positively correlated with age, aging does not equal disability. In 2005 it was estimated that 10.3 million Americans needed long-term care, of which 42 percent were under age 65. This under-65 age group includes individuals such as children with intellectual disabilities, young adults with spinal cord and traumatic brain injuries, and persons with serious mental illnesses (Centers for Disease Control and Prevention, 2009).

In fact, in the national health care debate which occurred during the Clinton administration, several of the proposed health-care-plan models included long-term care services for individuals of all ages, based on a beneficiary's need for assistance in performing activities of daily living, severe cognitive impairment, or profound intellectual disability. Despite the failure of those legislative proposals to move forward, they clearly introduced the principle that any public insurance model for long-term care will be based on need-for-service criteria rather than age-based ones.

Policy Needs

The importance of age-based programs for our nation's oldest old is beyond dispute. For the vast majority of individuals aged 85 or older, Social Security is their largest source of income, and virtually all elderly persons gain access to health care coverage (i.e., physician and hospital services) through Medicare. To a large extent, the success of these programs lies in the decision to design them based on social insurance principles. Inherent in both programs is the concept of providing universal protection to older citizens against a loss of income in old age through compulsory participation, in order to pool resources and share risk. It has long been recognized that universal programs avoid the stigmatization and stereotyping that occurs with means-tested programs. Moreover, the decision to make these programs age based can be fully justified because, for the majority of Americans, both income and access to health care insurance are derived from employment.

While these age-based programs have improved the aggregate well-being of older people, they do not adequately address the wide variation in well-being that is to be found within America's aging population, notably, those of advanced old age. Relative to the young old, the oldest old are both poorer and in worse physical health. Riley, Kahn, and Foner (1994) offer the concept of *structural lag* as a framework for understanding the mismatch between rapidly changing human lives (especially the phenomenon of longer and healthier lives) and social institutions. This concept is instructive in assessing the fit between population dynamics and policy design. For example, one of the basic assumptions at the outset of the Social Security program is no longer true: that only a small percentage of Americans would survive to old age and that those who did would receive benefits for only a brief period of time. Similarly, when Medicare was introduced in 1965, little attention was focused on the demographic implications of the rise of the oldest old. Nor was it originally envisioned that Medicaid, a program designed to finance acute health care for low-income people of all ages, would become the primary third-party payer for nursing home care for a large segment of America's older population.

The aging of the baby boom generation has increasingly focused attention on meeting the long-term care needs of America's future oldest citizens. Undoubtedly, the sheer size of the baby boom cohort as it enters advanced old age will have a major impact on the nation's health and social service systems. Yet predicting the precise impact of this demographic shift on individuals, families, and the government is difficult, as the effects may be lessened or exacerbated by a number of social, economic, and health trends. For example, optimistic forecasts suggest that advances in medical technologies, surgeries, pharmaceuticals, and prevention will lead to declining disability rates and compressed morbidity in the older population and thus reduce the economic burden of long-term care. More pessimistic forecasts, however, suggest that the dramatic growth of the oldest old, the most disabled segment of the aging population, will overwhelm the long-term care system and lead to a rapid increase in expenditures for long-term care.

It is also important to underscore that even among these "elite survivors" to advanced old age, inequalities by gender, race, and social class exist (Crystal and Shea, 1990; Thorsland and Lundberg, 1994; Jefferys, 1996; Schoenbaum and Waidman, 1997; Dunlop et al., 2000). These inequalities are derived from the fact that, although the United States does a better job than other industrialized countries in maintaining preretirement income in old age, it has one of the least egalitarian systems of income distribution before retirement (Myles, 1988). Although medical advances are often touted as having a profound impact on late-life disability rates, the greatest gains in the prevention of chronic diseases may be achieved through a focus on early-life experiences. Childhood and young adulthood exposure to diseases, poverty, inadequate nutrition, and substandard housing are increasingly being linked to a number of morbidities in later life, including cancer, arthritis, and cardiovascular diseases (Blackwell, Hayward, and Crimmins, 2001). Although future cohorts of America's older population as a whole may be better off, a disproportionate share of older persons of color and older women may be left behind.

Indeed, long-term care in later life is most often about women's lives. As the data presented in this chapter suggest, women are more likely to be the consumers and providers of long-term care services as a result of both their longer life expectancy and their greater likelihood of assuming the caregiver role. Thus women are major stakeholders in the long-term care debate. With longer life expectancies, we might anticipate that the experiences and problems of the young old caring for the oldest old will become even more familiar in our society. Faced with their own diminishing physical strength and stamina, these older daughters and wives may face considerable challenges in caring for their frail family members. And as we look toward the future, the relatively low birth rate among baby boomers means that they will have fewer children to call on in their old age, as almost one-fifth of women in their early 40s have no children.

Conclusion

The inadequacies of our nation's long-term care system, including the fragmentation of services, the lack of continuity of care, and a funding bias toward institutional care, have been well documented (Kane, Kane, and Ladd, 1998; Coleman, 2002). Critics of the existing system emphasize the continuing dominance of a medical model of care in spite of considerable evidence supporting the importance of social and environmental approaches to the delivery of long-term care services. Yet despite widespread dissatisfaction with our current system, debate about long-term care policy seems to be primarily centered on short-term fixes to address specific hardships experienced by users and on growing concerns about public cost.

America's demographic shift toward becoming an older society, coupled with a cultural shift emphasizing the inclusion of persons with disabilities in all aspects of society, may, however, offer an opportunity to bring structural reform to our nation's long-term care system. The recently enacted Americans with Disabilities Act and the Supreme Court's *Olmstead* decision increasingly mandate that services, programs, and facilities promote independence, inclusion, and consumer empowerment for individuals of all ages with disabling conditions. As this chapter emphasizes, age is associated with, but not defined by, disability. More than half of the people with chronic disabilities living in the community are under the age of 65, and almost all Americans are unprotected against the catastrophic health care costs associated with a chronic and severely disabling condition. While the oldest old have much to gain through a shift toward a social insurance model of long-term care, the best way to achieve this policy objective may be through a functionally based or disability-based program, rather than an age-based program. This social insurance approach, rather than fueling the fires of a "generational equity debate," emphasizes a lifelong, intergenerational sharing of and paying for the costs of long-term care.

References

Alzheimer's Association. 2008. Alzheimer's disease facts and figures. *Alzheimer's and Dementia* 4 (2): 1–41.

Arno, P. S., C. Levine, and M. M. Memott. 1999. The economic value of informal caregiving. *Health Affairs* 18 (2): 182–88.

Barer, B. 1994. Men and women age differently. *International Journal of Aging and Human Development* 38 (1): 29–40.

Binstock, R. H. 1994. Changing criteria in old-age programs: The introduction of economic status and need for services. *Gerontologist* 34 (6): 726–30.

Blackwell, D. L., D. Hayward, and E. M. Crimmins. 2001. Does childhood health affect chronic morbidity in later life? *Social Science and Medicine* 52 (8): 1269–84.

Bookman, A., and M. Harrington. 2007. Family caregivers: A shadow workforce in the geriatric health care system? *Journal of Health Politics, Policy and Law* 32 (6): 1005–41.

Callahan, D. 1987. *Setting Limits: Medical Goals in an Aging Society.* New York: Simon & Schuster.

Camacho, T., W. Strawbridge, R. Cohen, and G. Kaplan. 1993. Functional ability in the oldest old. *Journal of Aging and Health* 5 (4): 439–54.

Centers for Disease Control and Prevention. 2002. *Health, United States, 2002: With Chartbook on Trends in the Health of Americans.* DHHS Publication No. 1232. Hyattsville, Md.: Centers for Disease Control and Prevention, National Center for Health Statistics.

———. 2008. Web-Based Injury Statistics Query and Reporting System (WISQARS). National Center for Injury Prevention and Control. http://www.cdc.gov/injury/wisqars/index.html [retrieved January 11, 2009].

———. 2009. Health Data Interactive. National Center for Health Statistics. www.cdc.gov/nchs/hdi.htm [retrieved January 11, 2009].

Coleman, E. A. 2002. Challenges of systems of care for frail older persons: The United States of America experience. *Aging Clinical and Experimental Research* 14 (4): 233–38.

Congressional Budget Office. 1999. *Projections of Expenditures for Long-Term Care Services for the Elderly* (March). Washington, D.C.: Congressional Budget Office.

Crystal, S., and D. Shea. 1990. Cumulative advantage, cumulative disadvantage, and inequality among elderly people. *Gerontologist* 30 (4): 437–43.

Dunlop, D. D., L. M. Manheim, J. Song, and R.W. Chang. 2002. Gender and ethnic/racial disparities in health care utilization among older adults. *Journals of Gerontology, Series B: Social Sciences* 57 (4): S221–33.

Elo, I. T., and S. H. Preston. 1994. Estimating African-American mortality from inaccurate data. *Demography* 31 (3): 427–58.

Federal Interagency Forum on Aging-Related Statistics. 2001. *Older Americans, 2000: Key Indicators of Well-Being*. Washington, D.C.: Federal Interagency Forum on Aging-Related Statistics.

———. 2006. *Older Americans, 2006: Key Indicators of Well-Being*. Washington, D.C.: Federal Interagency Forum on Aging-Related Statistics.

———. 2008. *Older Americans, 2008: Key Indicators of Well-Being*. www.agingstats.gov/agingstatsdotnet/Main_Site/Data/Data_2008.aspx [retrieved January 3, 2008].

Gabrel, C. S. 2000. Characteristics of elderly nursing home current residents and discharges: Data from the 1997 National Nursing Home Survey. *Advance Data No. 312* (April 25). Washington, D.C.: Centers for Disease Control and Prevention, National Center for Health Statistics.

Gibson, M. J., and A. Houser. 2007. Valuing the invaluable: A new look at the economic value of family caregiving. www.aarp.org/research/ppi/ltc/care/articles/ib82_caregiving.html [retrieved March 11, 2008].

Gonyea, J. G. 2008. Multigenerational bonds, informal care and baby boomers: Current challenges and future prospects. Pp. 213–32 in R. B. Hudson (ed.), *Boomer Bust? Economic and Political Dynamics of the Graying Society*. Westport, Conn.: Praeger Publications.

Harris, T. M., R. Kovar, R. Suzman, J. Kleinman, and J. Feldman. 1978. Longitudinal study of physical ability in the oldest old. *American Journal of Public Health* 79 (6): 698–702.

Hudson, R. B. 1978. The "graying" of the federal budget and its consequences for old age policy. *Gerontologist* 18 (5, part 1): 428–40.

Jefferys, M. 1996. Social inequalities in health: Do they diminish with age? *American Journal of Public Health* 86 (4): 474–75.

Johnson, N. E. 2000. The racial crossover in comorbidity, disability, and mortality. *Demography* 37 (3): 267–83.

Kane, R. A., R. L. Kane, and R. C. Ladd. 1998. *The Heart of Long-Term Care*. New York: Oxford University Press.

Lawler, K. 2001. Aging in place: Coordinating housing and health care provision for America's growing elderly population. Working Paper W01-03, Joint Center for Housing Studies, Harvard University.

Longino, C., Jr. 1988. A population profile of very old men and women in the United States. *Sociology Quarterly* 29 (4): 559–64.

Myles, J. 1988. Postwar capitalism and the extension of Social Security into the retirement wage. Pp. 265–92 in M. Weir, A. Orloff, and T. Skocpol (eds.), *The Politics of Social Policy in the United States*. Princeton, N.J.: Princeton University Press.

National Council on Aging. 2000. *Myths and Realities 2000 Survey Results*. Washington, D.C.: National Council on Aging.

Neugarten, B. 1974. Age groups in American society and the rise of the young-old. Pp. 187–98 in F. Eisele (ed.), *Political Consequences of Aging*. Annals of the American Academy of Political and Social Science, vol. 415. Philadelphia: American Academy of Political and Social Sciences.

O'Brien, E. 2005. *Long-Term Care: Understanding Medicaid's Role for the Elderly and Disabled*. Henry J. Kaiser Family Foundation, Kaiser Commission on Medicaid and the Uninsured. www.kff.org/medicaid/upload/Long-Term-Care-Understanding-Medicaid-s-Role-for-the-Elderly-and-Disabled-Report.pdf [retrieved January 11, 2009].

Purcell, P. 2007. *Income and Poverty among Older Americans in 2006*. Washington, D.C.: Congressional Research Service, Library of Congress. http://digitalcommons.ilr.cornell.edu/key_workplace/312/ [retrieved January 7, 2009].

Riley, M. W., R. L. Kahn, and A. Foner (eds.). 1994. *Age and Structural Lag: Society's Failure to Provide Meaningful Opportunities in Work, Family, and Leisure*. New York: Wiley.

Robertson, A. 1991. The politics of Alzheimer's disease: A case study of apocalyptic demography. Pp. 429–42 in M. Minkler and C. Estes (eds.), *Critical Perspectives on Aging: The Political and Moral Economy of Growing Old*. Amityville, N.Y.: Baywood.

Robine, J. M., J. P. Michel, and F. R. Herrmann. 2007. Who will care for the oldest people in our ageing society? *British Medical Journal* 334 (7593): 570–71.

Santos-Eggimann, B. 2002. Evolution of the needs of older persons. *Aging Clinical and Experimental Research* 14 (4): 287–92.

Schoenbaum, M., and T. Waidman. 1997. Race, socioeconomic status, and health: Accounting for race differences in health. *Journals of Gerontology, Series B: Social Sciences* 52 (special issue): 61–73.

Suzman, R., and M. W. Riley. 1985. Introducing the "oldest old." *Milbank Quarterly* 63 (2): 177–86.

Thompson, E., Jr. 1994. Older men as invisible men in contemporary society. Pp. 1–24 in E. Thompson, Jr. (ed.), *Older Men's Lives*. Thousand Oaks, Calif.: Sage Publications.

Thorsland, M., and O. Lundberg. 1994. Health and inequalities among the oldest old. *Journal of Aging and Health* 6 (1): 51–69.

Treas, J., and V. Bengtson. 1982. The demography of mid- and late-life transitions. *Annals of the American Academy of Political and Social Science* 464 (Nov.): 11–21.

U.S. Bureau of the Census. 2000. *Projections of the Resident Population by Age, Sex, Race, and Hispanic Origin, 1999–2100* (January). Washington, D.C.: U.S. Department of Commerce, U.S. Bureau of the Census.

———. 2001. *Census 2000 Demographic Profile*. Washington, D.C.: U.S. Department of Commerce, U.S. Bureau of the Census.

———. 2003. *Current Population Survey, 2002 Annual Social and Economic Supplement*. Washington, D.C.: U.S. Department of Commerce, U.S. Bureau of the Census.

U.S. Bureau of Labor and U.S. Bureau of the Census. 2002. *Current Population Survey, 2002 Annual Demographic Survey, March Supplement*. Washington, D.C: U.S. Department of Commerce, U.S. Bureau of the Census, for the U.S. Bureau of Labor.

U.S. Department of Health and Human Services. 2009. *Paying for LTC*. National Clearinghouse for Long-Term Care Information. www.longterm care.gov/LTC/Main_Site/Paying_LTC/Costs_Of_Care/Costs_Of_Care .aspx [retrieved March 1, 2009].

Zedlewski, S., and T. McBride. 1992. The changing profile of the elderly: Effects on future long-term care needs and financing. *Milbank Quarterly* 70 (2): 247–76.

10. Caregiving and the Construction of Political Claims for Long-Term Care Policy Reform

Sandra R. Levitsky, Ph.D.

Providing care for elderly people has historically been understood to be a *family* responsibility—and the responsibility of women, in particular (Harrington, 2000). But over the course of the last half-century, increased longevity and dramatic changes in the provision of health care, household structure, and women's participation in the labor force have created what many observers (Glenn, 2000; Harrington, 2000; Garey et al., 2002) have dubbed a "crisis in care": the demand for care of the young, the old, and the infirm is growing at precisely the same time as the supply of private care within the family is substantially contracting. Today, more families are shouldering the responsibilities of caring for older—and sicker—people than at any time in our nation's history (Koren, 1986; Glazer 1988; Stevens, 1989; Abel, 1991). While there are a range of market-based supportive services to help contemporary families with long-term care provision—such as in-home supportive services, adult day care, or nursing home care—conventional health insurance policies generally do not cover these services, and most U.S. families do not have (and cannot afford) long-term care insurance (Harrington Meyer, 2005). Medicare provides acute care coverage for most of the nation's elderly people, but little assistance for people with chronic illnesses, and Medicaid provides long-term care assistance only for the very poor.

Despite the well-documented effects of the contemporary care crisis on economic security,[1] gender equity,[2] class equity,[3] and the physical and mental health of family care providers,[4] the U.S. public has shown remarkably little appetite for translating their private care dilemmas into political demands for policy intervention. Paid time off from work, tax credits, caregiving stipends, state-subsidized home care, respite care, child care, adult day care, and other support services could all dramatically affect the quality of life for family caregivers, but these are rarely discussed as political priorities in public discourse.

In this chapter, I consider why the economic, physical, and emotional challenges of providing chronic care for a family member have not produced more salient political demands for aggressive policy intervention. Drawing on data from a qualitative study of nearly 180 family caregivers—specifically, individuals caring for adult family members diagnosed with dementia, cancer, or similar chronic diseases—I analyze how, and under what conditions, family caregivers reconceptualize *private* long-term care dilemmas as *political grievances*. Claims for policy intervention in matters of social welfare do not, I will argue, emerge whole cloth from the appearance of unmet needs. Longstanding and deeply held beliefs about family responsibility for long-term care do not easily give way, even in the face of stresses on family or work life. Instead, beliefs in family responsibility play an important role in shaping how caregivers conceptualize solutions to their long-term care dilemmas. The evidence from this study suggests that caregivers who see themselves as being unable to meet the perceived care needs of their family members *do* in many cases imagine public policy solutions for their problems, but these solutions call for only a minimal role for government, and leave intact the assumption that families should bear the primary costs of care.

In what follows, I draw on social movement theory to lay out a framework for tracing how ordinary individuals construct political claims for public policy reform. I then elaborate on the research design and methodologies used in this study. My analysis of the development of political claims for long-term care policy reform—a process I will refer to as *grievance construction*—takes place in three parts. First, I analyze how individuals come to reinterpret longstanding care provision practices as *harms* or *injustices* requiring policy intervention. Second, I explore when, and under what conditions, participants shift responsibility for care dilemmas from the family to the market or the government. Finally, I examine the political claims that emerge from these processes of grievance construction, seeking to understand why family caregivers faced with unmet long-term care needs imagine only a limited role for government in assisting families with the strains of contemporary care provision.

Theoretical Framework for Analyzing Grievance Construction

Social movement researchers have long sought to explain how it is that people overcome resignation or quiescence during particular historical moments to challenge longstanding social conditions, practices, or modes of thought. To understand the subjective work involved in transforming individual political consciousness, social movement theorists have relied on the concept of collective action frames. *Collective action frames* refer to sets of beliefs and meanings that shape our understandings of our circumstances, including what kinds of action are imaginable, which targets are appropriate for blame, and what political concepts (such as *rights* or *entitlements*) may be employed in a given context (see, e.g., Snow et al., 1986; Snow and Benford, 1988; Steinberg, 1999; Ferree et al., 2002). *Legitimating frames* are interpretations of one's circumstances that largely reflect and reinforce the status quo; they have a taken-for-granted quality, an inevitability or naturalness that leads to acceptance, rather than critique, of one's circumstances (Gamson, Fireman, and Rytina, 1982). By contrast, *injustice frames* are interpretations of experiences or conditions that support the conclusion that some moral principle has been violated and ought to be redressed. Social movement theorists generally view the adoption of injustice frames as a necessary—if insufficient—condition for political mobilization (Moore, 1978; McAdam, 1982; Turner and Killian, 1987; Gamson, 1992). Researchers in a variety of fields have developed strikingly similar frameworks for analyzing the shifts in political consciousness that are involved in injustice framing. In what follows, I elaborate them as a single approach to studying the construction of political claims (see Marshall, 2003; Jones, 2006).

The first, and arguably the most critical, stage in grievance construction is the process of redefining—or *naming* (Felstiner, Abel, and Sarat, 1980–81)—as *unjust* or *unfair* those conditions or practices previously seen as acceptable or tolerable. William Gamson (1995, p. 91) argues that to inspire mobilization for change, the evaluation of harm must be something more than a cognitive or intellectual judgment about what is equitable; rather, it must be a *hot cognition*, "the kind of righteous anger that puts fire in the belly and iron in the soul." Naming an injury, then, requires attention to the emotional valence attached to an individual's perception that some standard or principle has been violated. Social movement scholars generally understand anger and indignation to be *high-activation emotions*, motivating people to challenge the conditions that they perceive as injurious (Jasper, 1998; Britt and Heise, 2000). By contrast, emotions such as shame or guilt or embarrassment are considered *low-activation emotions*, tending to paralyze rather than mobilize individuals to act (Taylor, 2000). The quality or degree of emotions individuals attach to social conditions depends in part on what or who they perceive to be responsible for the injury (Ferree and Miller, 1985).

Thus the second shift in political consciousness requires a target against which these emotions can be usefully vented—what Felstiner, Abel, and Sarat (1980–81) refer to in their framework for grievance construction as *blaming*. Gamson (1992) observes that while these targets can be anything from corporations or government agencies to individuals or groups, an injustice frame requires some degree of *concreteness*. To the extent that individuals see only impersonal or abstract forces as responsible for suffering—nature, bad luck, God, "the system"—they are more likely to accept the status quo and make the best of things. If reification and excessive abstraction act as impediments to grievance construction, so too can *internalization* of blame; people who blame themselves for a situation are less likely to see it as injurious (Felstiner, Abel, and Sarat, 1980–81; Britt and Heise, 2000). Thus individuals must have a way of seeing the cause of their injury as the result of specific, identifiable forces external to themselves (Ferree and Miller, 1985).

Finally, individuals must specify a remedy, or *claim*—that is, some course of action to ameliorate the perceived harm (Felstiner, Abel, and Sarat, 1980–81; Gamson, 1992). At any given time or place, individuals have a range of available solutions to problems in their everyday lives (see also Ewick and Silbey, 1998; Mansbridge, 2001). These solutions include, but are not limited to, those promoted by political parties, interest groups, and social movement organizations. They may also include public policies designed for other purposes or constituencies, or policies adopted by other countries. In what follows, I will argue that in constructing solutions to long-term care problems, individuals draw on those models that closely accord with their previously existing beliefs about long-term care. By integrating a new need for governmental assistance into a belief system that privileges family or market responsibility for health care, caregivers construct political claims that challenge existing social arrangements, but they do so within a welfare state framework that imagines only a minimal role for the government in assisting families with long-term care.

Research Design and Methodology

Studying grievance construction is difficult because it is a subjective process, requiring techniques for observing how individuals evaluate their experiences or conditions while minimizing their reactivity to researcher suggestion (Felstiner, Abel, and Sarat, 1980–81). To address this concern, my study employed a three-stage observational design: (1) nonparticipant observation of support group meetings for individuals caring for adult family members with dementia, cancer, or similar chronic diseases; (2) focus group discussions involving the same caregiver support groups; and (3) one-on-one interviews with group participants.

Over a four-month period in the fall of 2004, I observed 68 meetings (each 1–2 hours in length) of 14 different support groups for family caregivers in Los Angeles. The support groups provided a setting in which to look at how caregivers described—and sought solutions to—problems involving care provision as they arose in their everyday lives. To control for variability in caregiving experiences across diseases or disabilities, support groups were limited to two specific classes of diseases: dementia and cancer.[5] In total, 158 family caregivers participated in this stage of the study.

In the second phase of the study, I led nine of these support groups in focus group discussions about specific legislative initiatives involving long-term care. The purpose of these meetings was to observe how participants related their personal caregiving experiences to larger sociopolitical issues of the provision of long-term care. Eighty support group members participated in this phase of the study. I then conducted one-on-one, in-depth interviews with 66 support group participants (as well as interviews with 13 caregivers who had not joined support groups) to elicit more intensive discussions about their caregiving experiences, including their use (or nonuse) of supportive services and benefits, their political backgrounds, and their views of governmental, market, and family responsibilities for long-term care.

This multimethod approach was designed to compensate for the limitations of each individual method with respect to the issues of researcher reactivity and control. Nonparticipant observation provided a window into processes of grievance construction with little researcher reactivity, but it also minimized my control over the content of group discussions. Interviews maximized my control, but even the most carefully crafted questions ran the risk of influencing responses. Focus groups were something of a middle ground, permitting observation of the participants' interactions and the natural vocabulary with which they constructed meaning about specific issues posed to them.

To identify the conditions that give rise to political claims for long-term care policy reform, I conducted a comparative analysis of the needs, resources, and experiences of caregivers who relied exclusively on legitimating frames in talking about their care circumstances—reflecting the belief that families should care for their own, without intervention by the government—and caregivers who relied at least in part on injustice frames—challenging norms about family caregiving as unfair. Legitimating frames included references to family "responsibility," "duty," and "obligation," as well as expressions that naturalized the speaker's circumstances or made them seem inevitable: "That's life" or "That's what families do" or "I'm taking care of Mom the way she took care of her own mother." Injustice frames focused on explicit moral condemnations about family responsibility for care: "that's unfair" or "that pisses me off."

The data were also coded for references to *unmet care needs*, or instances in which caregivers sought assistance with care but encountered obstacles, such as a lack of information about available services or concerns about affordability, service quality, and accessibility. I also coded all references to *governmental intervention*, including regulation, subsidies for market-based services, and government-run long-term care services. These data, together with data on legitimating and oppositional frames, were analyzed to assess the conditions that shape caregivers' expectations for policy intervention in long-term care.

Injustice Framing among Family Caregivers

Legitimating Frames

In a country in which families provide 80 percent of long-term care (O'Brien and Elias, 2004), it should come as no surprise that caregivers in the present study uniformly demonstrated a tenacious commitment to the idea that it was their duty as family members to bear the primary burden of providing long-term care. The belief in family obligation is an archetypical example of a legitimating frame: most caregivers understood the provision of care for a family member—no matter what the cost—as the natural and normal thing to do. Indeed, for many, the idea that anyone else—and in particular the government—should bear responsibility for either the costs or the provision of care was simply inconceivable.

At the time of this study, Vincent[6] was caring for his mother, who had been bedridden for five years following a stroke. Vincent worked full time and cared for his mother before and after work. A Vietnam vet, he joked that caregiving was the most difficult tour of duty he had ever had, but he did it, he insisted, out of a sense of obligation:

> Because they brought me into the world, and my mom would do the same thing for me if I came back from overseas shot up or no legs or you know, something god forbid, that woulda happened. But I felt I owed it to her . . . That's what we were brought up with. From the time we were hatched, so to speak, that we were to take care of our older folks.

Asked why he has not hired any assistance with caregiving, Vincent acknowledged it was partly finances, but also a sense of obligation: "I think family would rather do it themselves. It's a matter of pride."

By conceptualizing their work as fulfilling a duty to their families, caregivers understood their situations as both natural and inevitable. Larry had given up his home to care for his parents, both of whom had been diagnosed with dementia. Complaining to his support group that his niece and nephew didn't seem to share his values about caring for family, he opined: "Because it's an obligation that they have to do! So you sacrificed your life to move back with Mom and Dad? So you do it. You just do it. You just make the best of it."

When caregivers experienced frustration or exhaustion or resentment about their circumstances, the family responsibility frame served to mediate those emotions, often transforming them into feelings of guilt or embarrassment. Caregivers felt guilty for not doing enough or for wanting a break, and they felt embarrassed when they admitted they needed help. One new participant illustrates the close relationship between frustration and guilt in the following confession to her dementia support group:

> I'm not a good caretaker, because of my resentment and anger. I lose my patience. "Is today Tuesday?" "Yes, today is Tuesday." Then a minute

later: "Is today Tuesday?" "Yes, today is Tuesday." And after a while I'm *screaming*! And you feel terrible. And you feel guilty. And you feel like you're not a good person.

By transforming high-activation emotions such as anger and resentment into low-activation emotions—resignation, shame, guilt—the family responsibility frame simultaneously legitimates and reinforces norms about family obligations for care provision.

It's important to emphasize that the family responsibility frame was used to some extent by *all* of the family caregivers in this study, including those who also adopted more oppositional perspectives. But what is remarkable here is not the strength of this commitment to family, but how hard it was for caregivers to imagine alternative social arrangements for long-term care. Caregivers whose feelings about their circumstances challenged or contradicted the expectations of family obligation struggled to find a language in which to articulate another view. The lack of a widely available discourse with which to challenge norms about family caregiving in the United States provides a useful opportunity to explore how, if at all, individuals come to question the widely held assumption that long-term care is exclusively the responsibility of family.

Injustice Framing

Naming the Harm or Injury. Most researchers agree that to (re)-evaluate deeply entrenched beliefs, individuals require some *trigger*—an unexpected event or piece of information that causes them to think about their basic values and how the world diverges from them in some important way (Jasper, 1998; Snow et al., 1998). Beliefs about family responsibility for care provision were not questioned—or even considered—by study participants unless or until they confronted some disparity between the care they felt obligated to provide their family members and their capacity—financially, emotionally, or physically—to satisfy that obligation. In other words, in the case of long-term care, the harm or injury lies in the belief that care provision is in some key respect falling short—that there are financial, physical, or emotional obstacles that caregivers simply cannot overcome on their own.

In many cases involving chronic care, particularly for dementia, caregivers reached a point where they could not personally provide all of the care they perceived to be required by the care receiver. Many worked outside the home on a full- or part-time basis, some had child care responsibilities, some maintained separate households in other parts of the city, state, or country, some had health problems themselves, and most simply needed to attend to other parts of their lives. While there are a wide variety of market-based supportive services available to help caregivers, many caregivers didn't know where to find these services, couldn't afford the services they needed, or faced transportation or language barriers in accessing needed services.

Of the 79 caregivers in the interview sample, 47 (or 60%) described themselves as successfully meeting the perceived care needs of their family members. These caregivers included those whose family members needed relatively little assistance (typically because their conditions had not yet significantly deteriorated), those who had ample resources with which to find and/or purchase supportive services, those who had significant assistance in care provision from other family members, and those who obtained supportive services at low or no cost through California's means-tested Medicaid program. In all of these cases, caregivers still faced the emotional and physical challenges of providing care to a family member with a chronic disease or disability, but they experienced no disparity between the care they felt it was their duty to provide and their capacity to fill that obligation.

Not surprisingly, caregivers who described themselves as successfully meeting the care needs of their family members were substantially less likely to characterize their care obligations as unfair or unjust. Of these 47 caregivers, 32 (or nearly 70%) relied exclusively on the family responsibility frame when talking about their care circumstances, reflecting the belief that families should bear the full cost and burden of care provision, without the government's intervention. By contrast, caregivers who struggled to satisfy their perceived care obligations were far more likely to reevaluate taken-for-granted assumptions about family responsibility. As the following section elaborates, these perceptions of injury did not always lead to grievances, but without the perception of a divergence between expectations and reality—without the recognition of unmet care needs—grievance construction simply did not take place. Of the 79 caregivers in the interview sample, 32 (or 40%) mentioned unmet care needs. Of these, 26 (or more than 80%) relied on injustice framing in describing their caregiving dilemmas.

Blaming. If unmet needs created an opportunity to reevaluate deeply entrenched beliefs about family responsibility for care, how caregivers evaluated the discrepancy between their beliefs about family care provision and their capacity to provide that care depended critically on *who they blamed* for the divergence. To the extent that caregivers internalized the blame for their predicaments, they were likely to feel shame, guilt, or embarrassment—low-activation emotions that are unlikely to lead to injustice framing (Britt and Heise, 2000; Taylor, 2000). In these cases, beliefs about family responsibility again strongly influenced perceptions of personal responsibility for care problems. Some caregivers blamed themselves for not purchasing long-term care insurance when they had the opportunity. Others blamed themselves for not arranging their finances in ways that would legally qualify their care receiver for state Medicaid long-term care benefits. Most were just embarrassed that lack of income or poor health would stand in the way of meeting their care obligations to their family. In all of these cases, self-blame played a prominent role in *defusing* potential grievances. Similarly, caregivers who blamed impersonal or abstract targets for their frustrations—bad luck or "life"—were more likely to be resigned to the conditions in which they found themselves, with little sense of agency about or awareness of the structural conditions underlying their predicaments (Gamson, 1992).

High-activation emotions like anger or moral indignation require an attribution of blame to specific, identifiable forces external to the potential grievants (Ferree and Miller, 1985). Because care provision is so widely understood to be a family responsibility in the United States, the government was *not* a natural target for blame when most participants began caregiving. Indeed, many had never considered the role of the government (in any capacity) with regard to providing long-term care. That most caregivers wrestle with serious long-term care dilemmas without ever questioning the assumption that family should bear exclusive responsibility for providing care highlights the importance of *expectations* in injustice framing: we experience moral indignation only when our expectations for how we should be treated have been violated. Joan, who for 18 years had been caring for her husband, participated in a focus group discussion about public policy on long-term care. Silent for much of the discussion, she finally confided to the group that the idea of the government taking responsibility for the costs of long-term care was new to her:

I think . . . that as a caregiver, we don't feel any entitlement. We never stamp our feet and say this is ridiculous, someone should be paying for this . . . I mean, I just thought hey, it's the luck of the draw, isn't it? You know? . . . But if someone said, you know what? The government . . . I mean this whole discussion is like hey wow, that's another way to look at it, isn't it? Someone should be paying for this!

Joan's revelation to the group illustrates how the introduction of an alternative frame can create new expectations or, in Joan's words, a sense of entitlement. But where did caregivers derive these alternative views of long-term care responsibilities?

During the course of caregiving, study participants were exposed to a wide range of alternative models of care provision, all of which served as potential paradigms for assigning responsibility for care struggles to institutions other than the family. In evaluating these alternatives, caregivers were primarily drawn to those models that assimilated their need for assistance with previously existing beliefs about the respective responsibilities of the family, the market, and the government for care provision.

For a clear majority of grievants in this study, the most resonant model for assigning responsibility for care dilemmas to an institution other than the family was California's means-tested Medicaid program. California's Medicaid program offers relatively generous long-term care benefit packages for those who qualify for the program, including full prescription drug benefits, and coverage for adult day care, in-home supportive services, and nursing home care. Because the income and asset eligibility levels are so stringent, few caregivers in this study actually qualified for state assistance. But, importantly, many participants knew of somebody who did qualify for Medicaid. Stories about Medicaid benefits circulated within support groups and in friendship and neighbor networks, not only providing concrete examples of what the government *could* provide in the way of long-term care assistance, but also creating an expectation that certain types of services *ought* to be subsidized by the government and available to a wider segment of the U.S. population. It is typically in conversations about Medicaid that caregivers most clearly articulated an injustice frame.

Susanna was caring for her parents, both of whom had dementia. Despite working full time, she could afford to hire a caregiver to stay with her parents for only 4–6 hours a day. Her parents were unable to qualify for Medicaid benefits, as their pensions placed them just above the eligibility cutoff line. Susanna observed, angrily, in her interview:

> I have girlfriends at work say oh, just call up so-and-so, they can help you. [They'll say] my mother has 24-hour care . . . [But] they don't pay a penny because they get on welfare . . . You have to be poor all your life or whatever, not work. And then when you're older, you get all the benefits, and that's just not fair! I think that's very unfair. My parents both have worked all their lives, and Daddy had two jobs for 16 years. And now he can't qualify because supposedly they make too much money.

If the need for assistance with the costs or provision of long-term care changed the way many participants viewed the government's responsibility, it was notable that Medicaid proved to be a more resonant model than Medicare. In many ways, Medicare would seem to be the more likely model for assigning responsibility for chronic care dilemmas to the government: not only are social insurance programs generally more respected than means-tested "welfare" programs such as Medicaid (Cook and Barrett, 1992), but most participants or their family members qualified for and received Medicare benefits for acute health care. It seems plausible, then, that caregivers would make the argument that if Medicare pays for the costs of acute care, it should also do so for costs associated with chronic diseases like Alzheimer's or Parkinson's. But, remarkably, *no* caregivers in this sample referenced Medicare as a source for their injustice frames.

One reason the Medicaid model of social provision resonated more with caregivers than the Medicare model is that Medicaid more closely accords with American cultural beliefs about family responsibility for care provision. In the United States, Medicaid and Medicare represent two distinct approaches to the provision of social welfare. Medicare is based on a social insurance model in which the *government* takes primary responsibility for meeting certain social welfare needs (retirement income for example, or acute health care for senior citizens); Medicaid is rooted in a residualist or needs-based model, in which *families* or *individuals* take primary responsibility for meeting social welfare needs, and the government steps in only when a person's most basic needs are not being met. Of these two forms of social welfare provision, the underlying logic of Medicaid benefits arguably resonated with caregivers, because it provided them with a way of reconciling their need for governmental assistance with their deeply held

commitments to family. In other words, participants who assigned responsibility for long-term care dilemmas to the government believed
that it had a role in helping families with care responsibilities, but only
when traditional systems of family provision break down.

The importance of finding a model for care assistance that modified
but closely accorded with participants' preexisting beliefs about long-
term care provision can also be seen in the failure of international
systems of social welfare provision to serve as resonant models for
assigning responsibility for unmet care needs. Most European countries, as well as Australia, Japan, and Canada, offer a wide range of
public benefits for family care providers, ranging from free or subsidized home care, adult day care, and institutionalized care to tax credits and direct payment allowances for caregivers (Daly, 2001; Daly
and Rake, 2003). But when participants in support groups and focus
groups made references to how other countries approach the issue of
long-term care, they were typically met with comments about the perceived limitations of the health care systems in other countries—lower
quality of care, longer waits for services, and so forth. In general, participants understood the health care systems of other countries to be
so different from health care provision in the United States that international comparisons ultimately failed to resonate as a meaningful source of alternative understandings of long-term care. Of the 41
interview participants who articulated an injustice frame, only three
relied on international comparisons to do so.

Those participants who relied on sources of injustice frames other
than Medicaid similarly emphasized models that closely tracked their
preexisting beliefs about care responsibilities. Five interview participants, for example, drew on their experiences with health insurance
companies in articulating an injustice frame. These caregivers—most
typically caregivers for cancer patients—reported constant struggles to
obtain coverage for various treatments and services and an ongoing
fear that their insurance companies would drop their care receiver at
the slightest misstep. In these cases, participants either assigned responsibility to the government for regulating the health care insurance
industry—leaving intact their more fundamental assumption that the
insurance market, rather than the government, should bear responsibility for the costs of health care—or they blamed their health insurance companies directly.

Notably, no participants assigned responsibility for unmet care needs to long-term care insurance companies. Participants in this study widely disparaged the long-term care insurance market for being unaffordable, inaccessible to people with diagnosed chronic diseases, and unreliable in delivering benefits to those who had obtained policies. In most cases, grievants viewed long-term care insurance as an ineffective tool for addressing the kinds of care crises that they routinely confronted.

Finally, some caregivers based their injustice frames on political or moral beliefs about the government's (or society's) responsibility to ensure the health and economic security of its citizens. Ten caregivers who identified themselves as "political liberals" emphasized that these were beliefs they held before their caregiving experiences, and they experienced little dissonance between their *need for* governmental assistance and their *expectations of* government in protecting the social welfare of its citizens.

In assigning responsibility for unmet long-term care provision needs, then, caregivers were exposed to a variety of government- and market-based models for assigning responsibility for unmet care needs, but they were primarily drawn to those models that closely accorded with preexisting beliefs about the responsibilities of the family, market, and government for care provision. As the next section elaborates, participants relied on a similar logic in constructing policy solutions, or *political claims*, for their unmet long-term care needs.

Claiming. The final shift in political consciousness necessary for grievance construction is the prescription of a *remedy*, some course of action to redress the perceived injustice (Snow and Benford, 1988). It is in the specification of solutions to care dilemmas that we see why caregivers' claims seem to call for an expanded role for the government in long-term care, yet lack the political force of claims for new rights or entitlements to long-term care.

Caregivers' claims for public provision were rooted in the specific care needs giving rise to their grievances. Those caregivers who struggled to afford adult day care for their care receivers argued for subsidized day care (or, less commonly, state-run day care centers). Those who needed help inside the home argued for subsidized home health care. While the form of policy intervention varied significantly, virtually all of the claims that emerged from processes of grievance construction reflected a substantially expanded view of the government's responsibility for long-term care provision. With the exception of those who identified themselves as political liberals and who held strong views of the government's responsibility for health care prior to caregiving, most of the grievants in this study had given little thought to the role of government in long-term care when they first began caregiving. That they now envisioned their care needs as the basis of claims for new or expanded systems of social welfare provision suggests a significant transformation in how they evaluated the need for, and importance of, the government in solving problems regarding long-term care.

And yet, importantly, grievants' claims for policy intervention bore the imprint of the grievance construction process in which they were forged: rather than justifying these claims on the basis of citizenship or market participation—as U.S. social insurance programs usually are—grievants in this case justified their claims for intervention on the basis of *need*. They spoke of getting "help" or "assistance" from the government, language that, in the United States, is associated with means-tested public assistance programs. This understanding of public long-term care provision as being based on need rather than citizenship or market participation accords closely with the logic participants used in attributing blame: to conceptualize policy solutions to their long-term care problems, participants required a way of reconciling their need for governmental assistance with deeply-held beliefs about family responsibility for providing care. The social insurance model of public provision in most cases failed to supply such a framework, instead symbolically suggesting to many caregivers that the government would be taking over long-term care obligations that more properly belonged to the family. Ruth, a caregiver for both of her parents, captures this concern that relying on the government for more than needs-based benefits might be perceived as abandoning one's responsibilities to one's family:

> I have mixed feelings about it . . . I'm definitely believing in home support services, definitely believe people need to have assistance with respite care and caregiving . . . So I'm much more for the government helping people out with these things. But I also can't say that I totally believe that I don't have any responsibility in this. So . . . I think what I would like for people to do, for government to do, is to help people when they need help.

A needs-based model, characterizing care provision as primarily a family responsibility, with the government supplying assistance only when families need it, presented caregivers with a way of accepting an expanded role for government in long-term care provision without in any way diminishing their own commitments to family.

But calling for governmental intervention on the basis of need rather than as a matter of right or entitlement has important consequences for the development of political demand. Needs-based claims represent a passive form of making political claims. There is, as others have argued before (Scheingold, 1974; Williams, 1987; Waldron, 1996), a critical qualitative difference between *asking for help* and *demanding one's rights*. Claims of rights demand a degree of attention and dignity in U.S. political discourse that claims of need, long associated with charity, rarely garner (Gordon, 1994; Gilliom, 2001). As Jeremy Waldron (1996, p. 94) once wryly observed, "the experience of our century has not shown that officials are galvanized to action by the discovery that somebody needs something, even to survive." Because needs-based claims are structured more on the perceived failure of individual family caregivers to take care of their own than on the failure of the nation to take care of its own, needs-based claims are always a half-step away from the demobilizing possibilities of shame, guilt, and embarrassment.

Conclusion

U.S. families find themselves on uncertain new terrain: caught between longstanding and deeply held beliefs about family responsibility for long-term care on the one hand, and shifting demographic, economic, and social realities on the other, Americans have not arrived at any consensus about whether, or to what extent, the government should bear responsibility for care provision. In this chapter, I have sought to illuminate how family caregivers who are navigating this new landscape imagine a role for government. Faced with strains on finances, work, family life, and the health of the care provider, when, if at all, do family caregivers reconceptualize care provision as a *social* responsibility—as a problem that might be ameliorated through the intervention of the government?

One of the most striking findings here is the remarkable persistence of the belief in family responsibility for care provision. The belief in taking care of one's own, of handling long-term care problems within the family, and the fear and guilt of being viewed as a "bad" son or daughter or deficient spouse for seeking help with care, all reinforce an understanding of caregiving as a private and individual—rather than a public or social—responsibility. So pervasive is this understanding of care provision as a family responsibility that the possibility of assistance from the government did not occur to most caregivers in my study until they faced some disparity between the care they felt obligated to provide and their capacity to satisfy those obligations.

Importantly, however, these beliefs in family responsibility do not merely prevent or delay turning to the government for assistance; *they shape the very solutions caregivers imagine from the government for their unmet care needs.* Thus, while social insurance programs such as Social Security and Medicare remain unequivocally popular forms of public provision, caregivers in this study were reluctant to embrace policy alternatives that might appear (even symbolically) to detract from their commitments to family. They instead imagined policy solutions that were modeled after Medicaid, a means-tested program that allocates primary responsibility for health care to the family, rather than the government. This is not to say that Medicaid itself should—or could—serve as a programmatic solution to the long-term care problems of the middle class. Medicaid was never intended to be the primary source of public funding for long-term care assistance. But these findings emphasize the important point that regardless of how difficult long-term care provision has become for contemporary American families, and no matter how striking the presence of their unmet health care needs, Americans remain uncomfortable with the idea of fully reallocating the costs of long-term care to the government.

At the same time, it should be emphasized that participants' claims for means-tested policy intervention were *not* an endorsement of a purely residualist social welfare policy. While participants believed that the government should assist families with care provision only when they cannot meet their basic needs, they nevertheless held an expansive definition of "need," one that envisioned not just the poor, but the middle class, as appropriate beneficiaries of public provision. Calls for expanded long-term care benefits for the middle class represent a striking rebuttal to policy makers who seek to limit the government's role in social welfare provision to that of a safety net only for the very poor. Because Medicaid is the only public program to offer substantial assistance with the costs of long-term care, this means-tested program has been used more frequently in recent decades by middle-class families with substantial chronic care needs who have no choice but to spend down their assets in order to qualify their care receiver for governmental assistance for nursing home care (O'Brien and Elias, 2004). Concerns among fiscal conservatives that Medicaid is evolving into a "middle-class entitlement" (Burwell, 1991; Moses, 1996) have resulted in a wide range of legislative initiatives designed to make it more difficult for the non-poor to use Medicaid as a safety net. The findings from this study suggest that not only is it true that public expectations *are* evolving toward a middle-class entitlement, but also that, paradoxically, the means-tested benefits provided under the Medicaid public assistance program are serving as the very foundation for these expectations.

Finally, it is important to note that caregivers' solutions were constructed largely independently of the influence of social reform organizations. Participants were largely unaware of advocacy organizations seeking public policy reforms for long-term care. While many knew of larger organizations like AARP or the Alzheimer's Association, few caregivers demonstrated any awareness of the specific policy solutions these organizations were promoting with regard to long-term care (Levitsky, 2006). While I address the role of advocacy organizations more fully elsewhere (Levitsky, 2006), it is worth considering here how advocacy organizations might influence the construction of grievances if they were better able to reach their isolated constituencies. Would advocacy organizations have helped caregivers in this case to construct political solutions that more fundamentally challenged the paradigm of family provision of care? Based on interviews with activists from state and national advocacy organizations pursuing long-term care public policy reform, evidence suggests that in the current political context, advocacy organizations are actually proffering more conservative policy alternatives than the ones caregivers imagine on their own. Because policy makers today on both sides of the political aisle express concern about the economic viability of *existing* systems of social provision (most notably, Social Security and Medicare), reform advocates are sharply constrained in the range of policy solutions they can credibly seek for *new* social problems such as long-term care provision. As a consequence, most advocacy organizations are currently pursuing modest, incremental, market-based reforms that bear little resemblance to the needs or expectations of caregivers for an expanded safety net for the middle class. The irony of this is that if reformers could mobilize this growing constituency, they could potentially transform the politics of social provision in ways that might make caregivers' imagined solutions a political reality.

Notes

1. Caregivers must cope with the financial expenses of caregiving, but working caregivers (who now constitute a majority of all caregivers) typically face additional stresses—and costs—relating to missed work and lost job and career opportunities (U.S. Department of Health and Human Services 1998; England and Folbre, 1999).

2. See Glenn (2000) and Fraser (1997). If the emotional and physical responsibilities of care provision fall disproportionately on women, so too do the economic costs of caregiving (Harrington Meyer 1994; Wabakayashi and Donato, 2005).

3. A growing body of literature considers the global consequences of the market for paid care, as women from poor countries leave their own families to work as care providers in richer countries (Hondagneu-Sotelo, 2001; Ehrenreich and Hochschild, 2002; Hochschild, 2003).

4. Researchers have linked caregiving stress to substantially increased rates of depression (Poulshock and Deimling, 1984), physical health problems (Archbold, 1982; Schulz and Beach, 1999), and greater alcohol and psychotropic drug use (Alzheimer's Association and National Alliance for Caregiving, 1999; George and Gwyther, 1986).

5. The burden of caregiving is well known to be greatest among those caring for patients with dementia (Dunham and Dietz, 2003). This burden is exacerbated by the fact that the costs of supportive services for patients with dementia are rarely covered by Medicare or private health insurance policies and can be as much as three times greater than the costs of caring for people with other chronic diseases or disabilities. By contrast, the costs of caring for patients with cancer are more frequently covered by health insurance policies. The sample of cancer caregivers thus provided a useful comparative group for examining the extent to which the costs of care provision influence the development of political consciousness.

6. All names of caregivers used in this chapter are pseudonyms.

References

Abel, E. K. 1991. *Who Cares for the Elderly? Public Policy and the Experiences of Adult Daughters.* Philadelphia: Temple University Press.
Alzheimer's Association and National Alliance for Caregiving. 1999. *Who*

Cares? Families Caring for Persons with Alzheimer's Disease. Washington, D.C.: Alzheimer's Association and National Alliance for Caregiving.

Archbold, P. J. 1982. An analysis of parent caring by women. *Home Health Care Services Quarterly* 3 (2): 5–26.

Britt, L., and D. Heise. 2000. From shame to pride in identity politics. Pp. 252–68 in S. Stryker, T. J. Owens, and R. W. White (eds.). *Self, Identity, and Social Movements.* Minneapolis: University of Minnesota Press.

Burwell, B. 1991. *Middle-Class Welfare: Medicaid Estate Planning for Long-Term Care Coverage.* Cambridge, Mass.: SysteMetrics.

Cook, F. L., and E. J. Barrett. 1992. *Support for the American Welfare State: The Views of Congress and the Public.* New York: Columbia University Press.

Daly, M. 2001. Care policies in Western Europe. Pp. 33–65 in M. Daly (ed.), *Care Work: The Quest for Security.* Geneva, Switzerland: International Labour Office.

Daly, M., and K. Rake. 2003. *Gender and the Welfare State: Care, Work, and Welfare in Europe and the USA.* Malden, Mass.: Blackwell.

Dunham, C. C., and B. E. Dietz. 2003. "If I'm not allowed to put my family first": Challenges experienced by women who are caregiving for family members with dementia. *Journal of Women and Aging* 15 (1): 55–69.

Ehrenreich, B., and A. Hochschild (eds.). 2002. *Global Woman: Nannies, Maids, and Sex Workers in the New Economy.* New York: Henry Holt.

England, P., and N. Folbre. 1999. The cost of caring. *Annals of the American Academy of Political and Social Science* 561 (1): 39–51.

Ewick, P., and S. S. Silbey. 1998. *The Common Place of Law.* Chicago: University of Chicago Press.

Felstiner, W., R. L. Abel, and A. Sarat. 1980–81. The emergence of disputes: Naming, blaming, claiming . . . *Law and Society Review* 15 (3–4): 631–54.

Ferree, M. M., W. A. Gamson, J. Gerhards, and D. Rucht. 2002. *Shaping Abortion Discourse: Democracy and the Public Sphere in Germany and the United States.* New York: Cambridge University Press.

Ferree, M. M., and F. D. Miller. 1985. Mobilization and meaning: Toward an integration of social psychological and resource perspectives on social movements. *Sociological Inquiry* 55 (1): 38–61.

Fraser, N. 1997. *Justice Interruptus.* New York: Routledge.

Gamson, W. A. 1992. *Talking Politics.* New York: Cambridge University Press.

———. 1995. Constructing social protest. Pp. 85–106 in H. Johnston and B. Klandermans (eds.), *Social Movements and Culture.* Minneapolis: University of Minnesota Press.

Gamson, W. A., B. Fireman, and S. Rytina. 1982. *Encounters with Unjust Authority*. Chicago: Dorsey Press.

Garey, A. I., K. V. Hansen, R. Hertz, and C. L. MacDonald. 2002. Care and kinship. *Journal of Family Issues* 23 (6): 703–15.

George, L. K., and L. P. Gwyther. 1986. Caregiver well-being: A multidimensional examination of family caregivers of demented adults. *Gerontologist* 26 (3): 253–59.

Gilliom, J. 2001. *Overseers of the Poor: Surveillance, Resistance, and the Limits of Privacy*. Chicago: University of Chicago Press.

Glazer, N. Y. 1988. Overlooked, overworked: Women's unpaid and paid work in the health services' cost crisis. *International Journal of Health Services* 18 (1): 119–37.

Glenn, E. N. 2000. Creating a caring society. *Contemporary Sociology* 29 (1): 84–94.

Gordon, L. 1994. *Pitied but Not Entitled: Single Mothers and the History of Welfare, 1890–1935*. Cambridge, Mass.: Harvard University Press.

Harrington, M. 2000. *Care and Equality*. New York: Routledge.

Harrington Meyer, M. 1994. The impact of family status on income security and health care in old age: A comparison of Western nations. *International Journal of Sociology and Social Policy* 14 (1/2): 53–73.

———. 2005. Decreasing welfare, increasing old age inequality: Whose responsibility is it? Pp. 65–89 in R. B. Hudson (ed.), *The New Politics of Old Age Policy*. Baltimore: Johns Hopkins University Press.

Hochschild, A. 2003. *The Commercialization of Intimate Life: Notes from Home and Work*. Berkeley: University of California Press.

Hondagneu-Sotelo, P. 2001. *Domestica: Immigrant Workers Cleaning and Caring in the Shadows of Influence*. Berkeley: University of California Press.

Jasper, J. M. 1998. The emotions of protest: Affective and reactive emotions in and around social movements. *Sociological Forum* 13 (3): 397–424.

Jones, L. 2006. The haves come out ahead: How cause lawyers frame the legal system for movements. Pp. 182–96 in A. Sarat and S. A. Scheingold (eds.), *Cause Lawyers and Social Movements*. Stanford, Calif.: Stanford University Press.

Koren, M. J. 1986. Home care—who cares? *New England Journal of Medicine* 314 (14): 917–20.

Levitsky, S. 2006. Private dilemmas of public provision: The formation of political demand for state entitlements to long-term care. Ph.D. diss., Department of Sociology, University of Wisconsin–Madison.

Mansbridge, J. 2001. The making of oppositional consciousness. Pp. 1–19 in J. Mansbridge and A. Morris (eds.), *Oppositional Consciousness*. Chicago: University of Chicago Press.

Marshall, A.-M. 2003. Injustice frames, legality, and the everyday construction of sexual harassment. *Law and Social Inquiry* 28 (3): 659–89.

McAdam, D. 1982. *Political Process and the Development of Black Insurgency, 1930–1970.* Chicago: University of Chicago Press.

Moore, B., Jr. 1978. *Injustice: The Social Bases of Obedience and Revolt.* White Plains, N.Y.: M. E. Sharpe.

Moses, S. A. 1996. Medicaid stifles LTC ins. purchases. *National Underwriter* (Aug. 5), S9.

O'Brien, E., and R. Elias. 2004. *Medicaid and Long-Term Care.* Washington, D.C.: Henry J. Kaiser Family Foundation, Kaiser Commission on Medicaid and the Uninsured.

Poulshock, S. W., and G. T. Deimling. 1984. Families caring for elders in residence: Issues in the measurement of burden. *Journal of Gerontology* 39 (2): 230–39.

Scheingold, S. A. 1974. *The Politics of Rights: Lawyers, Public Policy, and Political Change.* New Haven, Conn.: Yale University Press.

Schulz, R., and S. Beach. 1999. Caregiving as a risk factor for mortality: The caregiver health effects study. *JAMA: Journal of the American Medical Association* 282 (23): 2215–19.

Snow, D. A., Jr., and R. D. Benford. 1988. Ideology, frame resonance, and participant mobilization. Pp. 197–217 in B. Klandermans, H. Kriesi, and S. Tarrow (eds.), *From Structure to Action: Comparing Social Movement Research across Cultures.* Greenwich, Conn.: JAI Press.

Snow, D. A., Jr., D. M. Cress, L. Downey, and A. W. Jones. 1998. Disrupting the "quotidian": Reconceptualizing the relationship between breakdown and the emergence of collective action. *Mobilization: An International Journal* 3 (1): 1–22.

Snow, D. A., Jr., E. B. Rochford, S. K. Worden, and R. D. Benford. 1986. Frame alignment processes, micromobilization, and movement participation. *American Sociological Review* 51 (4): 464–81.

Steinberg, M. W. 1999. The talk and back talk of collective action: A dialogic analysis of repertoires of discourse among nineteenth-century English cotton spinners. *American Journal of Sociology* 105 (3): 736–80.

Stevens, R. 1989. *In Sickness and in Wealth: American Hospitals in the Twentieth Century.* New York: Basic Books.

Taylor, V. 2000. Emotions and identity in women's self-help movements. Pp. 271–99 in S. Stryker, T. J. Owens, and R. W. White (eds.), *Self, Identity, and Social Movements.* Minneapolis: University of Minnesota Press.

Turner, R. H., and L. M. Killian. 1987. *Collective Behavior,* 3rd ed. Englewood Cliffs, N.J.: Prentice-Hall.

U.S. Department of Health and Human Services. 1998. *Informal Care-*

giving: Compassion in Action. Washington, D.C.: U.S. Department of Health and Human Services.

Wabakayashi, C., and K. M. Donato. 2005. The consequences of caregiving: Effects on women's employment and earnings. *Population Research and Policy Review* 24 (5): 467–88.

Waldron, J. 1996. Rights and needs: The myth of disjunction. Pp. 87–109 in A. Sarat and T. R. Kearns (eds.), *Legal Rights: Historical and Philosophical Perspectives.* Ann Arbor: University of Michigan Press.

Williams, P. 1987. Alchemical notes: Reconstructing ideals from deconstructed rights. *Harvard Civil Rights-Civil Liberties Law Review* 22 (1): 401–33.

III. Public Policies on Aging

11. Social Security

Political Resilience in the Face of Conservative Strides

Andrea Louise Campbell, Ph.D., and Ryan King, S.B.

In early 2005, a 30-year effort on the part of conservatives to transform the structure of Social Security seemed poised for success. Long skeptical of the public pension program, conservatives had waged a protracted war against it. They first attacked the program directly, and then, after that tactic failed, they devised a new, more promising strategy of providing a private-sector alternative: individual accounts into which a portion of workers' payroll taxes would be deposited and then managed and owned by them. At this point, one of their own, George W. Bush, a long-time proponent of privatization, chose to make the introduction of Social Security individual accounts the central aim of his domestic agenda, barnstorming the country spreading his message. According to a Pew Research Center for the People and the Press (2004) poll, 54 percent of Americans supported private accounts, including 61 percent of those under age 45, precisely those who would benefit from this new structure.[1] Democrats failed to offer an alternative, and Republicans excoriated them for having "no ideas" (Toner and Rosenbaum, 2005).

Yet by late spring of the same year, the president's reform initiative appeared dead before it had even arrived. Labor unions, AARP, and congressional Democrats stood in unified opposition to individual accounts. Despite the president's entreaties, public support waned. More devastatingly, congressional Republicans failed to take up the reform gauntlet; Social Security reform, at least this version of it, was not to be in 2005.

Nonetheless, the very fact that individual accounts were part of the national conversation was a triumph for their proponents (Teles and Derthick, 2009). Once the pet idea of a small band of conservative think-tank analysts and academics, individual accounts were, if briefly, even embraced by some moderate Democrats as likely components of an eventual Social Security overhaul. The world-wide financial crisis that began in 2008, and the ensuing stock market declines, have unquestionably diminished the appeal of equity investing, and the safety of the traditional Social Security annuity looks good to many in light of 401(k) retirement account losses (Reno and Lavery, 2009).[2] But it seems unlikely that the menu of reform options in the future will not include some form of individual accounts, a testimony to the long-term strategizing and success of these conservative thinkers.

Fiscal Challenges Facing Social Security

The litany of challenges confronting the Social Security system in the future are familiar to most policy analysts by now. Given the actuarial predictability of the program, there is little disagreement about the size and scope of the program's long-term shortfall. Although the Social Security trust fund is accruing resources currently, thanks in part to program changes enacted through major reforms in 1983, a shift in the country's demographics in the near future will fundamentally alter the program's fortunes. Throughout its life, Social Security has generally enjoyed favorable demographic conditions, with an ever-expanding workforce supporting a smaller retiree contingent. However, the impending retirement of the baby boom generation will lead to the proportion of the population over age 65 increasing from 2005's 12 percent to 20 percent by 2030. In addition, improvements in life expectancy also increase the number of years that retired baby boomers are expected to draw on Social Security resources, and the number of workers aged 18 to 64 will shrink, due to the low fertility rates of the 1960s (Diamond and Orszag 2004). While the labor force grew at an average of 2.1 percent per year during the 1970s and 1980s, it fell to an average of 1.1 percent per year from 1990 to 2008 and is expected to drop to 0.4 percent after 2050 (Board of Trustees, 2009). Additionally, the rapid growth in the workforce due to rising female employment is expected to level off. Ultimately, a decline in the worker/beneficiary ratio from 3.3 in 2004 to 2.1 in 2035 will strain the system, necessitating tax increases, benefit cuts, or other kinds of reform in order to keep the program solvent in its current form.

The Social Security Board of Trustees and the Congressional Budget Office have both modeled the future of Social Security in response to growing concerns about its ability to withstand this influx of retirees.

Because of the funding structure created by the 1983 amendments to the Social Security Act and the future budget surpluses it will generate,[3] the trust fund is expected to increase to $6 trillion by 2026. In 2017, expenditures will begin to exceed payroll taxes and taxes on benefits, and in 2027 expenditures are expected to exceed payroll taxes, taxes on benefits, and income from interest on the existing principal. From 2027 onward, Social Security will run an annual budget deficit and gradually draw down the trust fund until the fund is exhausted in 2041 (Social Security Advisory Board, 2006). After 2041, expected program income from current workers will cover roughly 75 percent of scheduled benefits. Serious as it is, this situation is much less dire than that confronting Medicare. After an initial bump due to baby boomer retirement, Social Security spending as a percentage of gross domestic product (GDP) levels off. In contrast, Medicare spending, which is driven both by demographics and by the rising costs of health care in general, continues to grow faster than GDP and threatens to crowd out the rest of the federal budget (Congressional Budget Office, 2007).

Principal Ideas for Reform

For all of Social Security's actuarial predictability, how to reform it is highly contested. Two main camps have emerged. On one side are those who wish to preserve the current system and who advocate a series of incremental changes to the present structure that would bring it into long-term actuarial balance. On the other side are those who wish to transform the program, partly or wholly, into a system of private accounts in which program participants would have individual ownership rights and would make their own investment decisions. There is some disagreement about what the two approaches mean for future retirement incomes and national savings; the more profound source of disagreement, however, is ideological and reflects the fundamental debate in U.S. politics about the role of the individual versus that of the government in insuring against life's vagaries.

Incremental Change

One vision for Social Security's future entails preserving Social Security's basic structure while tweaking the benefit and revenue sides of the equation in order to bring the program into long-term actuarial balance. This is the approach advocated by AARP and by liberal economists Peter Diamond and Peter Orszag, among others. Proponents of incremental change view Social Security as a form of social insurance in which the risks of old age, disability, and low earnings are pooled across society, with workers subsidizing the retired, the able-bodied subsidizing the disabled, and the affluent subsidizing low earners.

AARP's (2006) Public Policy Institute, for example, has calculated the percentage of the long-term trust fund shortfall that would be met by each of a number of options, such as raising the cap on wages taxed, raising the normal retirement age, or gradually reducing benefits for high earners, among other steps.[4] Various combinations of these reforms could be assembled to meet the shortfall in a way that would spread the pain of reform across income groups and generations, in much the same way as the 1983 Social Security Amendments did.[5]

The Diamond/Orszag (2004) plan similarly makes changes within the existing framework to achieve long-term solvency and expand benefits for particular groups. Their plan addresses several challenges to Social Security that have emerged as the system has developed. First, because life expectancy has grown far beyond that of the 1930s, they propose to index Social Security to future improvements in life expectancy, with equivalent reductions in benefits and increases in payroll taxes. Second, they note that with increased income inequality, more and more earnings have escaped the Social Security tax; thus they seek to restore the taxable earnings base from its present 85 percent of aggregate wages to the 90 percent that obtained in the early 1980s. Third, a contributing factor to Social Security's long-term shortfall is the *legacy debt*, incurred when early cohorts received benefits despite paying little into the system. To address this problem, Diamond and Orszag advocate folding government employees into the program, imposing a legacy tax on earnings above the taxable maximum, and introducing a legacy charge on benefits and taxes beginning in 2023. In sum, the Diamond/Orszag plan would increase Social Security revenues by a total of 2.69 percent of the taxable payroll, with 2 percent going to addressing the 75-year actuarial imbalance and the remaining 0.69 percent financing increased benefits for at-risk groups.

Both of these approaches maintain Social Security's structure as a defined-benefit program. They also preserve the risk-pooling social insurance characteristics of the program, viewing Social Security as a safety net rather than as an investment. In addition, these proposals maintain and in some cases enhance the redistributive aspects of the current program.

Individual Accounts

An alternative vision for Social Security's future changes the basic structure of the program, allowing individuals to invest a portion of their current 6.2 percent payroll taxes—2 percent or 4 percent under most such proposals—into a personal account.[6] Workers would direct the investments in these individual accounts and would be able leave them to heirs, unlike current Social Security benefits. But with individual ownership comes individual risk: the size of the retirement benefits funded by this defined-contribution portion of Social Security would vary with the market performance of the chosen investments, and the amount invested would depend on individuals' wages, with no redistribution from high to low earners as in the traditional system.

The Origins and Political Rise of Individual Accounts

That this alternative vision for Social Security both attained a place and may still remain on the national agenda is a remarkable achievement, decades in the making, for a group of conservative thinkers who have long sought to reduce the size and scope of the U.S. welfare state and to wean individuals from governmental provision (Teles and Derthick, 2009).

For many years, Social Security policy making was dominated by a tightly knit community centered around the Social Security Administration, organized labor, and the tax-writing committees of the House and Senate (Derthick, 1979). This community shaped and protected the payroll-tax-financed nature of Social Security, satisfying the preferences of both liberals and fiscal conservatives by steadily expanding Social Security benefits, especially during election years (Tufte 1978), while increasing payroll taxes to match these benefit expansions and, therefore, seeming to keep the program in check (Derthick, 1979; Zelizer, 1998). In the face of the program's enormous popularity—surveys in the 1930s through 1950s found support levels among the public above 80 and even 90 percent (Schiltz, 1970)—skeptics of Social Security kept quiet.

Opponents of the traditional program gradually became bolder, beginning in the 1960s when Barry Goldwater suggested that Social Security be made voluntary, and again in the early 1980s when the Reagan administration attempted to cut benefits for early retirees. The firestorm that greeted the latter proposal proved to conservatives that direct attacks on the program were likely to fail, and instead they adopted a new strategy of creating attractive private alternatives to the government's program.

Key to this new path was the creation of a new community of conservative thinkers, centered around a set of well-endowed and active think tanks that could wrest the policy agenda away from the older Social Security establishment (Teles and Derthick, 2009). These think tanks, such as the Heritage Foundation, founded in 1973, and the Cato Institute, created in 1977, became places to foster technical expertise on Social Security to match that on the liberal side and to develop political strategies more likely to gain traction than did direct attacks on a popular program with a large and mobilized constituency base.

Conservatives settled on two basic tactics. One was to raise doubts in the public mind about the value associated with the traditional program and the certainty of future benefits. Commentators began publicizing the low rate of return that Social Security payroll tax contributions earned, downplaying the social insurance and safety net characteristics of the program and instead defining it as an investment, and a poor one at that.[7] They also began questioning the long-term viability of the program, targeting younger voters in particular by raising fears that they were paying substantial payroll taxes for a program that would not be there for them when they retired. Indeed, the percentage of Americans saying they were "very confident" in the future of the Social Security System dropped from 22 percent in 1975 to 9 percent in 1983, while those who were "not too confident" or "not at all confident" climbed from 37 percent to 64 percent (Bowman, 2005).[8]

The second tactic was to support the development of private alternatives, such as 401(k) retirement plans and Individual Retirement Accounts (IRAs). The political utility of these retirement savings vehicles was twofold. One was that they could undermine support for Social Security by allowing individuals to amass potentially sizable retirement savings outside of the governmental program, thereby reducing their dependence on Social Security and providing self-direction and higher returns. The other was that their eventual widespread use allowed conservatives to "analogize" private accounts in Social Security (Teles and Derthick, 2009, 271): as the public became accustomed to these private alternatives, individually directed accounts in Social Security would seem a familiar and popular extension.

The success of this conservative strategy is evidenced in the remarkable rise of private accounts on the political agenda. One significant moment came in 1997, when the 1994–96 Social Security Advisory Council released its report.[9] Advisory councils had for many years been creatures of the old Social Security establishment (Teles and Derthick, 2009). However, this council included a number of proponents of individual accounts and, for the first time, the council failed to reach a consensus on a long-term strategy for the program. Six council members advocated a "maintain benefits" approach that would preserve the current structure of the program and address the long-term shortfall with a 2045 increase in the payroll tax, a small decrease in benefits, and the possibility of investing part of the Social Security trust fund in the stock market. But seven council members supported some form of private accounts, two advocating an additional 1.6 percent payroll tax on employees that would be invested in an individual account (an *add-on proposal*) and five advocating a diversion of 5 percent of the employee share of the payroll tax into personal security accounts (a *carve-out proposal*; Kollmann, 1997).

The carve-out proposal in particular was a stunning development. In its wake, a number of private account proposals were developed, including some from Democratic lawmakers and groups like Senator Daniel Patrick Moynihan and the Progressive Policy Institute, the think tank of the Democratic Leadership Council associated with President Clinton. These proposals typically diverted a smaller percentage of the payroll tax to personal accounts—usually 2 percent rather than 5—but, importantly, they asserted that individual accounts were in keeping with "New Democratic" thinking (Teles and Derthick, 2009). Indeed, when Clinton urged the nation to "save Social Security first" in the face of an aging population in his 1998 State of the Union address, and then traveled the country discussing different proposals for reform, he used rate-of-return language himself and asserted that the government or individuals should invest directly in the market. "If there's any way we can get a higher rate of return in a market economy, while minimizing the risk, whether it's in either one of these approaches, we ought to go for it," he said in July 1998 (Stevenson, 2005). By the final years of the Clinton presidency, "saving Social Security first" was less about market investment and more about reducing Republican pressure to use the emerging budget surpluses for tax cuts. But the private account idea had clearly moved from fringe notion to mainstream proposal. However, no major changes in Social Security were enacted during the remainder of the Clinton presidency, as the Monica Lewinsky matter and other events put a stop to most domestic policy making.

The next occupant of the White House was someone who had been thinking about Social Security privatization for a long time, as early as his unsuccessful 1978 run for Congress, at least by some accounts. Like tax cuts, private accounts were "always there," according to Allan Hubbard, with whom George W. Bush attended business school and who later became a top economic advisor in the Bush White House (Stevenson, 2005). Stevenson's article also noted that Bush was intrigued by privatization in Chile, as well as by a 1981 plan in which workers in several Texas counties were allowed to opt out of Social Security and contribute a similar amount of earnings to a private investment program instead. As he began his presidential run in the late 1990s, Bush continued to meet with advocates of private accounts. Such accounts were viewed as a way not only to reduce the scope of the governmental program, a longstanding conservative goal, but also to soften the blow of the benefit cuts likely needed to bring Social Security into long-term solvency, a "sweetener" to counterbalance the "bitter medicine" of benefit reductions (Chait, 2005). Bush declared private accounts to be one of his top three policy goals in 1999 and, on assuming the presidency, appointed a commission to devise private investment proposals.

Chaired by Senator Moynihan and AOL-Time Warner Chief Operating Officer Richard D. Parsons, the 2001 President's Commission to Strengthen Social Security was staffed entirely by private account supporters, including several members with Cato Institute connections (Confessore, 2001). Indeed, the May 2001 executive order creating the commission stipulated that "Social Security payroll taxes must not

be increased" and that "modernization must include individually con-
trolled, voluntary personal retirement accounts," foreordaining the
commission's recommendations.[10] The commission released its final
report in December 2001, presenting three models for modifying Social Security, all featuring personal accounts.[11] However, the 9/11 ter-
rorist attacks intervened, and Social Security reform was pushed into
Bush's second term.

On reelection, Bush claimed a mandate for entitlement reform and
made transforming Social Security the centerpiece of his domestic
agenda. In his 2005 State of the Union address, he described the program as heading toward "bankruptcy," but he ruled out an increase
in payroll taxes to shore up the system. Instead, he asserted that the
"best way" to preserve the program for younger workers was through
voluntary private accounts, into which up to 4 percent of taxable
earnings could be invested. His plan envisioned a centralized system to
manage personal retirement accounts, similar to the federal employee
retirement program called the Thrift Savings Plan (TSP). Money from
personal accounts would be withdrawn through a mix of annuities
and lump sums, regulated to ensure that individuals remained above
the poverty line. Shortly after his January State of the Union address,
Bush began traveling the country to sell his plan.

The Failure of the Privatization Drive

Despite a considerable investment by President Bush, however, the
private account idea failed. No legislation changing the structure of
Social Security was considered by Congress, and eventually the administration dropped the idea. By late 2005, both Social Security reform generally and private accounts specifically were off the agenda.
Nor do they appear at all to be under serious consideration as the
Obama administration contemplates Social Security reform in 2009.
In February 2009, private account advocate Senator Lindsey Graham
(R-SC) said that "the carve-out account is off the table" (Calmes,
2009). What happened? Three factors help explain why privatization
failed in 2005.

First, public opinion never crystallized in support of private accounts. Although President Bush may have felt that upon reelection
he had a mandate to change Social Security, the American public dis-
agreed, 51 percent to 35 percent, according to a NBC News/*Wall*

Street Journal poll (Hickey 2005). Moreover, privatization was never popular among the voters for whom Social Security is the most salient issue, the elderly. Despite repeated reassurances that any changes would not affect current beneficiaries, poll after poll showed that support for privatization fell monotonically with age. Figure 11.1, for example, shows that in May 2005, those aged 65 or older were far more likely than their younger counterparts to follow news of "George W. Bush's proposal to deal with the Social Security system" closely and to have heard "a lot" about it, but they were also far less supportive of private accounts. Majorities among the age cohorts of people under 45 approved of private accounts—57 percent overall compared with just 26 percent among seniors—but, unfortunately for the President, the former didn't care much about the issue—only 23 percent of those under 45 followed the issue closely and 31 percent had heard a lot about it, compared with 53 percent and 60 percent among seniors.[12] Moreover, support for private accounts fell over time, particularly among the group for whom this was a salient issue, senior citizens. Figure 11.2 compares support for private retirement accounts in Pew polls of December 2004 and May 2005. Support among all groups eroded, but it declined the most among respondents aged 65 or older, whose support fell 15 percentage points in just five months.[13] These poll results hardly reassured skeptical members of Congress.

Second, both organized labor and AARP launched aggressive campaigns against privatization (Pear, 2004; Greenhouse, 2005). Labor unions used their financial muscle as joint trustees of huge pension assets to threaten financial service companies and force them to withdraw support from lobbying groups backing individual accounts. For AARP, opposition to privatization provided a much-needed "easy issue" after years of politically fraught stances, allowing the group to regain its voice in Washington in a way its members supported.

In 1987, the organization had backed the Medicare Catastrophic Coverage Act, an expansion of Medicare that would have capped out-of-pocket expenses for Medicare beneficiaries, in addition to covering some preventative services like mammograms and adding a modest prescription drug benefit. The legislation proved enormously unpopular with seniors, who objected to the new benefits (which some already had through former employers or private insurance) and to the new premiums and tax surcharges required to fund it (which some would have to pay and others erroneously thought they would). Congress

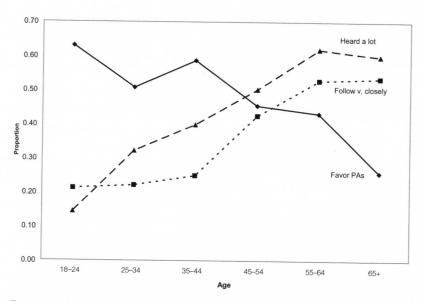

Figure 11.1. Private Account Favorability and Salience, by Age. Source: Data from the Pew Research Center for the People and the Press (2005).

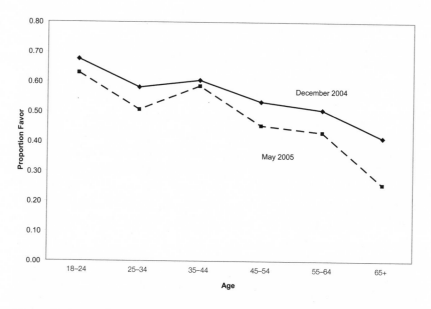

Figure 11.2. Declining Support for Private Accounts Over Time. Source: Data from the Pew Research Center for the People and the Press (2004, 2005).

repealed this act 17 months after passing it, with AARP losing much credibility on Capitol Hill as a representative of senior views (Himelfarb, 1995).

A chastened AARP kept a low profile for a number of years. It re-emerged in aging policy with its endorsement of the Medicare prescription drug legislation in 2003. Although the organization viewed the legislation as flawed, the opportunity to secure $400 billion in new drug benefits over ten years was too good an opportunity to pass up, particularly because the budget surplus that had once made a benefit expansion seem affordable had vanished by that point. AARP did withhold its endorsement until Republican framers made a few changes—increasing subsidies both to low-income seniors and to employers to preserve equivalent retiree drug benefits (Barry, 2003)—but it then endorsed the bill immediately before the roll-call vote, providing skeptical congressmen with the political cover they needed to vote for what was widely perceived as an imperfect piece of legislation. Although some AARP members protested the group's endorsement of the drug bill—and 40,000 resigned in protest—their reaction was not nearly as negative as with the Medicare Catastrophic Coverage legislation.

Critics alleged nonetheless that AARP was now too cozy with Republican interests and that it should not have endorsed the flawed Medicare Modernization Act (MMA) of 2003, but instead pushed harder for a better benefit. Opposition to Social Security privatization helped counteract these accusations and provided an opportunity for AARP to promote a stance popular among its large and diverse membership: both high- and certainly low-income seniors oppose any change to Social Security's basic structure (and many nonseniors realize that they will never save enough on their own for retirement, so they embrace Social Security's safety net as well; see Reno and Lavery, 2009). It was an easy and politically useful stance for the group to take.

In December 2004, in advance of the president's State of the Union address calling for private accounts, AARP announced a $5 million, two-week advertising campaign, including full-page advertisements in more than 50 newspapers, entitled "Social Insecurity." The ads highlighted the risks associated with private accounts and asserted that modest changes rather than wholesale reform would ensure the long-term viability of the program (Pear, 2004). We cannot know with certainty, but it seems likely that these ad campaigns contributed to declining public support for private accounts.

A third reason for the failure of privatization was due to tactical missteps on Bush's part. Bush's early decision—already reached by mid-1999—to prioritize tax cuts over Social Security reform undermined the fiscal and political prospects for the latter (Teles and Derthick, 2009). In one sense, the emphasis on tax cuts was not surprising. Opposition to federal income taxes was the one issue potent enough to knit together the various strands of the conservative movement—social conservatives, fiscal conservatives, and libertarians—who otherwise had competing policy priorities (Morgan, 2007). However, using the budget surplus that emerged in the late 1990s to fund tax cuts meant that those funds would not be available to finance the transition to private accounts. The fiscal dilemma is this: transitioning from the current Social Security system to private accounts means going from a pay-as-you-go system in which current payroll tax dollars pay current benefits to a prefunded system in which current payroll tax dollars fund equity investments that will provide future benefits. Because the same payroll tax dollars cannot be used for both purposes, the problem of financing the transition arises (Kosterlitz, 2005). Having used the money for tax cuts, Bush was left with no plausible way to fund the transition to private accounts, further undermining support for the reform.

A second tactical mistake was in presenting reform as a presidential initiative and failing to draw in sympathetic members of Congress. That the idea was never a congressional one is evidenced by comments from Senator Lindsey Graham (R-SC), a supporter of private accounts (quoted in Calmes, 2005): "[Bush] jumped out with a very big idea that he ran on, but he didn't lay the political groundwork in the Senate or the House. He ran on it. We didn't. He's not up for election again. We are." As public support for privatization declined, members of Congress also had less and less reason to support it.

Finally, with congressional support failing to emerge, Bush decided to take his campaign for Social Security privatization directly to the voters. This proved troublesome, however, because it increased the delay in introducing a bill and consumed valuable postelection momentum. Moreover, Bush struggled to articulate exactly what the problems were with the existing Social Security program, infamously replying to a media request to elaborate on the crisis that he shouldn't "negotiate with [him]self." After coaching from Republican consultant Frank Luntz, Bush shifted the emphasis in his speeches from "privatization" to "personal savings accounts," from "wealth" to "nest egg," and from the elderly maintaining existing benefits to the young gaining more freedom and earnings potential (Toner, 2005b). These changes in framing failed to convince the public, however. The long campaign allowed time for privatization opponents to argue that individual accounts did little to solve the program's long-term fiscal problems, problems that wouldn't come to a head for three decades anyway. The issue continued to be a low-salience one for younger voters, and there was no "American Association of Young People" to reinforce the president's message about the advantages of private accounts for such workers. Instead, the main voice on the issue continued to be AARP's, which used the first half of 2005 to hammer home its antiprivatization message to its well-mobilized constituency.

Weak public support, strong AARP and union opposition, and tactical mistakes on Bush's part undermined congressional prospects for privatization. Among Democrats, the privatization push had the effect of unifying a minority party that had often been in disarray. Previously, Democrats had lent crucial support to Republican initiatives such as the No Child Left Behind education reform (Sen. Ted Kennedy), the war in Iraq (Sen. Joe Lieberman), and the Bush tax cuts (Sen. Zell Miller). With privatization, too, Democrats had been split and some professed support for individual accounts. By Bush's second term, however, a number of Democratic supporters of private accounts, such as Congressman Charlie Stenholm and Senators Charles Robb and John Breaux, had left office (Beinart, 2005).

By 2005, problems had also emerged in many of the policy areas that moderate Democratic votes had helped pass. Increasing polarization in Washington, and a feeling among some Democrats that they had been duped by the administration on education, tax cuts, and the war, unified them in opposition to Bush's plans. Moreover, with Bush's popularity slipping, there was little Democratic incentive to cooperate with him. That Bush followed his 2005 State of the Union proposals on Social Security privatization with a two-day tour in the "red" states of North Dakota, Montana, Nebraska, Arkansas, and Florida— all states with Democratic senators—further infuriated party members (Calmes, 2005). Party leadership vowed not to be suckered again, and they enforced the party line, eliminating any chance for Bush to gain allies from across the aisle and maintaining a filibuster option in the Senate. In addition, Democrats decided simply to oppose privatization without offering an alternative of their own. This was an intentional strategy that helped stifle the issue; a plan of their own would have lent credence to Bush's assertion that Social Security was in fact facing a crisis. A competing plan would have also increased the amount of attention the public and media paid to Social Security privatization. The simpler and more effective political strategy was to "just say no" (*Economist*, 2005b).

If privatization unified Democrats, it had the opposite effect on Republicans, who splintered over the reform. As early as February 2005, House Republican Campaign Committee Chairman Tom Davis said that 30 percent of House Republicans were "already inclined to oppose Mr. Bush" on Social Security (Hickey, 2005). One source of controversy was the sheer expense of funding the transition to private accounts. Bush lost some conservative support when he floated the idea of financing the transition with borrowing, which would increase the budget deficit. This idea was shot down almost immediately, but not before making erstwhile supporters wonder just how expensive these private accounts would be. Then came policy features added in fruitless attempts to attract Democratic support. The final straw for many on the Right was Bush's February 16, 2005, announcement that although he opposed raising payroll tax rates, he would consider raising the maximum taxable earnings level. Tom Delay, the Republican House Majority Leader, responded that "I, for one, am one of those that didn't come here to raise taxes" (*Economist*, 2005a). Conservative commentator Stephen Moore (2005) called this a "strategic blunder of the first order" that left "even the strongest advocates of Social Security personal accounts . . . wondering what hefty price will have to be paid to enact them." Conservatives argued that increasing the payroll tax cap meant a 12.4 percent marginal tax on all income between the current and the new cap, a move that would undo the Bush income tax cuts at that income level (Roberts, 2005).

Although Republican lawmakers may have been sympathetic with the idea of individual accounts in principle, the electoral logic they confronted continued to worsen. Their conservative bases were unhappy about any possible tax increases necessary to finance the transition. Other constituents—conservative red states tend to have older and poorer populations than more liberal blue states (Barnes,

2005)—were never enamored with individual accounts to begin with. As early as February 2005, Republican House Speaker Dennis Hastert was warning that "you can't jam change down the American people's throat" (Toner 2005a). With the Social Security shortfall projected for the early 2040s, the main crisis confronting Republicans was a political one presented by the president's proposal, not a fiscal one. And in this instance, electoral logic trumped ideology.

Conclusion

The failure of Social Security private accounts demonstrates the importance of program structure and the sequencing of policy and political events (Pierson, 2004). Social Security's pay-as-you-go structure created the problem of financing the transition to individual accounts. The existence of a budget surplus in the late 1990s created a once-in-a-generation opportunity: a brief moment where there was a possibility of covering the transition costs. Instead, Bush decided to prioritize tax cuts, thus foreclosing his best chance for individual accounts. If he had privatized Social Security first, he may have succeeded.

By pushing for Social Security privatization earlier, he might also have attracted moderate Democratic support, just as he did with other initiatives in his first term—such as No Child Left Behind, the Iraq war, and tax cuts. But precisely because those other initiatives came first, and because Democrats later felt duped for supporting them, the political waters were irretrievably poisoned and the possibilities for bipartisan reform of Social Security extinguished.

Beyond the barriers to change that these political choices created, individual account reform represented only a slim upside for the public. Consider the contrast between Social Security reform and two reforms that did pass during the Bush presidency: tax cuts and the 2003 Medicare Modernization Act, creating the prescription drug benefit for senior citizens. In both of those instances, conservatives achieved at least some of the reforms they sought—reduced tax progressivity in the one instance and enhanced privatization of the Medicare system in the other.[14] At the same time, reform was politically feasible because the nonaffluent got something as well: tax cuts (albeit much smaller ones than the rich received, but tax cuts nonetheless) and a new prescription drug benefit (as imperfect as it was). But Social Security reform proved far less politically appealing. The supposed sweetener for long-term benefit reduction—individual accounts—proved more risky to and less popular among the public than conservatives had hoped, especially the public for whom Social Security is a salient issue, senior citizens.

In the end, individual accounts were buried this time around for political and electoral reasons. Beyond the technical fiscal problems that transition costs presented, members of Congress had little incentive to push through a controversial reform to a cherished program, especially one with a well-mobilized and adamant constituency. Although a majority of younger people support individual accounts, the issue is a low-salience one for them. The ordinary Americans most focused on this issue—senior citizens—were precisely the subpopulation most opposed to the reform. Presidential insistences that this reform would not affect current retirees fell on deaf ears. Ultimately, the president had the support neither of congressional Democrats, who unified in opposition, nor of Republicans, who could see no advantage in championing a reform that, while ideologically appealing, solved a problem that would only hit decades hence with a solution that at the present moment incensed both their conservative base and, especially, their crucial senior constituents. Electoral concerns trumped the ideological desire to reform Social Security.

Notes

1. Author calculations from a Pew Research Center for the People and the Press poll (2004).

2. See Barabas (2006) on the relationship between the level of the stock market and support for individual accounts; support for privatization is higher when the domestic stock market is rising and falls when equity markets decline.

3. Although talk of trust fund bankruptcy is dramatic, it is also inaccurate, in that public trust funds, unlike their private counterparts, can be shored up by new tax revenues, if Congress were to so choose (Marmor 2000).

4. The AARP's (2006) options include the following (percentages refer to the proportion of the trust fund shortfall that each would address): raise the cap on taxed wages from its current $90,000 to $120,000, and introduce a 3 percent surcharge on earnings greater than $120,000 (43% reduction in the total shortfall); raise the cap on taxed wages to its historical level (currently only 85% of wages are taxed, while 90% were in the past), which would raise the income ceiling to which the Social Security payroll

tax is applied from about $90,000 to $140,000 per year (43% shortfall reduction); raise the age to receive full benefits to 70 by the year 2083 (38% shortfall reduction); reduce benefits for new retirees, gradually, by 5 percent (26% shortfall reduction); index the benefit levels, based on increases in average longevity at age 65 (25% shortfall reduction); raise the payroll tax by 0.5 percent (i.e., 0.25% each on employees and employers; 24% shortfall reduction); increase the number of work years included in benefit calculations from 35 to 38 (16% shortfall reduction); invest 15 percent of the trust fund in a total stock market index fund (15% shortfall reduction); lower the benefits for high-wage workers (11% shortfall reduction); and include all newly hired state and local government employees among those whose wages are taxed (9% shortfall reduction).

5. The 1983 Social Security Amendments raised the retirement age from 65 to 67 by the year 2027, delayed the 1983 cost-of-living adjustment for six months, introduced taxation of Social Security benefits for high-income recipients, and sped up scheduled increases in payroll taxes (Light, 1985).

6. Some private account proposals, such as the plan advocated by Michael Tanner of the Cato Institute (2004), would allow individuals to invest their entire 6.2 percent payroll tax in a private account. Note that we use the terms "individual accounts," "private accounts," and "personal accounts" interchangeably, although these terms have been used by different groups and have evolved over time. Opponents use the terms "private accounts" and "privatization"—less popular among the public—and proponents use the terms "individual accounts"—and, later, "personal accounts"—to foster support.

7. For example, a Heritage Foundation issue brief (Beach and Gareth, 1998) asserted that "Social Security's inflation-adjusted rate of return" is especially low for two-income households with children and for younger African American men: it is just 1.23 percent for an average household of two 30-year-old earners with children, where each parent made just under $26,000 in 1996, and it is negative for African American males born after 1959.

8. The percentage of Americans feeling "somewhat confident" fell from 41 percent to 25 percent over the same period. Confidence was particularly low during the early to mid-1980s, when a much-publicized shortfall in the program's trust fund led to rescue legislation through the 1983 Social Security Amendments. By 2000, 11 percent were "confident" in the future of the Social Security system, 39 percent were "somewhat confident," and 47 percent were "not too confident" or "not at all confident" (Bowman, 2005).

9. The Social Security Act required the Secretary of Health and Human Services to appoint an advisory council every four years to review its key

programs. In 1994, when the Social Security Administration was made an independent agency, a permanent seven-member Advisory Board was established.

10. Executive Order 13201, May 2, 2001. www.presidency.ucsb.edu/ws/index.php?pid=61491/.

11. This report, revised on March 19, 2002, is available at http://gov info.library.unt.edu/csss/index.htm.

12. Author calculations from a Pew Research Center for the People and the Press poll (2005).

13. Author calculations from ibid. and from a Pew Research Center for the People and the Press poll (2004).

14. The 2003 Medicare reforms increased the role of private firms in Medicare by providing its new prescription drug benefit through private, stand-alone insurance plans that beneficiaries purchase outside of Medicare, and by increasing the incentives for beneficiaries to leave Medicare altogether and join private managed-care plans (called Medicare Advantage) for all of their health care.

References

AARP. 2006. Social Security: A Background Briefing (May 15). http://as sets.aarp.org/www.aarp.org_/articles/money/Social_Security/socialsecu ritybackgroundbriefing_v5.pdf.

Barabas, J. 2006. Rational exuberance: The stock market and public support for Social Security privatization. *Journal of Politics* 68 (Feb.): 50–61.

Barnes, F. 2005. A Social Security quagmire? *Weekly Standard* (May 2).

Barry, P. 2003. "An opportunity we can't let pass": AARP backs Medicare bill after bargaining improves provisions for retirees, poor. *AARP Bulletin Today* 44 (December): 3–4.

Beach, W. W., and G. E. Davis. 1998. *Social Security's Rate of Return.* Heritage Foundation Center for Data Analysis Report 98-01 (Jan. 15). www.heritage.org/research/socialsecurity/cda98-01.cfm.

Beinart, P. 2005. Boomerang. *New Republic* (Jan. 31): 6.

Board of Trustees. 2009. *2009 Annual Report of the Board of Trustees, the Federal Old-Age and Survivors Insurance and Federal Disability Insurance Trust Funds.* House of Representatives, 111th Cong., 1st sess., House Document 111–41, May 12. Washington, D.C.: U.S. Government Printing Office. www.ssa.gov/OACT/TR/2009/tr09.pdf.

Bowman, K. 2005. *Attitudes about Social Security Reform.* AEI Public Opinion Study (Aug. 2). American Enterprise Institute. www.aei.org/pa per/14884.

Calmes, J. 2005. Lost appeal: How a victorious Bush fumbled plan to revamp Social Security. *Wall Street Journal* (Oct. 20), A1.

———. 2009. Obama finds resistance in his party on addressing Social Security. *New York Times* (Feb. 23), A15.

Chait, J. 2005. Blocking move. *New Republic* (Mar. 21): 18.

Confessore, N. 2001. Commission impossible. *American Prospect* (Dec. 17).

Congressional Budget Office. 2007. *The Long-Term Budget Outlook* (Dec). www.cbo.gov/doc.cfm?index=8877/.

Derthick, M. 1979. *Policymaking for Social Security*. Washington, D.C.: Brookings Institution.

Diamond, P. A., and P. R. Orszag. 2004. *Saving Social Security: A Balanced Approach*. Washington, D.C.: Brookings Institution.

Economist. 2005a. A hard sell: Social Security reform (Feb. 26).

———. 2005b. Looking for a plan: The Democrats (June 11).

Greenhouse, S. 2005. Labor unions enter Social Security debate. *New York Times* (Mar. 17), C2.

Hickey, R. 2005. A battle Progressives can win: Bush's privatization splinters Republicans and unites Democrats. *American Prospect* (Jan. 14).

Himelfarb, R. 1995. *Catastrophic Politics: The Rise and Fall of the Medicare Catastrophic Coverage Act of 1988*. University Park: Pennsylvania State University Press.

Kollmann, G. 1997. *Social Security: Recommendations of the 1994–1996 Advisory Council on Social Security*. Congressional Research Service Report for Congress (May 7). www.policyarchive.org.

Kosterlitz, J. 2005. Inside the new Social Security accounts. *National Journal* (Jan. 8).

Light, P. 1985. *Artful Work: The Politics of Social Security Reform*. New York: Random House.

Marmor, T. R. 2000. *The Politics of Medicare*, 2nd ed. New York: Aldine de Gruyter.

Moore, S. 2005. Read my lips: The sequel? Bush opens the door to a big tax increase. *Weekly Standard* (Mar. 7).

Morgan, K. J. 2007. Constricting the welfare state: Tax policy and the political movement against government. Pp. 27–50 in J. Soss, J. S. Hacker, and S. Mettler (eds.), *Remaking America: Democracy and Public Policy in an Age of Inequality*. New York: Russell Sage Foundation.

Pear, R. 2004. In ads, AARP criticizes plan on privatizing. *New York Times* (Dec. 30), A16.

Pew Research Center for the People and the Press. 2004. *Pew Research Center Poll: Typology* (December 1–16, 2004). Study no. Pew/PSRAI Poll #2004-TYPO, available from the Roper Center for Public Opinion Research at http://roperweb.ropercenter.uconn.edu/.

———. 2005. *Pew Research Center Poll: May News Interest Index* (May

11–15, 2005). Study no. Pew/PSRAI Poll #2005-05NII, available from the Roper Center for Public Opinion Research at http://roperweb.roper center.uconn.edu/.

Pierson, P. 2004. *Politics in Time: History, Institutions, and Social Analysis*. Princeton, N.J.: Princeton University Press.

Reno, V. P. and J. Lavery. 2009. *Economic Crisis Fuels Support for Social Security: Americans' Views on Social Security* (August). Washington, D.C.: National Academy of Social Insurance.

Roberts, P. C. 2005. Private accounts: Right idea, wrong time; Why a long-time advocate isn't backing Bush's plan. *Business Week* (Mar. 7): 39.

Schiltz, M. E. 1970. *Public Attitudes toward Social Security, 1935–65*. U.S. Social Security Administration, Office of Research and Statistics, Research Report No. 33. Washington, D.C.: U.S. Government Printing Office.

Social Security Advisory Board. 2006. *Annual Report 2005*. Washington, D.C.: U.S. Government Printing Office.

Stevenson, R. W. 2005. For Bush, a long embrace of Social Security plan. *New York Times* (Feb. 27), section 1, 1.

Tanner, M. 2004. *The 6.2 Percent Solution: A Plan for Reforming Social Security*. Cato Institute, SSP No. 32 (February 17). http://www.cato.org/ pub_display.php?pub_id=1618.

Teles, S. M., and M. Derthick. 2009. Social Security from 1980 to the present: From third rail to presidential commitment—and back? Pp. 261–90 in B. J. Glenn and S. M. Teles (eds.), *Conservatism and American Political Development*. New York: Oxford University Press.

Toner, R. 2005a. Hastert warns not to hurry overhaul of Social Security. *New York Times* (Feb. 12), A13.

———. 2005b. Its "private" vs. "personal" in debate over Bush plan. *New York Times* (Mar. 22), A16.

Toner, R., and D. E. Rosenbaum. 2005. The '06 vote is echoing in the Social Security war. *New York Times* (June 24), A16.

Tufte, E. R. 1978. *Political Control of the Economy*. Princeton. N.J.: Princeton University Press.

Zelizer, J. E. 1998. *Taxing America: Wilbur D. Mills, Congress, and the State, 1945–75*. Cambridge: Cambridge University Press.

12. Medicare
Deservingness Encounters Cost Containment
Kimberly J. Morgan, Ph.D.

Medicare is the largest public health insurance program in the United States, providing coverage to approximately one out of every seven people. It is also a major source of income for many health care providers, insurers, medical technology firms, and pharmaceutical companies. These facts alone often make Medicare policy a high-stakes affair, but political conflict over the program has intensified in recent years. Since the 1990s, U.S. politics have become increasingly polarized and contentious, with fierce debates over the role of the government in the economy, how to reform the health care system, and the future of entitlement policy (given the aging of the population). Medicare has been enmeshed in these larger disputes, which have begun to produce some real changes in the Medicare program, perhaps portending greater reforms in the years ahead.

This chapter offers an overview of Medicare, exploring some of the main issues facing the program and the political dynamics around it. Cost control has been a major concern throughout the program's existence, generating a perennial search for ways to rein in spending. The fiscal squeeze on Medicare explains why policy makers have, at times, stood firm against powerful provider groups and clamped down on reimbursements. It also helps explain why a group viewed as highly deserving—senior citizens—has hardly seen much expansion in the generosity of the program, although the creation of a prescription drug benefit in 2003 did fill a major gap in coverage. Now, faced with the imminent retirement of the baby boom generation, there are calls for a fundamental reform of Medicare to ensure the program's long-term sustainability. As this chapter will show, however, Medicare's real problem is that it is hostage to trends in the larger health care system over which program officials have little control. Real Medicare reform requires system-wide health care reform to contain the forces fueling the high cost of medical care. Barring that, policy makers will face difficult decisions about how to preserve a program that is highly popular with beneficiaries, of vital importance to their health and well-being, and a major source of income to many health-related industries and professions.

This chapter first provides some background on the Medicare program and then notes three elements in it that are distinctive when viewed from a cross-national perspective. The remaining sections build on those distinctive features to help make sense of some of the main issues facing Medicare and the politics around the program.

Background on the Medicare Program

The population covered by Medicare consists largely of senior citizens. Most of today's 45 million beneficiaries are people over the age of 65 who themselves (or whose spouses) paid the Medicare payroll tax on at least ten years of earnings, but there are also 7 million people under age 65 who receive Medicare coverage because they are permanently disabled, suffer from end-stage renal disease, or have amyotrophic lateral sclerosis (Lou Gehrig's disease). While most beneficiaries are generally healthy, more than a third have three or more chronic conditions and nearly 30 percent have a cognitive or mental impairment of some kind (Kaiser Family Foundation, 2009). Most people covered by Medicare have modest incomes: nearly half of the beneficiaries have incomes below 200 percent of the federal poverty line, and those who are black, Hispanic, or under the age of 65 have high poverty rates (Kaiser Family Foundation, 2009).[1] In short, Medicare serves a generally healthy and non-poor population, but it also covers a large concentration of chronically ill and low-income people.

Medicare has four parts, each of which has distinct benefits and financing arrangements. Medicare Part A is paid for primarily through payroll taxes and covers inpatient hospital services, a limited amount of care provided by skilled nursing facilities or home health care agencies, and hospice care. Part B, financed through beneficiary premiums and general revenues (mostly income taxes), covers physician services, outpatient care, and durable medical equipment, among other items. Part D is the prescription drug benefit that, like Part B, is voluntary and paid for through a mix of beneficiary premiums and general revenues. The Part D benefit is provided entirely by private insurance plans that must meet certain standards but may otherwise structure their benefits package as they wish. Finally, Part C, also known as Medicare Advantage, offers beneficiaries an option to enroll in a private managed care plan that covers parts A, B, and (almost always) D. The plans are financed by a mix of general revenues, payroll taxes, and beneficiary premiums.

Although Medicare provides a fairly comprehensive package of benefits, there are significant limits to what and how much the program covers. Medicare pays for only a limited amount of long-term care, leaving most beneficiaries to either finance this care on their own or impoverish themselves so as to become eligible for state Medicaid programs. Outside of some Part C plans, Medicare does not cover vision, dental, or hearing-related services. There is also significant cost-sharing in Parts A, B, and D—through deductibles, premiums (for parts B and D), and copayments—and little in the way of catastrophic coverage. There is no limit on out-of-pocket costs each year in Parts A and B, and there is a sizeable coverage gap in Part D—the *doughnut hole*—during which beneficiaries have to pay 100 percent of drug costs before catastrophic coverage begins. In the standard drug benefit for 2009, for instance, after covering $2,700 in total drug costs ($896 of which is paid by the beneficiary in the form of a $295 deductible and a subsequent 25% copayment), there is a $3,454 coverage gap, during which the enrollee has to pay 100 percent of his or her prescription drug costs. Catastrophic coverage then kicks in, but the enrollee continues to pay 5 percent of costs above that level (Kaiser Family Foundation, 2009). The high degree of Medicare cost-sharing renders its benefits package less generous than that typically found in the private sector or enjoyed by federal employees (Yamamoto, Neuman, and Strollo, 2008). For that reason, beneficiaries often rely on supplemental Medigap policies (which they purchase at additional cost), the extra coverage in some Medicare Advantage plans, employer-provided retiree benefits, or Medicaid to cover program gaps. About 11 percent of recipients depend solely on Medicare (Kaiser Family Foundation, 2009).

Distinct Features of Medicare

When viewed in cross-national perspective, the Medicare program is unique in a number ways. First, as is evident from the above discussion, the program exists principally to provide coverage for people over the age of 65. No other country in the world limits its public health insurance coverage by age, and virtually all advanced industrialized states assure health coverage for the entire population. The United States went down this unusual path because of the political opposition that regularly surfaces against efforts to enact a system of national health insurance (NHI). In the 1930s, President Franklin Roosevelt dropped health insurance from his social policy proposals for fear that the antipathy of the medical profession might jeopardize the larger package of reforms. After the Second World War, attempts to enact NHI were repeatedly stymied, and employer-provided health insurance filled the gap, albeit imperfectly. Narrowing their ambitions, NHI advocates decided to push for health insurance for senior citizens, a "deserving" group that was also an undesirable market for insurers, a burden on employer-sponsored insurance plans, and a source of uncompensated care for many hospitals and physicians (Marmor, 2000; Quadagno, 2005). Following an electoral landslide that reelected Lyndon Johnson and swept in a large Democratic majority in Congress, Medicare was created in 1965.

A second distinctive aspect of Medicare concerns its relationship with the larger health care economy. The creation of Medicare grafted a public financing system onto a private world of health care delivery in which government interference was intended to be minimal. In and of itself, this is not so unusual: many countries have public insurance programs that contract with private providers rather than set up a national health service in which health care workers are public employees. In the United States, however, public authority over the private system is especially limited. Medicare covers a large but still limited portion of the population, and while public, health-related subsidies are significant—through the large tax subsidies to employer-provided health insurance, for instance—there is no oversight or coherent management of the health care system as a whole. The consequence for Medicare is that the program is very much affected by trends in private health care, but policy makers have only limited control over this larger environment within which the program is embedded.

The third cross-nationally distinctive element of Medicare concerns the role that Congress plays in managing the program. In most industrialized countries, executive agencies and their appointed ministers are deeply involved in social policy making, not parliaments. In the

United States, by contrast, Congress has had a dominant influence over Medicare since its creation. Although the impetus for Medicare initially came from reformers operating within the executive branch, the crucial barrier to the bill's passage was Wilbur Mills, the chair of the House Ways and Means Committee and one of the most powerful members of Congress. Mills had a decisive impact on the legislation, most notably in the program's hybrid structure (Parts A and B), and in the creation of an additional program, Medicaid, that provides health insurance for the poor, including poor senior citizens (Marmor, 2000). Since that time, members of Congress have been intimately involved in Medicare, whether it be in drafting payment policy, crafting program expansions, or pressuring the Centers for Medicare and Medicaid Services (CMS) on behalf of provider interests located within their congressional districts or states (Vladeck, 1999; Oberlander, 2003).

These three aspects of the Medicare program help shed light on both the major issues facing Medicare and the politics around the program.

The Problem of Cost Control

A perennial feature of Medicare politics—struggles over how to contain program spending—is largely a reflection of the program's vulnerability to trends in the larger health care economy. Medicare's financial stability is intimately connected with that of the health care system as a whole, and debates over how to deal with medical inflation inevitably color debates over the future of Medicare—and vice versa. For decades, the dominant divide has been over greater governmental regulation of health care versus market-based reforms. Neither side has yet gained enough power to fully implement its vision of reform, but each approach has shaped aspects of the Medicare program.

The Long-Term Sustainability of Medicare

One of the major issues facing Medicare today is its long-term financial sustainability. In 2008, Medicare accounted for about 13 percent of the federal budget and about 19 percent of all national health spending. In the coming decade, Medicare spending is forecast to grow by well over 7 percent a year, several percentage points above average annual economic growth (Keehan et al., 2008). The trustees of the trust funds that finance Parts A and B publish annual reports filled with even gloomier news about the long-run sustainability of the program. The Boards of Trustees (2008) report forecasts that Part A spending will grow faster than income to the trust fund over the next ten years and that the trust fund will be exhausted by 2019. Spending on all parts of Medicare is expected to exceed the annual growth in wages and the economy, rising from 3.2 percent of the gross domestic product (GDP) in 2007 to 7 percent in 2035, and 10.8 percent in 2082.[2]

As Marmor (2000) has argued, the rhetoric around trust fund bankruptcy is frequently misleading, given that the Medicare (and Social Security) trust funds are not the equivalent of private trust funds, but are accounting devices meant to cordon off funds for each program. The Hospital Insurance trust fund that finances Part A cannot go bankrupt unless the federal government adamantly refuses to raise payroll taxes or shift other funds to cover program costs. Medicare's long-term viability is thus a political question and not an actuarial one. The relative lack of concern about the Part B program, which is financed differently, is revealing about how Medicare's past financial crises are a product of its financing structure (Oberlander, 2003). In Part B, beneficiary premiums and general revenues are automatically adjusted to cover higher costs, whereas raising the Part A payroll tax requires specific congressional action. Given Congress's reluctance to increase taxes of any kind (Campbell and Morgan, 2005b), Part A has suffered various financing "crises," but Part B has not. The somewhat manufactured nature of these crises aside, it is clear that both programs are expensive and growing ever more so. The Congressional Budget Office (2008) projects that Medicare and Medicaid will be the main source of long-term growth in federal spending.

Trends in Medicare spending are closely linked to the forces generating medical inflation throughout the entire health care system. Although it is frequently claimed that demographic aging will be the main driver of higher entitlement spending, the Congressional Budget Office (2008) argues that demographics will be significant but not the main cause of higher Medicare spending. Rather, per beneficiary cost increases are the bigger problem, which in turn reflect the forces fueling medical inflation in the rest of the economy. And what is behind medical inflation? As one *Health Affairs* article put it succinctly, "It's the prices, stupid"—Americans pay higher prices for medical care than people in other advanced industrialized countries (Anderson et al., 2003). Although Medicare has often held down annual spending increases below that of private insurers, annual Medicare spending still exceeds the rate of economic growth (Boccuti and Moon, 2003; White, 2008). Thus, as long as annual health care spending continues expanding faster than the economy, Medicare will steadily enlarge its claim on the nation's economic resources.

The Impact of the Cost Issue on Medicare Politics

The issues of cost control and Medicare's relationship to the larger health care system have dominated debates around the program since its creation. The 1965 law creating Medicare injected a large amount of public financing into the private system of health care finance and delivery in the United States, but it did not question the organization of that system. Instead, to gain the acquiescence of providers leery of federal intervention in the medical sphere, the 1965 law explicitly promised that the government would stay out of the practice of medicine. Moreover, given the statutory promise that the government would reimburse hospitals for their "reasonable costs" in providing services and physicians for their "reasonable charges"—without questioning the utility of those services or the fees charged—the early Medicare program suffered from, and contributed to, a rapid run-up in medical inflation. Policy makers scrambled to contain program spending in the short term, but the cost overruns added urgency to wider debates that had begun in the 1970s about how to contain medical inflation in the health care system as a whole.

These debates, often characterized as being about "competition versus regulation," have shaped Medicare politics and policy making ever since. For the pro-competition side, advocates have argued that the high cost of medical care reflects flaws in the health care marketplace that impair competition, leading to higher prices, lower-quality care, and a limited choice of insurance plans. These advocates favor transforming the entire health care system, including Medicare, so that consumers have more power to choose health plans and the kind of care that they receive. Employer-sponsored health insurance would be abolished and replaced with tax credits that help people purchase their own insurance plans, and Medicare would become a system of subsidized private insurance plans that compete for beneficiaries' business (Enthoven, 1980; Pauly, 2008).

On the other sides are advocates of regulation, who argue that health care will never be equivalent to other market goods because of the patient's limited information about medical conditions and treatments; the irregular and unpredictable need for care; and because of health care's positive externalities, among other things (Marmor, Boyer, and Greenberg, 1983). These proponents believe that what is needed, if anything, is more federal involvement in managing the health care system, in setting the terms of provider payment, and in assuring universal coverage. In the case of Medicare, reformers on this side advocated replacing Medicare's retrospective, largely unquestioning reimbursement of provider charges with a system of prospective payment that establishes in advance the fee schedules for services.

Until recently, pro-competitive reform ideas have held less sway over Medicare than have regulatory approaches. Although the Reagan administration came into office vowing to enact a market-based reform of Medicare, it instead embraced a prospective payment system (PPS) that imposes government-determined prices on providers. Fiscal imperatives explain the turnabout: faced with large and growing federal budget deficits in the 1980s, the administration had to set aside its market-reform agenda and find ways to immediately tamp down Medicare spending (Oliver, 1991; Oberlander, 2003). A similar method of payment was extended to physicians in 1989, with the adoption of a resource-based relative value scale to determine reimbursements, as well as the extension of the PPS to all outpatient/post-acute services in 1997.[3]

By the 1990s, however, pro-competitive forces had gained greater political power. The Republicans elected to Congress in the 1990s, led by Speaker Newt Gingrich, were determined to not only cut federal spending, but also to enact market-based reforms that would fundamentally alter the architecture of federal entitlements. Yet, lacking sufficient support to convert Medicare into a system of competing private plans, Republicans and some centrist Democrats aimed to at least augment the role of these plans in the program. For decades, beneficiaries could choose to receive Part A and Part B benefits through a private HMO that receives payments from the federal government. The Balanced Budget Act (BBA) of 1997 attempted to expand the use of these plans by allowing a larger array of insurance products that would compete for beneficiaries' business and by altering the formula for reimbursement. The law also created a Bipartisan Commission on the Future of Medicare in 1998 to consider long-term reform objectives. Although unable to reach the supermajority required to send on proposals to Congress and the president, the commission further advanced the idea of a *premium support* model for Medicare, whereby the government would subsidize premiums and beneficiaries would choose between private insurance plans.

The pro-competitive vision attained its greatest success in the 2003 Medicare Modernization Act (MMA) that added a prescription drug benefit (Part D) to the program. The drug benefit is provided entirely by private plans, making this the first time beneficiaries must sign up with a private insurer to receive a portion of their Medicare benefits. In most states, seniors now choose from about 50 different drug plans that vary in their formularies and cost-sharing requirements. Part C, previously called Medicare+Choice, was relabeled Medicare Advantage, and subsidies to these plans were increased to lure back the insurers who found the subsidies inadequate after the 1997 BBA and had been exiting from the program. To some observers, the MMA thus represented an important advance of market-based principles in Medicare (Jost, 2005; Krugman, 2007), although not all conservatives were convinced that there was enough reform in the law to justify expanding a federal entitlement. Discontent over this issue still festers among conservatives and is indicative of their determination to enact fundamental changes in the program.

Today the question is what role private plans will play in Medicare from here on out. Medicare Advantage enrollment has increased sharply, rising from 13 percent of all beneficiaries in 2003 to 23 percent in 2008 (Zarabozo and Harrison, 2009). The fact that these plans receive payments beyond what it costs to cover a beneficiary in the traditional program has drawn much criticism (MedPAC, 2008), making at least some cuts in these subsidies likely.[4] The larger issue concerns whether or not Medicare will steadily move toward a system of competing private plans, eliminate these plans altogether, or continue the current hybrid approach. Related to this are questions about the ability of Medicare beneficiaries to effectively navigate the plethora of plan choices now available to them; whether private plans provide better quality care than traditional Medicare; and whether these plans will ultimately yield budgetary savings.

Debates over these questions have been fierce, reflecting the tendency of analysts and politicians to see Medicare as a proving ground for their larger reformist aims. To some degree, Medicare has always been a vessel in which reformers pour their hopes for a national health policy. As a compromise measure for advocates of national health insurance, reformers initially viewed the program as a step along the path to universal coverage. This was precisely the fear of market-based advocates, who sought to stave off what seemed to be an inevitable march toward government-run health insurance for all. These reformers have instead tried to use Medicare to demonstrate the effectiveness of consumer-choice reforms in improving social programs while containing federal spending. On the other side, those who favor greater governmental authority over the health care system hold up traditional Medicare as a program that works and that can be a model for national health care—"Medicare for All" (Mayes and Berenson, 2006; Schlesinger and Hacker, 2007).

In recent years, some analysts have tried to take a different tack, advocating a new payment system that they believe would produce both lower costs and higher-quality care—the holy grail in health care reform. Once again, the problems facing Medicare are representative of those in the health care system as a whole: both the cost and the quality of care that people receive vary widely across geographic regions and among providers (Wennberg, Fisher, and Skinner, 2002). In regions where services are more expensive, the quality of care is no better—and frequently is worse—than that found in lower-cost areas. More generally, many providers fail to follow the best clinical practices. These facts have generated calls for a new approach to Medicare reimbursement that would reward efficient, high-quality care (Fisher et al., 2009). What remains to be seen is whether such reforms can be adopted, succeed, and serve as a model for the rest of the health care system, as their advocates hope.

In sum, Medicare has been buffeted by trends in the larger health care system, of which it is an integral part. As long as health care spending continues to grow at a rapid clip, Medicare will also experience high rates of cost increases. One consequence has been on-going debates over how best to deal with the high cost of health care, arguments that have spilled over into Medicare and are exerting a powerful influence on policy making.

Congress and Medicare Politics

Given the dominant role of Congress in managing Medicare policy, program politics are intimately bound up with the nature of Congress as an institution. Perhaps most important is the relationship between Congress and the large number of Medicare claimants, including providers and beneficiaries, who have a substantial stake in Medicare coverage and payment policy. Here, we can see both permissive and restrictive tendencies in Medicare policy, as Congress has been vulnerable to the lobbying of these groups but has also stood firm against them when fiscal imperatives demand it.

The Mixed Influence of Medical Interest Groups

As the single largest source of income for many doctors, hospitals, and other health care providers (Vladeck, 1999), Medicare is a major force in the larger health care system. When Medicare squeezes reimbursements, as it has under the PPS, this shrinks provider margins and may induce cost-shifting to other payers (Mayes and Berenson, 2006). Moreover, decisions over Medicare payment policy—such as what treatments the program covers and what compensation is received for them—often influence the practices of other insurers. Given the large stake that providers, medical suppliers, pharmaceutical companies, and other medical interest groups have in the program, it is hardly surprising that they are deeply engaged in lobbying policy makers. Since the 1970s there has been an explosion in the number of health-related interest groups; one estimate holds that, at the turn of the millennium, there were more than 1,100 such organizations active in national politics (Heaney, 2004). Some are among the most revered (or feared) lobbying groups in Washington, including not only physicians, hospitals, and the pharmaceutical industry, but also AARP, the main advocate of beneficiaries.

How effective have these groups been at promoting their interests? There generally are two views on this question, ones which reflect distinct visions about the nature and autonomy of the U.S. government. For some, Medicare typifies the kind of government capture at which well-paid lobbyists have long proven adept (Etheredge, 1998). In this view, Medicare, and indeed any system of government-sponsored health insurance, will fall victim to the pressures of powerful provider interests seeking to protect their monopoly power, high fees, and control over clinical practices (Enthoven, 1980). By contrast, others cite the experience of the Medicare PPS to argue that the U.S. government is capable of holding firm against provider interests and keeping down costs (Mayes and Berenson, 2006). Oberlander (2003), for instance, argues that the adoption and extension of prospective payment techniques have come at the expense of powerful groups such as hospitals and physicians. One lesson he takes from Medicare's experience is that the U.S. government can be fairly autonomous vis-à-vis organized interests, with policy making shaped by the ideologies and goals of elected officials rather than being dictated by powerful lobbyists.

The record of Congress in managing Medicare provides sustenance to both views. As was noted earlier, the influence of Congress over Medicare policy making is one of the program's distinctive elements; in most other countries, the executive branch agencies that direct health care policy stand atop more centralized, parliamentary systems of government. This limits the access of interest groups to government ministries, and decisions often are reached through corporatist bargaining with a relatively small number of actors. In the permeable U.S. Congress, by contrast, there are 535 points of potential influence—albeit not all of them equally effective. The U.S. political context is perhaps especially hospitable to small, well-organized groups that, through persistent, low-visibility lobbying, can get policy changes of sole benefit to them. These groups can have considerable weight, particularly if said groups are located in a member's district.

At the same time, however, some believe the power of Congress vis-à-vis interest groups has been strengthened over the past three to four decades, owing to a number of developments. The adoption of a congressional budget process has centralized political authority in Congress in the hands of key committee officials and the party leadership. It also created a vehicle for enacting controversial changes: must-pass reconciliation bills that are huge, packed with large numbers of complex provisions, and surrounded by a sense of urgency over the need to reduce government deficits (Smith, 2002). Finally, political polarization—the widening ideological gap between the two parties—has spurred the centralization of authority within the party leadership, counteracting some of the traditional fragmentation of U.S. political parties. As party members have become more similar in their political orientations, they have been more willing to delegate policy making powers to the leadership in the hope that the latter can muster enough votes around legislation that meets both electoral and programmatic objectives (Rohde, 1991; Sinclair, 1995). This has enabled a more unified, but at times highly partisan, approach to Medicare as leaders seek to meet the electoral and programmatic objectives of their members.

Medicare has shown that both dynamics—permissive and restrictive—have at times been at work in the relationship between Congress and organized interests. The record of prospective payment shows that fiscal constraints have often stiffened the spine of legislators on provider payment issues (Oberlander, 2003). At the same time, however, persistent lobbying by providers has often eroded the bite of these policies. CMS administrators have long complained about how much time the agency spends fielding phone calls from members of Congress concerned about narrow provisions affecting a hospital or medical supplier or other interest located in their district. A deeper problem lies in congressional unwillingness to enforce cuts in physician reimbursements that they themselves created. The 1997 BBA enacted a mechanism, the *sustainable growth rate*, to trim physician payments if they exceed a certain benchmark. So far, however, the cuts have been imposed only once—in 2002—and the resulting outcry from physicians led Congress to raise reimbursement rates. Nearly every year since, Congress is supposed to reimpose the limits, yet short-term fixes keep delaying the cuts. In brief, if fiscal crises have at times enabled Congress to withstand interest group pressures, in less dire moments persistent and vocal lobbying by providers can nibble away at congressional determination.

The Mixed Influence of Medicare Beneficiaries

Policy makers have also shown both permissive and restrictive tendencies toward Medicare beneficiaries. Given the size of the senior citizen population, their presence in every state and congressional district in the nation, and their high levels of political participation, one might expect politicians to be responsive to the needs of this group (Campbell, 2003). Legislators have certainly sought to shield seniors from cuts to Medicare, reflecting the well-known tendency of *blame avoidance* that features strongly in entitlement politics (Weaver, 1986). This is one reason why the prospective payment system has proven so attractive, as it has enabled policy makers to trim program spending without having to impose direct cuts on beneficiaries. Even if the lower payments ultimately degrade the quality of care given or lead some physicians to refuse to see Medicare patients, it is difficult to directly trace these developments to actions taken by members of Congress (Arnold, 1990).

There have also been periods of intensified political competition around Medicare that create openings for program expansions. The 2003 MMA that added Part D to Medicare was the culmination of one such moment: the Clinton administration launched the call for a prescription drug benefit to counter the Republican push for market-based reform of the program. This set off a competitive spiral, with extensive media coverage of the plight of senior citizens lacking drug insurance and political battles over which party could best respond to this group. With Democrats pummeling the Republican majority in Congress for their failure to add a drug benefit to Medicare, Republicans hastened to develop their own plan. Contrary to their long-standing push for cuts in federal spending in general and restraint on entitlement spending in particular, Republicans crafted and passed the largest expansion in Medicare (or any domestic social program) since the Great Society: an expanded entitlement estimated to cost $400 billion over 10 years (Campbell and Morgan, 2006).

However, such episodes have been the exception, and not the rule, in Medicare policy making. Despite the fact that Medicare has long had significant coverage gaps, between 1965 and 2003 the generosity of Medicare coverage hardly changed. Even the 2003 reform left seniors with significant cost-sharing, due to the doughnut hole. Still more problematic for seniors is the high cost of long-term care, yet this issue has largely been absent from the political radar screen (Campbell and Morgan, 2005a). The exceptional nature of the MMA highlights a general puzzle: why haven't entrepreneurial politicians regularly exploited the political popularity of Medicare and the hefty size of its constituency to promote continual expansions of the program? One way to help make sense of this puzzle is to explore a final dimension of the Medicare program: its generational politics.

Generational Conflict over Old Age Entitlements

The third distinctive aspect of Medicare—the age basis of its entitlement—has proven to be a mixed blessing when it comes to program politics. Social policy analysts have long assumed that, because of its wide constituency of beneficiaries, Medicare is a politically secure program. Even though it provides insurance only to a portion of the population, an intergenerational bargain is embedded in the program: working people pay taxes today to enable health insurance for senior citizens, and these workers will in turn be entitled to benefits once they retire, also paid by younger generations. However, one might expect that providing an age-defined group with benefits that are denied to everyone else could antagonize the rest of the population. Certainly this has been the dynamic around public assistance programs, which are seen as taxpayer subsidies of nonworking, nontaxpaying people.

Indeed, by the late 1970s, the intergenerational bargain underpinning Medicare and Social Security appeared to be coming under stress, and some began questioning the nation's age-based entitlements. Some analysts raised concerns about the apparent graying of the federal budget—the high proportion of public dollars being spent on senior citizens through Social Security, Medicare, Medicaid, and other social programs (Hudson, 1978). The very success of these programs in reducing poverty among senior citizens fueled questions about why the federal government was providing benefits to a group that was doing fairly well (Oberlander, 2003). The political obstacles to reforming these entitlements spurred the creation of groups such as Americans for Generational Equity (AGE) in the 1980s, followed by the Concord Coalition and the Third Millennium in the 1990s. These groups—and various political analysts—argued for an overhaul of federal entitlements as a way to tackle the mounting pile of federal debt and prepare the country for the impending retirement of the baby boom generation. Among the proposed reforms are means-testing federal entitlements such as Social Security and Medicare, a move that critics claim would undermine the broad base of support for these programs.

An uglier version of these arguments tagged senior citizens as "greedy geezers" who were unfairly benefiting from the hard labors of younger people (Quadagno, 1989). This rhetoric gained some currency following the legislative debacle over the 1988 Medicare Catastrophic Coverage Act (MCCA)—a law that capped total beneficiary spending in the event of high medical costs but instituted an income-related premium on seniors to pay for this. Although most seniors would have benefited from the new policy, a small number managed to ignite a firestorm through misleading claims about how many beneficiaries would have to pay high premiums. After a well-publicized popular outcry, which included images of senior citizens surrounding Ways and Means Chair Dan Rostenkowski's car in protest, the bill was repealed in 1989. The episode contributed to a view of senior citizens as a politically powerful group that was determined to make younger generations foot the bill for their retirement.

Arguments about generational equity appear to have made few inroads into mass public opinion. Surveys regularly show continued strong public support for Social Security and Medicare and opposition to extensive cuts in these programs as a way to shore up their long-term viability (Cook and Barrett, 1992; Campbell and Morgan, 2005b). One study shows a drop in support for social spending on seniors during the 1990s, but finds that this is not a result of reduced sympathy for older people (Silverstein et al., 2000). Instead, declining faith in government programs is found to indirectly undermine support for old age entitlements, although majority opinion still strongly favors these programs.

If anyone has been influenced by the discourse of generational fairness, it appears to be political elites. Several studies have documented a strikingly large gap between these elites and the mass public when it comes to entitlement policy (Cook and Barrett, 1992; Page and Barabas, 2000). In part this is due to the realities of governing: policy makers better understand the budgetary issues faced by a program such as Medicare and must find ways to contain program spending lest they be forced to enact tax increases, which the general public also does not favor. But it additionally reflects concern about the balance of spending on different age groups that has been influenced by the language of generational equity. As Cook and Barrett (1992) show, members of Congress who doubt the effectiveness of programs such as Medicare often voice concerns about the aging of the population or the unfair burden of old age entitlements on younger generations.

Such views have shaped the parameters of the policy debate over federal entitlement programs, and they even had some influence over Medicare policy. As Quadagno (1989) documents, the founder of AGE, David Durenberger, was influential in requiring that the MCCA's catastrophic benefit be financed entirely by higher premiums paid by senior citizens rather than by imposing higher taxes on the working population. This measure was precisely what sparked the revolt against the MCCA and led to its repeal (Himelfarb, 1995). More recent Republican attempts to introduce income-related provisions into Medicare were more successful. The 2003 MMA provides additional subsidies to low-income beneficiaries to help them with premiums, deductibles, and other cost-sharing for the drug benefit, whereas higher-income beneficiaries—people with incomes greater than $85,000 for an individual and $170,000 for a couple—now pay Part B premiums that are graduated according to income. In 2009, these premiums ranged from $134.90 to as high as $308.30 a month, well above the $96.40 paid by other beneficiaries. This marks a major change in the Medicare program and has raised questions about whether the higher premiums will start to unravel support for the program among higher-income recipients (Jost, 2005). It does move the program closer the vision enunciated by the Concord Coalition and others for a means-tested system of federal entitlements.

Conclusion

What is the image of Medicare politics that emerges from the above portrayal? It is one of highly complex, multifaceted politics, characterized by both moments of dynamism and change and long periods of stability and stagnation. There are periods when policy makers seem highly (some would say hopelessly) responsive to the concerns of beneficiaries or narrowly based interests, yet there are other times when they hold the line against such pressures. In recent years, generational conflict around this age-specific entitlement appears to have intensified, yet this is largely an elite and not a mass phenomenon. There is strong public support for Medicare as it is currently provided, an attitude that seems to protect this program against major cuts, yet Medicare has experienced some significant market-based reform in recent years.

The future of the Medicare program hinges on what happens in the larger health care system. Many have argued that addressing Medicare's problems, particularly those of cost control, requires fundamental health system reform along the lines of either full market-based reform or greater expansion of governmental authority over the provision of and payment for health care. The failure of either side to achieve their goals has left Medicare hostage to larger forces in the health care system over which its program officials have limited control. This has led to various stop-gap measures, such as trimming provider payments or raising beneficiary premiums, but such measures cannot assure the program's long-term viability. It is hard to predict what path policy makers will take as program costs continue to mount, but it is clear that there are no easy choices and no easy politics of reform.

Notes

1. For instance, 37 percent of African American beneficiaries have incomes below 100 percent of the poverty line, as do 33 percent of Hispanics and 35 percent of people under age 65 (Kaiser Family Foundation, 2009).

2. This forecast is based on intermediate assumptions made by the actuaries about demographic and economic circumstances.

3. The Resource-Based Relative Value Scale (RBRVS) calculates payments for services based on the work and resource costs that go into providing the service.

4. In 2008, in a rare instance of Congress overriding a presidential veto, the Medicare Improvements for Patients and Providers Act made modest cuts to Medicare Advantage subsidies.

References

Anderson, G. F., U. E. Reinhardt, P. S. Hussey, and V. Petrosyan. 2003. It's the prices, stupid: Why the United States is so different from other countries. *Health Affairs* 22 (3): 89–105.

Arnold, R. D. 1990. *The Logic of Congressional Action.* New Haven, Conn.: Yale University Press.

Boards of Trustees. 2008. *2008 Annual Report of the Boards of Trustees of the Federal Hospital Insurance and Federal Supplemental Medical Insurance Trust Funds.* www.cms.hhs.gov/reportstrustfunds/downloads/tr2008.pdf [retrieved February 2, 2008].

Boccuti, C., and M. Moon. 2003. Comparing Medicare and private insurers: Growth rates in spending over three decades. *Health Affairs* 22 (2): 230–37.

Campbell, A. L. 2003. *How Policies Make Citizens: Senior Political Activism and the American Welfare State.* Princeton, N.J.: Princeton University Press.

Campbell, A. L., and K. J. Morgan. 2005a. Federalism and the politics of old-age care in Germany and the United States. *Comparative Political Studies* 38 (Oct.): 887–914.

———. 2005b. Financing the welfare state: Elite politics and the decline of the social insurance model in America. *Studies in American Political Development* 19 (2): 173–95.

————. 2006. The Medicare Modernization Act and the new politics of Medicare. Presented at the American Political Science Association Annual Meeting, August 31–September 3, Philadelphia, Penn.

Congressional Budget Office. 2008. *Accounting for Sources of Projected Growth in Federal Spending on Medicare and Medicaid.* Economic and Budget Issue Brief (May 28). Washington, D.C.: Congressional Budget Office.

Cook, F. L., and E. J. Barrett. 1992. *Support for the American Welfare State: The Views of Congress and the Public.* New York: Columbia University Press.

Enthoven, A. 1980. *Health Plan: The Only Practical Solution to the Soaring Cost of Medical Care.* Reading, Mass.: Addison Wesley.

Etheredge, L. 1998. The Medicare reforms of 1997: Headlines you didn't read. *Journal of Health Politics, Policy and Law* 23 (3): 573–79.

Fisher, E. S., M. B. McClellan, J. Bertko, S. M. Lieberman, J. J. Lee, J. L. Lewis, and J. S. Skinner. 2009. Fostering accountable health care: Moving forward in Medicare. *Health Affairs* 28 (2): w219–31.

Heaney, M. T. 2004. Identity, coalitions, and influence: The politics of interest group networks in health policy. Ph.D. diss., University of Chicago.

Himelfarb, R. 1995. *Catastrophic Politics: The Rise and Fall of the Medicare Catastrophic Coverage Act of 1988.* University Park: Pennsylvania State University Press.

Hudson, R. B. 1978. The "graying" of the federal budget and its consequences for old-age policy. *Gerontologist* 18 (5, part 1): 428–40.

Jost, T. S. 2005. The most important health care legislation of the millennium (so far): The Medicare Modernization Act. *Yale Journal of Health Policy, Law, and Ethics* 5 (Winter): 437–99.

Kaiser Family Foundation. 2009. *Medicare: A Primer.* www.kff.org/medicare/upload/7615-02.pdf [retrieved February 2, 2009].

Keehan, S., A. Sisko, C. Truffer, S. Smith, C. Cown, J. Poisal, M. K. Clemens, and the National Health Expenditure Accounts Projections Team. 2008. Health spending projections through 2017: The baby-boom generation is coming to Medicare. *Health Affairs* 27 (2): w145–55.

Krugman, P. 2007. The plot against Medicare. *New York Times* (Apr. 20), A23.

Marmor, T. R. 2000. *The Politics of Medicare*, 2nd ed. New York: Aldine de Gruyter.

Marmor, T. R., R. Boyer, and J. Greenberg. 1983. Medical care and pro-competitive reform. Pp. 239–61 in T. R. Marmor (ed.), *Political Analysis and American Medical Care.* Cambridge: Cambridge University Press.

Mayes, R., and R. A. Berenson. 2006. *Medicare Prospective Payment and the Shaping of U.S. Health Care.* Baltimore: Johns Hopkins University Press.

MedPAC. 2008. *Report to the Congress: Medicare Payment Policy.* Testimony before the Subcommittee on Health of the Committee on Ways and Means, U.S. House of Representatives, March 11. Washington, D.C.: Medicare Payment Advisory Commission.

Oberlander, J. 2003. *The Political Life of Medicare.* Chicago: University of Chicago Press.

Oliver, T. R. 1991. Health care market reform in Congress: The uncertain path from proposal to policy. *Political Science Quarterly* 106 (3): 453–77.

Page, B. I., and J. Barabas. 2000. Foreign policy gaps between citizens and leaders. *International Studies Quarterly* 44 (3): 339–64.

Pauly, M. 2008. *Markets without Magic: How Competition Might Save Medicare.* Washington, D.C.: AEI Press.

Quadagno, J. 1989. Generational equity and the politics of the welfare state. *Politics and Society* 17 (3): 353–76.

———. 2005. *One Nation Uninsured: Why the U.S. Has No National Health Insurance.* Oxford: Oxford University Press.

Rohde, D. W. 1991. *Parties and Leaders in the Postreform House.* Chicago: University of Chicago Press.

Schlesinger, M., and J. S. Hacker. 2007. Secret weapon: The "new" Medicare as a route to health security. *Journal of Health Politics, Policy and Law* 32 (Apr.): 247–91.

Silverstein, M., T. M. Parrott, J. J. Angelelli, and F. L. Cook. 2000. Solidarity and tension between age groups in the United States: Challenges for an aging America in the 21st century. *International Journal of Social Welfare* 9 (4): 270–84.

Sinclair, B. 1995. *Legislators, Leaders, and Lawmaking: The U.S. House of Representatives in the Postreform Era.* Baltimore: Johns Hopkins University Press.

Smith, D. G. 2002. *Entitlement Politics: Medicare and Medicaid, 1995–2001.* New York: Aldine de Gruyter.

Vladeck, B. C. 1999. The political economy of Medicare: Medicare reform requires political reform. *Health Affairs* 18 (1): 22–36.

Weaver, R. K. 1986. The politics of blame avoidance. *Journal of Public Policy* 6 (4): 371–98.

Wennberg, J. E., E. S. Fisher, and J. Skinner. 2002. Geography and the debate over Medicare reform. *Health Affairs Web Exclusive* (Feb. 13): w96–114. http://content.healthaffairs.org/.

White, C. 2008. Why did Medicare spending growth slow down? *Health Affairs* 27 (3): 793–802.

Yamamoto, D., T. Neuman, and M. K. Strollo. 2008. *How Does the Benefit Value of Medicare Compare to the Benefit Value of Typical Large Employer Plans?* Medicare Issue Brief (Sept.). Henry J. Kaiser Family Foundation. www.kff.org/medicare/upload/7768.pdf [retrieved February 2, 2009].

Zarabozo, C., and S. Harrison. 2009. Payment policy and the growth of Medicare Advantage. *Health Affairs* 28 (1): w55–67.

13. The Politics of Aging within Medicaid

Colleen M. Grogan, Ph.D., and
Christina M. Andrews, M.S.W.

The U.S. health care system is often characterized as *two-tiered*, where the tiers are separate and unequal. Medicare, our universal health insurance program for elderly people, defines the upper tier, where recipients qualify for benefits without having to satisfy a means-test. Medicare is governed by uniform national standards, has strong public support, and is politically stable. Medicaid, our health care program for "the poor," defines the lower tier. Medicaid is a targeted, means-tested program that is often considered to be stigmatizing, institutionally fragmented, and politically vulnerable (Rosenberry, 1982; Brown, 1988; Kuttner, 1988; Grogan and Patashnik, 2003b).

Given the saliency of this two-tiered image, under a "veil of ignorance"[1]—that is, knowing nothing about the political history of these two programs—one would predict the following: that benefits under Medicare have substantially expanded under an arena of strong public support and political stability since its enactment in 1965, whereas Medicaid has suffered repeated periods of policy retrenchment under its stigmatizing, politically vulnerable umbrella. Yet, although one can find specific policy examples that fit this prediction, the general trend in both programs (at least since the mid-1980s) has been the reverse. While the recipient pool for Medicaid has exploded from roughly 18 million in 1970 to 52 million in 2004, the recipient pool for Medicare has remained largely constant over the last twenty-five years (Oberlander, 2003b).[2] The reasons behind this political puzzle are complex and are the subject of a much longer manuscript. We raise the point here, however, because acknowledgement of this trend reversal throws into question the usefulness of the two-tiered image for understanding the political evolution of these two programs.

One fundamental problem with the two-tiered image is that it fails to recognize that these programs typically contain contradictions in goals and purposes, as do most social welfare programs (Marmor, Mashaw, and Harvey, 1990; Grogan and Patashnik, 2003b). For example, the targeted Medicaid program often fails to serve those in greatest need and yet extends its reach to the middle class, while the universal Medicare program often provides extra benefits to low-income recipients. In thinking more generally about universal welfare state programs, Theda Skocpol labels the latter phenomenon "targeting within universalism." She points to Social Security as the leading modern example: while it benefits politically from being a universal program that provides a basic social entitlement to the middle class, it is also the nation's most effective antipoverty program, offering proportionately more generous pensions to retirees with a history of low earnings (Skocpol, 1995).[3]

Grogan and Patashnik (2003b) invert Skocpol's analysis and label the former phenomenon—extending benefits to a relatively large middle-class constituency within the context of a means-tested design—as "universalism within targeting." They note that middle-class participation in targeted programs is most likely when the programs involve the delivery of expensive goods and services like education or health care. As a result, the targeted program's threshold of means-tested income is set high enough so that a significant number of people from mainstream backgrounds qualify (see also Gilbert, 2001). Medicaid's incorporation of middle-class senior citizens residing in nursing homes is a good example of universalism within targeting (Grogan and Patashnik, 2003b).

Another reason for elderly middle-class participation in the targeted Medicaid program probably has to do with a positive social construction of the elderly. Schneider and Ingram (1997) argue that the political vulnerability associated with certain targeted programs is not inherent in means-testing per se, but rather stems from the provision of benefits to groups that are perceived to be undeserving. Thus, following this logic, it is likely that the political viability of incorporating members of the middle class within Medicaid also stems from the social construction of the targeted group, albeit in this case a group seen as being socially deserving.

In this chapter, we analyze the politics of Medicaid's incorporation of the middle class by examining the social construction of the elderly within the Medicaid context. Understanding this inclusion is important for two reasons. First, examining Medicaid's incorporation of the middle class and its associated politics opens the door to reexamining the political evolution (and possibilities) of targeted programs in general (not just Medicaid) as something other than pure policy retrenchment. As the enactment of targeted programs is much more the norm than the creation of universal programs in the United States, this reexamination seems worthwhile. Second, documenting the evolving social construction of the elderly within Medicaid allows us to consider whether various framings of social deservingness give rise to new political possibilities. In particular, despite repeated advocacy for long-term care expansions within Medicare, elderly middle-class incorporation may give rise to universal long-term care within Medicaid. This notion is not so far-fetched, especially if one considers that most universal programs in other countries began first as targeted programs, with incremental middle-class incorporation over time.

The framing of Medicaid's incorporation of the middle class in the United States, however, is complex. Although the generally positive construction of the elderly as socially deserving allowed universalism within targeting to occur under Medicaid, the enactment of Medicare alongside Medicaid, and the incorporation of other needy groups within Medicaid, has created multiple and conflicting frames of elderly deservingness. In our attempt to show that notions of elderly deservingness in relation to the program have changed over time, we document how the political constructions of the Medicaid program have changed as well—from a program that was universally described in rather stigmatizing ways as "welfare" to a program that is sometimes invoked today as a "core social entitlement."

To understand the social construction of the elderly and the political construction of Medicaid, we conducted a content analysis of selected congressional hearings (spanning from 1966 to 2008) concerning this program. Using the Congressional Universe database, we identified 944 hearings that had "Medicaid" as a subject heading. To choose hearings for content analysis out of this population of 944, we used various keyword title selections. In the early years of the program (1966–75), there were no hearings where Medicaid was the sole purpose of the discussion. It was much more common for Medicaid to be discussed as part of a larger hearing about both Medicare and Medicaid; 11 hearings fit that category during the 1966–75 period and all were reviewed. For the years 1976 through 1995, any hearing (from the 944) that included the term "Medicaid" (but not also "Medicare") was selected for review (46 hearings). To capture how the elderly were invoked under broader discussions of Medicaid, we also chose hearings with Medicaid as the subject heading combined with the term "elderly" (or aged/aging or seniors) in the title. During the 1966–95 period, 24 hearings met this criteria. Additionally, to concurrently track broader developments in the discourse related to long-term care policy, we identified five hearings that included "long-term care" in the title and had elderly and Medicaid as subject headings. This search process generated a total of 86 hearings selected for review.

A similar search process was conducted to identify hearings during 1996–2008 period: again using Medicaid as a subject heading, hearings were selected that had either "seniors" or "elderly" in the title or as a descriptor. However, due to the large number of hearings held specifically on Medicaid in the last decade (56 hearings met the search criteria), the two most relevant hearings from each year were chosen for review. For cases in which several hearings were relevant to our study's focus, three or more hearings held during a single year were included in the sample. In other instances, no relevant hearing was found. In total, 22 hearings conducted between 1996 and 2008 were included in the sample. All 108 hearings were reviewed to identify specific themes in the witnesses' testimony, with a focus on their social construction of the elderly and the political construction of the Medicaid program.

The first section of this chapter is an overview of Medicaid's legislative origins, to explicate how this means-tested program expanded to incorporate the elderly middle class.[4] In the second section, we elaborate on the three distinct frames of elderly deservingness within Medicaid and discuss how various frames have been more salient at different points in time. In each of these sections we examine how the Medicaid program changed in ways that influenced the salience of the frame. Finally, we conclude by considering the potential of any one frame to dominate under the politics of Medicaid's universalism within targeting and the implications of various frames for Medicaid's future policy and political possibilities.

Medicaid's Political Origins and Development

Medicaid's creation in 1965 must be understood in the context of the long struggle to adopt universal health insurance in the United States.

By the late 1950s, liberal proponents of health care reform focused their attention on senior citizens, a clientele group that was viewed sympathetically and was already tied to the federal government through the Social Security system. In 1964, most informed observers thought Congress would adopt one of three alternative approaches to improve access to health care for elderly people: (1) a universal hospital insurance program based on Social Security (the King-Anderson bills of 1963 and 1964); (2) a voluntary physician services program supported by beneficiary premiums; or (3) an expansion of the means-tested Kerr-Mills program, which offered a wide range of health care benefits to the low-income elderly. Under the influence of Ways and Means Committee Chairman Wilbur Mills, the Social Security Amendments of 1965 combined all of these approaches into a single package. By all accounts, the creation of this massive three-layer cake took nearly everyone by surprise (Marmor, 1970; Stevens and Stevens, 1974). The first layer was Medicare Part A, a hospital insurance program based on the Social Security contributory model. The second layer was Medicare Part B, a voluntary supplementary medical insurance program funded through beneficiary premiums and federal general revenues. The third and final layer was the Medicaid program (originally called Part C), which broadened the protections offered to the poor under Kerr-Mills. The Kerr-Mills means-test was liberalized in order to cover additional elderly citizens, and eligibility among the indigent was broadened to include blind people, the permanently disabled, and adults in (largely) single-parent families and their dependent children.

Medicaid carried over two crucial provisions from Kerr-Mills that would profoundly influence its subsequent policy evolution: the concept of medical indigency and the inclusion of comprehensive benefits. Kerr-Mills had originally been drafted in 1959 as an alternative to the Forand bill, which proposed universal coverage for the elderly with a restricted benefits package (Marmor, 1970). Proponents of the Kerr-Mills approach argued that a means-tested program would be more efficient than a universal program, because it offered help to the most needy. They also stressed that this approach offered the truly needy more security than the Forand bill, because it provided comprehensive benefits—covering hospital, physician, and nursing home services. Although Kerr-Mills was a targeted program, it was designed to be distinct from welfare. Eligibility for benefits under Kerr-Mills was restricted to the *medically indigent*. These were older persons who needed assistance when they became sick because they had large medical expenses relative to their current income. Proponents emphasized that the "medically indigent should not be equated with the totally indigent" (Fein, 1998). The latter term refers in this case to those who receive cash assistance. The moral argument behind this expansion reasoned that the sick elderly should not have to become completely impoverished, and a medical indigency criterion would help prevent that. Both policy concepts—comprehensive benefits and medical indigency—were carried over from Kerr-Mills and enacted under the Medicaid program in 1965.

As mentioned above, the adoption of Kerr-Mills in combination with Medicare Parts A and B was completely unexpected, in part because means-tested Kerr-Mills (presented in 1964 bills as Eldercare) and universal Medicare offered fundamentally competing notions of social provision.[5] The principle of medical indigency was strategically included under Kerr-Mills, and subsequently under Eldercare bills, as an alternative to universalism. As a result, this concept—in light of the universality of Medicare—often confused policy makers. Yet by keeping the medical indigency idea in place, the seeds of middle-class reliance on Medicaid were planted.

Because Medicare covered only hospital and physician care services, Medicaid emerged as the most significant payer of nursing home care. As early as 1970, Medicaid was the dominant governmental purchaser in the nursing home market (table 13.1). In 1980, Medicaid spending on nursing home care ($8.8 billion) not only surpassed all other public sources combined ($0.7 billion), but it also slightly exceeded out-of-pocket payments for nursing home care ($7.4 billion). Medicaid nursing home expenditures rose rapidly during the 1990s. By 1997, Medicaid nursing home expenditures ($39.4 billion) greatly exceeded out-of-pocket payments for nursing home care ($25.7 billion). In that year, Medicaid picked up almost half (47%) of the $83 billion spent on nursing homes in the United States. By 2000, Medicaid payments for nursing home care had risen to $42 billion, representing 44 percent of the total expenditures ($95.3 billion). Since that time, Medicaid expenditures have continued to rise. However, the program's proportion of nursing home expenditures has remained relatively stable. In 2007, Medicaid covered roughly 42 percent ($54.8) of the nation's $131.3 billion in nursing home costs.

Table 13.1 Nursing Home Care Expenditures (in Billions), by Source of Funds, 1970–2007

Year	Total	Private			Public	
		Out-of-pocket	Private health insurance	Other private funds	Medicaid	All other public sources
1970	4.2	2.3	0.0	0.2	0.9	0.8
	(100)	(54)	(0)	(5)	(21)	(19)
1980	17.6	7.4	0.2	0.5	8.8	0.7
	(100)	(42)	(1)	(3)	(50)	(4)
1990	50.8	21.9	2.1	0.9	23.1	2.8
	(100)	(43)	(4)	(2)	(45)	(6)
2000	95.3	28.7	7.9	4.5	42.0	12.2
	(100)	(30)	(8)	(5)	(44)	(13)
2007	131.3	35.3	9.8	4.6	54.8	26.8
	(100)	(27)	(7)	(4)	(42)	(20)

Source: Data from the Centers for Medicare and Medicaid Services, 2007 historical data (www.cms
.hhs.gov/NationalHealthExpendData/).
Note: Percentages (shown in parentheses) may not add up to 100 due to rounding.

Not surprisingly, given demand and the spend-down provisions under Medicaid, many senior citizens who receive Medicaid do not have a history of poverty before entering a nursing home. Indeed, a summary of the literature on nursing home use indicates that approximately 60 percent of the people residing in nursing homes have Medicaid as a payment source on any given day. Somewhere between 33 and 40 percent of nursing home residents are eligible for Medicaid on admission. Only about one-third of those who do not have Medicaid as a payment source at the time they are admitted remain private payers throughout their stay. Two-thirds of such individuals eventually spend down their savings to Medicaid levels (Cohen, Kumar, and Wallack, 1993).

The significance of middle-class reliance on Medicaid raises an important question: why haven't the elderly claimed the Medicaid program as their own? In other words, why haven't they lobbied more persistently for Medicaid to be America's long-term care program? The answer to this question lies in the simultaneous creation of Medicare and Medicaid. Elderly people have always advocated for a Medicare

expansion approach, because Medicare is perceived to be "their program" and because it is seen as being more politically acceptable than
Medicaid. Indeed, notions of elderly deservingness within Medicaid
have been strongly influenced by the various possibilities for expansions within Medicare. As both the prospects for Medicare expansions
and the fortunes of elderly people have changed, and as Medicaid has
continued to expand over time, multiple frames of elderly deservingness within Medicaid have emerged.

Competing Frames of Elderly Deservingness within Medicaid

Three distinct social constructions of the elderly are apparent simultaneously and at different points in time during Medicaid's political evolution: elderly people as too deserving for a stigmatized means-tested
program such as Medicaid; elderly people as too well off relative to
other needy groups and therefore undeserving of Medicaid (in its for-
mat as a targeted program for the poor); and elderly people as deserving of Medicaid's social entitlement. Note that these various frames of
elderly deservingness under Medicaid depend not only on the social
construction of elderly people, but also on the political constructions
of the Medicaid program itself. Not only have notions of elderly deservingness in relation to the program changed over time, but political
constructions of the Medicaid program have changed as well—from
a program that was universally described as "residual" or as "stigmatized welfare" to a program that is consistently invoked today as a
"crucial safety net for the needy" and sometimes referred to as a "core
social entitlement" on a par with Medicare.

Elderly People as Too Deserving for Stigmatized Medicaid

Because the passage of both Medicare and Medicaid were unexpected,
and because policy makers did not give much thought to the ramifications of medical indigency, these individuals viewed Medicaid as a
relatively minor piece of the 1965 Social Security legislation, of much
less significance than Medicare. Governmental estimates of Medicaid's
future budgetary costs assumed that the program would not lead to
a dramatic expansion of health care coverage (Stevens and Stevens,
1974). For example, even supposing that all fifty states would implement the new program, the federal government projected Medicaid

expenditures to be no more than $238 million per year above what was then being spent on medical welfare programs. As it turned out, this expenditure level was reached after only six states had implemented their Medicaid programs. By 1967, thirty-seven states were implementing Medicaid programs, and spending was rising by 57 percent per annum (Congressional Research Service, 1993).

A key factor that explains Medicaid's early expenditure growth was the establishment of generous eligibility standards under various state Medically Needy programs. Known as Kerr-Mills (medical indigency) extensions, the Medically Needy programs allowed states to proffer Medicaid eligibility to persons with income levels above the regular Medicaid income criterion established by each state. A number of states were initially open-handed in where they set these levels. For example, under New York's Medically Needy enrollment standards, almost half of the state's population in 1966 could have qualified for Medicaid's comprehensive medical coverage, including access to prescription drugs and long-term care facilities (Stevens and Stevens, 1974).

New York State policy makers seem to have envisioned Medicaid as the stepping-stone to universal health care for its residents, which created a major branching point in U.S. health care policy. The federal government had to decide whether it should embrace this expansive vision of Medicaid or instead restrict program eligibility to a narrow clientele, and it chose the latter course, clamping down hard on New York's attempted liberalization. In 1967, only a year after the New York expansion began, Congress passed legislation lowering the Medically Needy eligibility level to 133-⅓ percent of the means-tested level of a state's Aid to Families with Dependent Children program.[6]

In halting New York's 1967 efforts, federal policy makers made a conscious decision to define Medicaid as a restricted welfare program, off-limits to the employed. "The House is moving toward a program where you provide medical care to those who can't pay, and expect people to pay it if they are working and can earn income," stated one conservative Senator in floor debate (U.S. Congress, 1967, p. 1547). Although elderly people—especially those in need of long-term care—are exempt from popular notions of a work requirement, this legislation did put strict limits on the generosity of Medically Needy programs, which in turn affected elderly people.

Perhaps more importantly, this policy retrenchment solidified an image of Medicaid as a stingy welfare program not worthy of elderly people. Indeed, we see this framing clearly in hearings throughout the 1970s and into the 1980s where Medicaid is discussed. During this period, in hearings where the topic under consideration is either long-term care or health issues of concern to the elderly more generally (e.g., Alzheimer's disease), Medicaid is either not mentioned, disregarded as inappropriate for the elderly, or quickly dismissed as a residual program unfit to meet the needs of elderly people. For example, in a 1970 Senate hearing on *Sources of Community Support for Federal Programs Serving Older Americans*, only one witness among the four who discussed concerns about nursing home coverage mentioned Medicaid, and then only in passing. After describing the details of Medicare nursing home coverage (or the lack thereof), he said "these shortcomings apply equally to Medicaid situations." Although by 1970 Medicaid already was the primary public payer of nursing home care, the other three witnesses similarly focused on the limitations in nursing home coverage under Medicare. Senator Long's earlier statement (U.S. Congress, 1967, p. 1547) provides some insight into the emergence of this view: "We were warned for many years if we didn't pass Medicare that the cost of the Kerr-Mills program, which is Medicaid, as I understand it, that was the genesis of it, was going to skyrocket. Now we have Medicare and we also have this Medicaid program. As I understand the House bill tried to hold the cost of the Medicaid program down." Despite the fact that nursing home care was clearly not covered under Medicare and applied only to the medically needy under Medicaid, there was a popular conception—against programmatic reality—that Medicare was for the elderly and should therefore suffice to take care of their needs.

In a 1981 hearing on the *Impact of Alzheimer's Disease on the Nation's Elderly*, several witnesses discuss the problem that nursing homes often reject patients with dementia, due to these individuals' lack of mental health coverage. Although this was clearly a limitation in Medicaid policy, almost all of the policy recommendations focused on amending Medicare policy.

In another hearing that dealt with the *Impact of Federal Budget Cuts on the Elderly* in 1981, Representative Claude Pepper, a long-time advocate for the elderly and chair of the committee, began his opening remarks by stating the deservingness of the elderly across the board (U.S. Congress, 1982). However, in turning to discuss the "less fortunate" elderly, he noted (p. 2): "In spite of Social Security, one-

sixth, more than 16 percent, of the elderly live below the poverty line
. . . They lack decent housing. Medicare pays only 38 percent of their
medical costs. They live under fear of serious disease when they would
not have the aid of Medicare. They wouldn't be eligible for Medicaid
because if you have anything at all to speak of, you are not eligible for
Medicaid." Although there were valid concerns about the elderly having to impoverish themselves to become eligible for Medicaid's long-
term care services, and no spousal protections were in place at this
time, by 1982 Medicaid nursing home expenditures greatly exceeded
out-of-pocket payments for nursing home care. Nonetheless, the Medicaid program was generally dismissed out-of-hand as too stingy and
too stigmatizing to be an acceptable reform strategy for elderly people.
There is little discussion about Medicaid reform under this framing;
instead, Medicare is viewed as the appropriate program to which to
devote advocacy efforts.

This framing of Medicaid also applied when policy makers considered health care expansions to nonelderly middle-class people. We see
it in health care reform proposals during this period, where Medicaid is similarly invoked as a residual program. For example, under
the National Health Plan Act (HR 5400/S 1812) presented in 1980,
proposed revisions to Medicaid are summarized as follows: "Services
available to low-income individuals under HealthCare would no longer be covered under Title XIX. Title XIX would continue as a residual program covering those services not under HealthCare." Under
the Health Care for All Americans Act (HR 5191/S 1720), "the bill
would make certain changes in the Medicare program . . . Medicaid would remain as a residual program." Indeed, Medicaid was referred to as a residual program in every health reform bill presented in
1980.

Despite the persistence of this residual frame, the Medicaid program
experienced significant changes during the 1980s that were difficult
to ignore. These changes allowed policy makers to view both the program and elderly people's relationship to it in a different light.

Elderly People as Too Well Off for
Medicaid's Needed Safety Net

In contrast to a policy retrenchment era for Medicaid during the
1970s, the program enjoyed an expansionary period during the 1980s.

In particular, there were two main enlargements: (1) greater coverage for children and pregnant women, and (2) coverage expansions for low-income elderly people financed by Medicaid.[7] However, the cumulative force of these policies over the 1980s created a new framing of the Medicaid program by the early 1990s. By this time, few described the program as residual. Instead, 20-plus years postenactment, Medicaid was recognized as a crucial safety net for many diversely needy groups. Under this new understanding of the program, and with the emergence of a relatively new rhetoric of the elderly as politically privileged (to the detriment of younger generations), elderly middle-class inclusion in Medicaid was often discussed as problematic. Elderly people were portrayed as too well off financially compared with other potential recipients of the crucially needed but limited resources provided under means-tested Medicaid. Below we first describe the two expansionary developments during the 1980s and then document the emergence of this new frame.

Expanded Coverage for Children and Pregnant Women. The federal government enacted incremental Medicaid expansions for children or pregnant women and infants in every year between 1984 and 1990 (Tanenbaum, 1995). By the end of this period, approximately 5 million children and half a million pregnant women had gained Medicaid eligibility (Rosenbaum, 1993).

The targeted expansions for pregnant women and children emphasized a message that Medicaid served the "deserving poor," not just people on welfare (or, more accurately, on cash assistance). Advocates for these Medicaid expansions also argued that extending Medicaid coverage to pregnant women and children was cost-effective (Tanenbaum, 1995). The health care costs associated with low-birth-weight babies rose dramatically during the 1980s, in part because technological improvements were allowing more and more babies of lower and lower birth weights to be saved. Advocates argued that increasing access to prenatal care through Medicaid would yield significant economic savings via higher birth weights and better infant outcomes. A similarly pragmatic argument was made for expanded coverage for children: inexpensive immunizations and well-child care were portrayed as prudent investments for a healthy population and a strong future workforce (Sardell, 1991).

Expansions for Low-Income Elderly People. Although the adoption of Medicare in 1965 successfully brought the aged into the mainstream of U.S. medicine, serious gaps in coverage remained twenty years later. As mentioned, Medicare did not (and still does not) cover most long-term care needs, nor did the program cover prescription drug expenses. In addition, the out-of-pocket costs associated with Medicare's copayments and deductibles could reach catastrophic proportions for many elderly people with serious medical conditions. Low-income seniors not covered under Medicaid spent, on average, one-quarter of their annual income on medical bills (Rosenbaum, 1993).

Given the Medicaid program's longstanding role in the long-term care sector, health reform advocates might have been expected to use it as the institutional vehicle for adopting catastrophic health care coverage. Instead, advocates for long-term care coverage primarily lobbied for Medicare expansions. The Medicare Catastrophic Care Act (MCCA) of 1988 was the federal government's response to this advocacy. The act expanded coverage to include outpatient prescription drug benefits and long-term hospital care. This represented the largest expansion to the Medicare program since its inception in 1965. To finance MCCA, however, the government made a sharp break from Medicare's social insurance tradition and required Medicare beneficiaries, rather than current workers, to shoulder the financial burden. In particular, Medicare beneficiaries were asked to pay special premiums, according to family income, to cover the cost of expanded benefits under MCCA. Controversy over this new financing scheme (and several other reasons)[8] ultimately led to MCCA's repeal just one year later. The irony of this repeal lies in two major expansionary policies that remained intact within the Medicaid program. The first provided protection against spousal impoverishment by increasing the amount of money that seniors in the community can retain when their institutionalized spouses receive Medicaid benefits. The second Medicaid expansion, also not repealed under MCCA, was the creation of the Qualified Medicare Beneficiary (QMB) program. This program requires the Medicaid program to buy into the Medicare program for low-income seniors and persons with disabilities. Specifically, since 1989 Medicaid has been required to pay Medicare Part B premiums and cover any deductibles or cost-sharing expenses for those elderly under 100 percent of the poverty line (in 1990, premium support was expanded to elderly people with incomes up to 120% of this line).

While budget constraints and a relatively large federal deficit were significant motivating factors behind MCCA's passage and its intragenerational financing scheme, a new rhetoric of intergenerational equity also contributed to its support in Congress. This new rhetoric emphasized two points: (1) that relatively few resources were devoted to children in need because of large public costs imposed by elderly people; and (2) that families were financially burdened due to transfers from the young to the old to support large, expensive, federal programs such as Social Security and Medicare (Cook et al., 1994). Several scholars have documented the emergence of the intergenerational equity theme during the 1980s around widespread discussions about the elderly more generally and about its particular importance in the passage and then the repeal of MCCA (Quadagno, 1989; Cook et al., 1994; Pierson and Smith, 1994). Not surprisingly, given the significant expansions that remained for elderly people within the Medicaid program after the MCCA's repeal, this intergenerational equity discourse also became infused into Medicaid's political discourse.

New Framing: Elderly People as Too Well Off and Overburdening Medicaid. Intergenerational equity concerns probably emerged first among state actors. Indeed, it has long been the case that while the elderly comprise less than 15 percent of Medicaid recipients, they account for more than 30 percent of the program's costs, in large part because of their nursing home care (Rosenbaum, 1993). In light of these statistics, in the 1980s some advocates for poor children began to argue that it was inappropriate for a disproportionate share of Medicaid dollars to support elderly people while younger people were struggling to pay for their health care (Benjamin, Newacheck, and Wolfe, 1991). With federal mandates that expanded benefits to both "cost-effective" pregnant women and children and the "expensive" elderly in the 1980s, representatives from the states started to voice concerns that they could not legitimately finance expansions to both groups; difficult choices needed to be made, or growing long-term care costs would result in fewer services for poor families. For example, a representative from the State Medicaid Directors' Association made the following remarks in her testimony before the Subcommittee on Health and the Environment for a 1987 hearing titled *Medicare and Medicaid Catastrophic Protection*: "Obviously, for the private payer, the spousal protections . . . are very desirable and very needed. As you reduce their share of the cost, you are again passing those increases onto the Medicaid program. I'm not suggesting that you not do it, only to keep in mind that those Medicaid budgets are being consumed by long-term care expenditures. Because state revenues and local revenues are not limitless, again choices have to be made. What we are seeing in effect is Medicaid by default becoming a long-term care budget and not being able to cover more of the primary health care needs of women, children, and families" (U.S. Congress, 1988, Matula, May 28, 1987, p. 433).

This intergenerational concern within Medicaid became even more heated as the benefit expansions for the elderly were implemented at the state level in the early 1990s. For example, in a federal hearing titled *Medicaid Program Investigation*, testimony from a state congressional representative from Michigan not only emphasized the disproportionate share of the Medicaid budget consumed by elderly people, but also suggested that such expenses were used inappropriately for expensive care during the last year of life. "Congressman, two-thirds of our health care dollars are spent in the last year of life, and two-thirds of those are spent in the last 90 days. This is the fastest-growing part of our population. We have a dramatically aging society spending more and more on health care. The health care share of our budget in Michigan has gone from 20 percent of the budget in 1980, to 26.8 percent in 1990. Medicaid is one of the major problems and you will hear across the country, 'Medicaid is eating up state budgets'" (U.S. Congress, 1992, Hollister, October 2, 1991, pp. 272–73).

These quotes are illustrative of concerns emerging from the states in federal discourse over the Medicaid program. In all the hearings discussing Medicaid during the early 1990s and continuing throughout the decade, representatives from the states mentioned the explosive costs of long-term care and how these costs forced them to choose between needy population groups. For example, many often mentioned the "truly" needy groups that Medicaid should cover—but cannot—due to expensive long-term care costs, groups such as working families without insurance. In North Carolina, the state Medicaid director's attempted to simplify the complexity of the Medicaid program by presenting the following symbolic image that sums up the way policy makers viewed the intergenerational tension within the program:

The Medicaid program is up a creek . . . In the creek are two islands. They are filled with people who need help with their medical bills.
One island contains infants, children, teenagers, their parents. This

island threatens to sink just by the sheer weight of the numbers of the people on the island, twice as many as occupy the second island.

The second island has fewer people, but they are all severely disabled or elderly. The weight of their problems is twice as great as those on the first island. This island, too, is sinking fast, but, ironically, there is a boat docked here at the second island named Medicare, the good ship Medicare. It should be carrying the elderly and disabled to shore, but it is so filled with holes it is of little use to the would-be patients. It does not go where the patients want to go.

The Medicaid program is the only available boat in the river, and its course is not clearly charted. Should it head toward the island and save the children and their parents or should it head in the opposite direction, tow Medicare's boat, and bring those patients aboard? The answer is it must do both. Its seating capacity is unlimited by law. (U.S. Congress, 1992, Matula, October 2, 1991, p. 303)

Note that in addition to emphasizing a dichotomous choice facing the states between taking care of the children versus the elderly, this image also points to Medicare as the culprit in creating this tension within Medicaid, and it concludes by arguing that Medicaid has no choice—it must take care of both populations. The conclusion leads to the questions of how Medicaid can possibly do both, and how the program might be restructured. Should Medicaid remain a means-tested program and therefore make hard choices between needy groups, or should Medicaid become something else to accommodate the diverse needs of program recipients as well as other groups that need help? Indeed, this dilemma foreshadows the third frame that began to emerge around this time, one that became most pronounced during the 1995 debate about the Republican proposal to restructure the Medicaid program into a block grant. This frame emphasizes Medicaid as a core social entitlement that appropriately includes the middle-class elderly who need long-term care. In contrast, the intergenerational equity frame implicitly paints Medicaid as a means-tested program that must choose between needy groups.

Elderly People as Deserving of Medicaid's Core Social Entitlement

Emergence of the Social Entitlement Frame. At the same time that the intergenerational equity frame was emerging from the states, there was another frame being developed that recognized the Medicaid program as a major social welfare program reaching into the middle class—far from its rhetorical beginnings that defined it as a residual program. For example, in a 1990 hearing titled *Medicaid Budget Initiatives*, Chairman Henry Waxman highlighted the middle-class aspect of Medicaid in his opening statement: "Most people who need nursing home care eventually find themselves dependent on Medicaid . . . It is absurd, and it is unacceptable that an individual could work hard for their entire life, set aside a fund for his or her retirement, then become—then have to be impoverished and go on welfare in order to take advantage of facilities and services and aids that flow from the Medicaid system. With the passage of Representative Kennelly's bill, my state and nine others are proposing to offer an alternative" (U.S. Congress, 1991, Waxman, September 10, 1990, p. 2).

Representative Kennelly's bill called for demonstration projects to develop private/public partnerships to encourage the middle-class elderly to purchase long-term care insurance. Under this bill, "if and when an individual exhausts his or her insurance and applies for Medicaid, each dollar that the insurance policy has paid out in accord with state guidelines will be subtracted from the assets Medicaid considers in determining eligibility. In other words, coverage of long-term care expenses by private insurance would count as asset spend-down for the purpose of Medicaid eligibility" (U.S. Congress, 1991, Kennelly, September 10, 1990, p. 23). Although Representative Waxman, as chair of the Subcommittee on Health and the Environment, expressed general support for Kennelly's bill in his opening remarks, he raised concerns about whether this bill would create a new category of Medicaid eligibility—one that expanded eligibility to middle-class (or even upper-income) elderly people by allowing Medicaid to be used to protect assets and to finance the transfer of wealth. Kennelly's response to Waxman's concerns puts at the forefront the issue of whether Medicaid is still a truly means-tested program or has expanded to something beyond that:[9]

First let me say that I think part of the reason you and I have different perspectives on this issue [whether her bill creates a new category of Medicaid eligibility] is that we start from very different points. You seem to see Medicaid solely as a means-tested entitlement for the poor. While I agree, I also see Medicaid as a program where, at least based on Connecticut figures, more than 40 percent of those who receive Medicaid long-term care services did not start out poor.

I hear of financial planners teaching seniors how to transfer their assets and access Medicaid benefits and I feel there ought to be a better way . . . Our society has changed markedly in the 25 years since the enactment of the Medicaid program to the point where many of those receiving Medicaid are not included in our traditional definition of "poor."

The current Medicaid long-term care program is a means-tested program in name only. The major asset most seniors possess is a house which is typically protected by Medicaid . . . Given the political pressures associated with the aging of the population, we are likely to see even more proposals to further increase the amount of assets exempted from Medicaid.

In that context, my proposal . . . may be the *only* proposal that has the potential of actually protecting Medicaid against further erosion of its means-tested origin. (U.S. Congress, 1991, Kennelly, September 10, 1990, p. 23, emphasis in the original)

This quote is important for two reasons: (1) as mentioned above, it shows that by 1990, Medicaid's mean-tested origins were openly questioned; and (2) it shows how intergenerational concerns fed into redefining the program. Representative Kennelly explicitly acknowledges the political power of the elderly in support of her bill requiring middle-class elderly people to purchase private long-term care insurance, with Medicaid as a type of stop-gap coverage. However, her statement that Representative Waxman views the Medicaid program as "solely a means-tested entitlement for the poor" is ironic, given that Waxman championed the Medicaid expansions for pregnant women and children throughout the 1980s. Waxman clearly envisioned Medicaid as a vehicle for expanding coverage to the uninsured, including working middle-class families. This is pure conjecture, but his knowledge of Medicaid's expansionary tendencies might explain why he was concerned about creating yet another eligibility expansion, in this case one to the potentially well-off elderly who might receive benefits at the expense of other groups he cared about. Indeed, Waxman's expansive view of Medicaid as a core social entitlement is stated clearly in a 1991 hearing investigating the Medicaid program:

Medicaid is an enormously important and enormously complex program. It is the major source of health care reform for the poor in this country, covering more than 28 million poor people, roughly half of whom are children. It is the single largest payer for maternity care . . . It is the single largest payer for nursing home care . . . It is the single largest payer for residential services for individuals with mental retardation . . . [The] program has been asked to solve almost every major problem facing this society, from infant mortality to substance abuse to AIDS to the need for long-term care . . . Despite all of the current interest in health care reform, nothing will be enacted tomorrow, . . . [and] the poor in this country, mothers and children, the disabled, the elderly will continue to rely on Medicaid for access to basic health care. (U.S. Congress 1992, Waxman, June 20, 1991, pp. 3–4)

Representative Waxman's last statement about Medicaid's role in discussions about national health care reform is noteworthy. In sharp contrast to health care reform proposals offered in the early 1980s (discussed above), where Medicaid was easily dismissed as a residual program, most health care reform bills in the early 1990s proposed expanding Medicaid to cover the uninsured (e.g., using Medicaid 1115 waivers) or expanding access to private insurance and leaving the Medicaid program intact. Few bills proposed eliminating the Medicaid program altogether.

Indeed, even during hearings about transforming the Medicaid program in 1995, Republican legislators in favor of a block grant for Medicaid went to great pains to stress that their goal was to strengthen and not dismantle the program. For example, in Chairman Bilirakis's opening statement, he said: "We all have very personal and compelling views about Medicaid. No one involved in this reform effort sees our objective as dismantling a program that is essential to millions of low-income Americans. In fact, we are motivated in this effort by the conviction that what we are doing will strengthen and preserve the Medicaid program for years to come, and that's our goal" (U.S. Congress, 1996, Bilirakis, August 1, 1995, p. 164). Liberals (or Democrats) might discard the sincerity of such statements as pure rhetoric, but it is important to note that the program had changed significantly enough that even conservative Republicans felt compelled to frame their argument in this way.

While Republicans moved from a residual frame to a frame that supported the necessity of the Medicaid program, Democrats and advocates of the program went a step further during the 1995 debate. For example, one advocate[10] concluded her written testimony, presented at a 1995 hearing, with the following summary of Medicaid's transformation over time: "Since its enactment in 1965, Medicaid has improved access to health care for the poor, pioneered innovations in health care delivery and community-based long-term care services, and stood alone as the primary source of financial assistance for long-term care. In implementing solutions to meet the crises of today, it is important not to undo the progress Medicaid has made in providing health and long-term care for tens of millions of low-income and elderly and disabled Americans" (U.S. Congress, 1996, Rowland, August 1, 1995, p. 177).

Even President Clinton recast Medicaid under this new frame of being a middle-class entitlement during the 1995 debates. It was not surprising that President Clinton sought to rally public opinion against the GOP budget package by arguing that it would entail huge cuts in spending for Medicare, education, and environmental protection—three federal programs with obvious appeal for middle-class voters. However, Clinton's explicit support for *Medicaid*, on a par with these other universal (i.e., middle-class) programs, was quite startling (Grogan and Patashnik, 2003b). In explaining why protecting Medicaid was so vital, Clinton emphasized that Medicaid was a key support for senior citizens residing in nursing homes; that many of these seniors were middle class before they depleted their resources; and that they had middle-class children and grandchildren. As Clinton stated in one address: "Now, think about this—what about the Medicaid program? You hardly hear anything about Medicaid. People say, Oh, that's that welfare program. One-third of Medicaid does go to help poor women and their poor children on Medicaid. More than two-thirds of it goes to the elderly and the disabled. All of you know that as well. [He added, in commenting on Republican proposals,] You think about how many middle-class working people are not going to be able to save to send their kids to college because now they'll have to be taking care of their parents who would have been eligible for public assistance" (*U.S. Newswire*, 1995).

Note the huge political significance of this frame: by 1995, Medicaid's long-term care role and financial protection policies were sufficiently recognized so that it was acceptable for the president, in a major public address, to explain Medicare and Medicaid as comprising a health care *package* for the mainstream elderly (Grogan and Patashnik, 2003b). In sum, Clinton sought to cast Medicaid as a broad social entitlement that incorporated the middle class.

Emphasizing elderly middle-class incorporation is an important aspect of the core social entitlement frame. During the 1995 hearings, all advocates for the elderly mentioned this incorporation of the middle class into Medicaid. For example, a representative from what was then called the American Association of Retired Persons (its official name is now just AARP) began her testimony by saying "I testify today on behalf of the almost 5 million older Americans who rely on Medicaid." She then continued: "Many who need long-term care start off as tax-paying middle-class Americans. They worked hard and saved" (U.S. Congress, 1996, August 1, 1995, Braun, pp. 288–89). Note the change in discussions about the elderly middle class with regard to Medicaid. In 1990, Representative Kennelly recognized the importance of Medicaid for the elderly middle class and offered a bill to keep them out of the program and preserve Medicaid's means-tested origins. In 1995, advocates, members of Congress, and the president mention the elderly middle class participating in Medicaid as a central reason why the program should be viewed as a core social entitlement.

This strategic recasting also found expression in the 1996 Democratic Party platform. It stated that securing both Medicare and Medicaid was a "duty for our parents, so they can live their lives in dignity," and prominently pledged to protect Medicaid in particular from devastating cuts that "would jeopardize the health care of children and seniors." Inspection of Democratic Party platforms from 1984, 1988, and 1992 reveals that the platforms either did not mention Medicaid (1984 and 1988) or discussed the program only in the context of welfare reform and encouraging work.

Also important in the 1996 Democratic platform is the effort to mention the importance of Medicaid to both children and the elderly—specifically downplaying the intergenerational tension. In contrast to the intergenerational frame which emphasized children, the disabled, and the elderly as separate and competing groups, many advocates presenting a core entitlement frame discussed these groups as a coalition coming together under Medicaid—all needing important and necessary health care services. For example, a representative from the Alzheimer's Association[11] began his remarks in the 1995 Medicaid transformation hearing with the following point: "You have assembled this panel to talk about Medicaid and the elderly. But before doing that, I want to make a broader point. Distinctions among 'categories' of Medicaid beneficiaries are arbitrary and potentially dangerous. The elderly need long-term care because of their disabilities; people with disabilities are aging; disabling illnesses like Alzheimer's and Parkinson's—generally considered diseases of aging—are striking younger people as well. That is why the Alzheimer's Association has always approached the long-term care issue as part of a coalition of aging, disability, and children's organizations that make up the Long Term Care Campaign" (U.S. Congress, 1996, August 1, 1995, McConnell, p. 261). This testimony by the representative from the Alzheimer's Association is also important because it illustrates how far the program's frame has shifted over time in relation to elderly people. In sharp contrast to the 1981 hearing on elderly people and Alzheimer's disease, in which representatives dismissed Medicaid out of hand, the representative in 1995 said: "My testimony will focus on Medicaid as a vital lifeline to long-term care, because that is what brings families dealing with Alzheimer's disease into the system" (ibid.).

Conservative Response to the Emerging Social Entitlement Frame. By 2000, efforts by Democrats to strategically recast Medicaid as a core social entitlement for elderly people had fostered significant concern among Republicans. Debate emerged within Congress over whether Medicaid was becoming a middle-class program—a development vehemently opposed by Republicans. As part of a series of hearings (spanning several years and culminating in 2005) concerning the Medicaid spending "crisis," Republicans sought to reveal the growing pattern of middle-class elderly reliance on Medicaid and to develop measures to curb it. Implicit within this struggle was an emerging conservative challenge to the core social entitlement frame that aimed to return Medicaid to its roots as "welfare medicine," consequently retaining the program's mission to serve only the nation's most economically vulnerable populations.

Concerns about the use of Medicaid by middle- and upper-income elderly people emerged within the context of rising Medicaid costs and a declining U.S. economy. Steady increases in Medicaid expenditures during the late 1990s created apprehension among policy makers— particularly fiscal conservatives—about the growing burden of the program's costs for state and national budgets. Indeed, Congress faced growing pressure to curb Medicaid growth, particularly from state governments hamstrung by increasing program costs, growing Medicaid enrollment, and—especially by 2002—serious fiscal stress. Moreover, many states began to openly acknowledge that home and community-based care (HCBC) approaches would not solve Medicaid's budget problems and were no longer considered the great panacea to *significantly* cut long-term care costs without compromising quality. Similarly, while Cash and Counseling demonstration programs continue to hold out hope for cost containment, deinstitutionalization, and individual empowerment, the evidence to date suggests that such programs are significantly limited in their reach and may only defer costs rather than providing long-term cost savings (Robert Wood Johnson Foundation, 2006).

With the program under pressure for greater fiscal austerity, the process of spending down to qualify for Medicaid emerged as an important area for reform, one with the potential to cut costs by limiting enrollment to only the most economically vulnerable seniors. While the tactic of divesting assets to qualify for Medicaid had long been acknowledged among policy makers,[12] this practice was again brought to the fore by Republicans and defined as a significant policy problem. In contrast to the social entitlement frame, which sought to redefine Medicaid as a program benefiting all seniors, this framing seeks to draw a stark distinction between the "truly needy" and those seniors who presumably can afford to pay for long-term care but avoid doing so and ultimately end up relying on Medicaid. Similar to the debate regarding the Medicaid block-grant transformation proposal in 1995, legislators who opposed the use of Medicaid by middle-class elderly people sought not to dismantle the program, but rather to limit its scope to only the most economically vulnerable seniors.

Yet these arguments went one step further, suggesting that any move to reframe Medicaid as a core social entitlement for elderly people would ultimately threaten the program's fiscal sustainability and, in so doing, compromise its ability to fulfill its primary role as a health care safety net intended for the nation's most vulnerable populations—both young and old. This theme is mentioned repeatedly during a series of hearings held in 2005 to address Medicaid's growing costs. For example, Representative Mike Ferguson (R-NJ) made the following opening statement during a hearing focusing on the need to reform long-term care financing under the Medicaid program: "This hearing will shed light on an issue that requires urgent attention as a new generation of Americans, the baby boomers, grow closer to retirement age and the Medicaid program continues to hemorrhage money. Medicaid, as it stands right now, is financially unsustainable. And without true reform, the Medicaid program may not be around for those in future years, for those who really need it" (U.S. Congress, 2005, Ferguson, April 27, 2005, p. 9). Mark McClellan, former administrator of the Centers for Medicare and Medicaid Services, reiterated this viewpoint succinctly, noting that "to make sure Medicaid remains secure and sustainable, we need to take steps to help individuals who can contribute to their long-term care costs to do so, and then we need to concentrate our Medicaid funds on people who have no alternatives" (U.S. Congress, 2005, McClellan, April 27, 2005, p. 21).

These hearings also inserted a new theme into the long-term care debate—that of personal responsibility for long-term care planning. In his opening remarks, Representative Nathan Deal (R-GA) states this clearly: "There are many other facets, obviously, of the Medicaid problem. But the one that I continue to harp on—and it is an essential ingredient that I think causes the problem and if we can fix it, we'll perhaps provide the solution—and that is the current absence of individual responsibility in the program as it is designed" (U.S. Congress, 2005, Deal, April 27, 2005, p. 2). This theme is significant, because it represents a shift in the policy debate over long-term care. For the first time, it suggested that the root of the long-term care problem is a lack of personal responsibility among citizens to prepare for their own long-term care needs. What is more, this view suggests a new political construction of Medicaid, one promoting government dependency by enabling middle-class citizens to avoid planning for their care during their years of economic productivity. This, in turn, leads to the need for economic dependency on the government in late life. As Representative Charlie Norwood (R-GA) stated in one such hearing: "It is impossible to talk about reformed Medicaid without addressing the funding of long-term care, which I understand is about 56 percent of the cost. Because Medicaid is an alternative, the program encourages people to avoid long-term care plans and rely instead on this free benefit . . . Moving away from such views would allow Medicaid to return to its proper mission. Because Medicaid is an alternative to private insurance, the program encourages people . . . to drop coverage, or avoid long-term care planning, and rely instead on this free Medicaid. Put simply, Medicaid discourages proper planning, and is quickly becoming a welfare program for middle-income families" (U.S. Congress, 2005, Norwood, April 27, 2005, p. 5).

What is more, this argument harkens back to the "private" solution to the long-term care challenge—introducing public incentives to persuade citizens to pay for their own care. Such policies, as Representative Deal put it, would fill a need for "something that will individually make us responsible for recognizing that this is not just something that somebody else is going to pay for" (U.S. Congress, 2005, Deal, April 27, 2005, pp. 2–3). Among the most prominent policy prescriptions for planning appropriately for potential long-term care needs are (1) the expansion of long-term care insurance partnership projects; (2) public incentives to private insurance companies to offer affordable long-term care insurance plans to citizens; and (3) the use of federally backed reverse mortgages. Proposals to encourage private long-term care insurance have been around for a long time. They were first introduced in the 1970s and—as discussed in the previous section—were at the heart of Representative Kennelly's proposal to maintain Medicaid as a means-tested program in the early 1990s. Nonetheless, the private-sector approach became more prominent during the 2000–2008 timeframe—it was the central alternative repeatedly positioned on the policy agenda and it was integral to the discussion surrounding the Deficit Reduction Act (DRA) of 2005.

The DRA was passed by a small margin in both the House and Senate and signed into law by President Bush in February 2006. A principal aim of the DRA was to reduce federal expenditures on entitlement programs. While the act's reach was not limited to Medicaid, its implications for the health care program were significant. The DRA sought to prevent enrollment in Medicaid by middle-class elderly people by extending the "look back" period for all asset transfers from three to five years, implementing stricter rules regarding the treatment of annuities, and barring eligibility for individuals with a home equity above $500,000. At the same time, the DRA included several measures designed to promote private alternatives to Medicaid with regard to financing long-term care. These included extending the option to establish long-term care insurance partnership programs to all states and providing states with greater flexibility to impose cost-sharing on beneficiaries (Kaiser Commission on Medicaid and the Uninsured, 2006).

Democratic Retreat from the Social Entitlement Frame. Whereas the late 1990s found Democrats proactively advocating for a new framing of Medicaid as a core social entitlement for elderly Americans, in recent years they have assumed a more defensive role. This retreat has been driven in part by the larger political context (as a reaction to a Republican administration), but also in part by a dramatic economic downturn and mounting pressure from state governments to control the cost of Medicaid. By 2000, Democrats increasingly avoided discussing Medicaid as a middle-class entitlement and instead returned to the more traditional rhetoric of Medicaid as a critical safety net for the nation's most vulnerable populations—lower-income women, children, seniors, and disabled people. Such references abound among Democrats and Republicans alike in hearings during this time.

Democrats have also become more cautious in their discussions about middle-class involvement in Medicaid. While the evidence suggests that some middle-class seniors do transfer assets to qualify for Medicaid, few (if any) Democrats have been willing to publicly acknowledge this or to openly question whether the incorporation of the middle class into the Medicaid program may be a positive development. Testimony given by Lois Capps (D-CA) is reflective of the kind of approach taken by many Democrats on the issue of middle-class spend-downs to achieve Medicaid eligibility: "Many proponents of change claim that wealthy seniors in large numbers are gaming the system and stealing from Medicaid. They argue that we must make dramatic changes to asset transfer limits in order to cut back on these practices. But there is, to my knowledge, nothing but anecdotal information to support these claims" (U.S. Congress, 2005, Capps, April 27, 2005, p. 14).

Another approach, illustrated by statements from Representative Henry Waxman (D-CA), attempts to more roundly attack the Republicans' assertion that middle-class reliance on Medicaid stems from perverse incentives built into the program for individuals to avoid personal responsibility for their long-term care. Waxman poses the following questions to Mark McClellan, former administrator of the Centers for Medicare and Medicaid Services:

> As a man familiar with Medicare, Medicaid, economics, and human nature, do you think people refuse to go out and buy private insurance because they're calculating on the fact that Medicaid is going to be available to them when they have long-term care needs?
>
> Or, you think it's more likely that they don't anticipate ever having those needs, they think Medicare maybe already covers it, they have other pressing economic demands on them, . . . they're not well informed, . . . and these policies exclude people who have underwriting problems and

there are no uniform standards in terms of information and coverage? (U.S. Congress, 2005, Waxman, April 27, 2005, p. 66)

Waxman clearly rejects the assertion that the Medicaid program creates incentives for middle-class citizens to avoid planning for long-term care. What is more, he suggests that even if the middle class was encouraged to finance their own care, they may face several challenges to doing so. However, like Capps, Waxman does not raise the question of whether extending eligibility to middle-class elderly people could be a solution to this problem.

Conclusion

This chapter documents how the various frames of elderly deservingness under Medicaid depend not only on the social construction of elderly people, but also on political constructions of the Medicaid program itself. Medicaid has clearly evolved away from its political frame as a residual program into a program that is either portrayed as a crucially necessary, means-tested program for many needy groups or as a core social entitlement that helps the needy and appropriately extends its reach into the middle class. Indeed, this is the critical question about Medicaid today: should we preserve its means-tested origins or should we allow (or encourage) the program to evolve into something more universal?

As Medicare continues to be stuck in gear, and the enactment of targeted programs (rather than the creation of universal programs) continues to be the norm in the United States, it is important to reexamine Medicaid's possibilities. While the factors that lead to passage or failure of a particular bill are always more complex than those that emerge from simply analyzing the elite discourse surrounding that bill, it is noteworthy that the framing of Medicaid as a core social entitlement that emphasized the incorporation of the elderly middle class was successful in fighting back Republican efforts in 1995 to transform the program into a block grant (which advocates viewed as a major policy retrenchment). This suggests that targeted programs, rather than suffering from an unchangeable, stigmatized rhetoric, can instead change and be recast in more politically acceptable ways. It also suggests that targeted programs can evolve over time from a negative frame into a more positive one and, with this new frame, perhaps become acceptable to middle-class groups. Indeed, despite repeated advocacy for long-term care expansions within Medicare, it is Medicaid that has changed most significantly in this regard.

While a shift in public discourse regarding the elderly and the Medicaid program has certainly occurred over time, the most recent period emphasizing "personal responsibility" suggests that parts of old frames can be reinvoked. While the residual frame is largely absent from political discourse about the elderly and Medicaid today, one can still find traces of it. When discussing the spend-down process, for example, policy elites often emphasize Medicaid as a stingy, inadequate program where the elderly must lose their dignity to become eligible, or—more recently—that forward-looking, responsible adults purchase private long-term care insurance. Moreover, despite the good intentions of diverse advocacy groups (representing children, the elderly, and the disabled) to present a united front, when budgets get tight at the state level, the intergenerational equity frame often rears its ugly head.

Besides partisan alignment, successful reform efforts often need a consistent and common frame (or theme). For example, the consistent use of the personal responsibility/private long-term care insurance frame under the Republican Bush administration led to the 2005 Deficit Reduction Act, which allows states to impose rules to restrict incorporating the middle class into Medicaid. In contrast, the social entitlement frame, if presented in a consistently united manner by the current Democratic Obama administration, could allow Medicaid to act as a stepping-stone to universal long-term care coverage. Unfortunately for reform advocates, such consistency is often difficult to maintain throughout the normal ebb and flow of budgetary politics, let alone through periods of significant financial crisis.

Notes

1. We use Rawls's (1971) phrase here.

2. One important exception to this stagnation theme is the expansion of prescription drug benefits under the Medicare Modernization Act of 2003. For more details, see Oberlander (2003a); Frakt, Pizer, and Hendricks (2008); and Sessions and Lee (2008).

3. Skocpol's essay was originally published in *The Urban Underclass*, edited by Christopher Jencks and Paul E. Peterson (Washington, D.C.: Brookings Institution, 1991).

4. This section draws heavily from two articles by Grogan and Patashnik (2003a, 2003b).

5. While unexpected, the adoption of both makes sense in hindsight, given the incentives of the key political actors at the time (for a further explanation, see Grogan and Patashnik, 2003a).

6. This bizarre fractional percentage to determine eligibility is a testament to Medicaid's complexity.

7. For more detail on these expansions, see Grogan and Patashnik (2003a).

8. For a book-length discussion that explains MCCA's passage and repeal, see Himmelfarb (1995).

9. This is taken from Kennelly's testimony and her prepared statement for the record, in which she responds to Chairman Waxman's questions and concerns about her bill.

10. The executive director of the Kaiser Commission on the Future of Medicaid.

11. The Alzheimer Association's senior vice president for public policy.

12. Back in 1993, Congress mandated that states tap the estates of the deceased to recover Medicaid nursing home costs. While a few states still implement such programs with vigor, most simply refuse to follow the law. Two years later, Republicans proposed making adult children financially liable for their parents' nursing home expenses, a bill that was quickly dropped after a CBS/*New York Times* poll found that even 68 percent of conservatives were opposed to the idea. In 1996, an obscure provision buried in a health reform bill made it a federal crime for a person to dispose of assets to become eligible for Medicaid. Despite support among federal leaders, the "Send Grandma to Jail" law (as it was called by the press at the time) was rejected by the states and eventually overturned.

References

Benjamin, A. E., P. W. Newacheck, and H. Wolfe. 1991. Intergenerational equity and public spending. *Pediatrics* 88 (1): 75–83.

Brown, M. K. 1988. The segmented welfare state: Distributive conflict and retrenchment in the United States, 1968–1984. Pp. 182–210 in *Remaking the Welfare State: Retrenchment and Social Policy in America and Europe*. Philadelphia: Temple University Press.

Cohen, M. A., N. Kumar, and S. S. Wallack. 1993. Simulating the fiscal and distributional impacts of Medicaid eligibility reforms. *Health Care Financing Review* 14 (4): 133–50.

Congressional Research Service. 1993. *Medicaid Source Book: Background Data and Analysis (A 1993 Update)*. Washington, D.C.: U.S. Government Printing Office.

Cook, F. L., V. W. Marshall, J. G. Marshall, and J. E. Kaufman. 1994. The salience of intergenerational equity in Canada and the United States. Pp. 91–129 in T. R. Marmor, T. M. Smeeding, and V. L. Greene (eds.), *Economic Security and Intergenerational Justice: A Look at North America.* Washington, D.C.: Urban Institute.

Fein, S. 1998. The Kerr-Mills Act: Medical care for the indigent in Michigan, 1960–1965. *Journal of the History of Medicine* 53 (3): 285–316.

Frakt, A. B., S. D. Pizer, and A. M. Hendricks. 2008. Controlling prescription drug costs: Regulation and the role of interest groups in Medicare and the Veterans Health Administration. *Journal of Health Politics, Policy and Law* 33 (6): 1079–106.

Gilbert, N., ed. 2001. *Targeting Social Benefits: International Perspectives and Trends.* New Brunswick, N.J.: Transaction.

Grogan, C. M., and E. M. Patashnik. 2003a. Between welfare medicine and mainstream entitlement: Medicaid at the political crossroads. *Journal of Health Politics, Policy and Law* 28 (5): 821–58.

———. 2003b. Universalism within targeting: Nursing home care, the middle class, and the politics of the Medicaid program. *Social Service Review* 77 (1): 51–71.

Himmelfarb, R. 1995. *Catastrophic Politics: The Rise and Fall of the Medicare Catastrophic Coverage Act of 1988.* University Park: Pennsylvania State University Press.

Kaiser Commission on Medicaid and the Uninsured. 2006. *Deficit Reduction Act of 2005: Implications for Medicaid.* Washington, D.C.: Henry J. Kaiser Family Foundation.

Kuttner, R. 1988. Reaganism, liberalism, and the Democrats. Pp. 99–134 in S. Blumenthal and T. B. Edsall (eds.), *The Reagan Legacy.* New York: Pantheon.

Marmor, T. R. 1970. *The Politics of Medicare.* New York: Aldine.

Marmor, T. R., J. L. Mashaw, and P. L. Harvey. 1990. *America's Misunderstood Welfare State.* New York: Basic Books.

Oberlander, J. 2003a. Medicare and the politics of prescription drug pricing. *North Carolina Medical Journal* 64 (6): 303–4.

———. 2003b. *The Political Life of Medicare.* Chicago: University of Chicago Press.

Pierson, P., and M. Smith. 1994. Shifting fortunes of the elderly: The comparative politics of retrenchment. Pp. 21–59 in T. R. Marmor, T. M. Smeeding, and V. L. Greene (eds.), *Economic Security and Intergenerational Justice: A Look at North America.* Washington, D.C.: Urban Institute.

Quadagno, J. 1989. Generational equity and the politics of the welfare state. *Politics and Society* 17 (3): 353–76.

Rawls, J. 1971. *A Theory of Justice*. Cambridge, Mass.: Belknap Press of Harvard University Press.

Robert Wood Johnson Foundation. 2006. *Choosing Independence: A Summary of the Cash and Counseling Model of Self-Directed Personal Assistance Services*. www.rwjf.org/pr/product.jsp?id=15916/.

Rosenbaum, S. 1993. Medicaid expansions and access to health care. Pp. 45–82 in D. Rowland, J. Feder, and A. Salganicoff (eds.), *Medicaid Financing Crisis: Balancing Responsibilities, Priorities, and Dollars*. Washington, D.C.: AAAS Press.

Rosenberry, S. A. 1982. Social insurance, distributive criteria, and the welfare backlash: A comparative analysis. *British Journal of Political Science* 12 (4): 421–47.

Sardell, A. 1991. Child health policy in the U.S.: The paradox of consensus. Pp. 17–53 in L. D. Brown (ed.), *Health Policy and the Disadvantaged*. Durham, N.C.: Duke University Press.

Schneider, A. L., and H. Ingram. 1997. *Policy Design for Democracy*. Lawrence: University Press of Kansas.

Sessions, S., and P. Lee. 2008. A road map for universal coverage: Finding a pass through the financial mountains. *Journal of Health Politics, Policy and Law*. 33 (2): 155–97.

Skocpol, T. 1995. Targeting within universalism: Politically viable policies to combat poverty in the United States. Pp. 250–74 in T. Skocpol (ed.), *Social Policy in the United States*. Princeton, N.J.: Princeton University Press.

Stevens, R. B., and R. Stevens. 1974. *Welfare Medicine in America: A Case Study of Medicaid*. New York: Free Press.

Tanenbaum, S. J. 1995. Medicaid eligibility policy in the 1980s: Medical utilitarianism and the "deserving" poor. *Journal of Health Politics, Policy and Law* 20 (4): 533–53.

U.S. Congress. 1967. *Social Security Amendments of 1967, Part 3*. Committee on Finance. Hearings, Senate, 90th Cong., 1st sess., September 20–22 and 26. Washington, D.C.: U.S. Government Printing Office.

———. 1982. *Impact of Federal Budget Cuts on the Elderly, Seattle, Wash*. Subcommittee on Health and Long-Term Care of the Select Committee on Aging. Hearings, House of Representatives, 97th Cong., 1st sess., November 14, 1981. Committee Publication No. 97-327. Washington, D.C.: U.S. Government Printing Office.

———. 1988. *Medicare and Medicaid Catastrophic Protection*. Subcommittee on Health and the Environment of the Committee on Energy and Commerce. Hearings, House of Representatives, 100th Cong., 1st sess., Serial No. 100-74, May 21, 27, 28 and June 2, 1987. Washington, D.C.: U.S. Government Printing Office.

————. 1991. *Medicaid Budget Initiatives*. Subcommittee on Health and the Environment of the Committee on Energy and Commerce. Hearings, House of Representatives, 101st Cong., 2nd sess., Serial No. 101-206, September 10 and 14, 1990. Washington, D.C.: U.S. Government Printing Office.

————. 1992. *Medicaid Program Investigation, Part 1*. Subcommittee on Oversight and Investigations of the Committee on Energy and Commerce. Hearings, House of Representatives, 102nd Cong., 1st sess., Serial No. 102-91, June 20, July 18, and October 2, 1991. Washington, D.C.: U.S. Government Printing Office.

————. 1996. *Transformation of the Medicaid Program, Part 3*. Subcommittee on Health and the Environment of the Committee on Commerce. Hearings, House of Representatives, 104th Cong., 1st sess., Serial No. 104-108, July 26 and August 1, 1995. Washington, D.C.: U.S. Government Printing Office.

————. 2005. *Long-Term Care and Medicaid: Spiraling Costs and the Need for Reform*. Subcommittee on Health of the Committee on Energy and Commerce. Hearings, House of Representatives, 109th Cong., 1st sess., Serial No. 109-24, April 27, 2005. Washington, D.C.: U.S. Government Printing Office.

U.S. Newswire. 1995. Remarks to representatives of senior citizens' organizations [President Bill Clinton speech]. (Sept. 15).

14. The Older Americans Act and the Aging Services Network

Robert B. Hudson, Ph.D.

Older Americans today are offered a broad range of community-based services through a network of federal, state, and substate regional agencies largely created through the Older Americans Act of 1965 (OAA). While the magnitude of the OAA programs pales in comparison with the other major aging-related enactments of that year—Medicare and Medicaid—the aging services network has become an institutionalized presence in the human services delivery system throughout the nation. Today this network is made up of the Administration on Aging in Washington, D.C., 56 state and territorial Agencies on Aging, and 655 substate Area Agencies on Aging, in addition to several thousand local service providers contracting with network agencies.

The birth and evolution of the aging services network is important for both policy and political reasons. Its financial support was long tied to funding under the OAA—which plateaued at roughly the $1 billion level[1] in the late 1980s and has risen only modestly since—and the network has struggled to address, much less meet, the encompassing set of policy objectives laid out in the act's Title I. Most challenging has been the imperative to at least nominally address the needs of all older Americans—no formal means-testing is allowed under the act—while targeting limited resources on populations of the old who are deemed to be especially vulnerable. Multiple and inconsistent mandates in the authorizing legislation have made realizing these divergent objectives more difficult yet. As a result, there has long been great variation in the strategies and successes among these several hundred individual agencies otherwise reified as a singular entity in the "aging network" parlance dating to the 1970s.

Yet despite limited resources and some ambiguity of purpose, network agencies have taken hold in most regions of the country. In a number of instances, they have become major players at the state and local levels in the design and implementation of home and community-based services (HCBS) for both seniors and, increasingly, younger adults with disabilities. An expanding number of state and area agencies are charged with community-based alternatives funded through Medicaid and state-only funding sources. Where the three major funding streams have come together, aging network agencies have become major players in the human services arena, a far cry from what they were in the immediate post-1965 years.

Viewed more broadly, the evolution of the OAA and the network reflects changing perceptions that public sector actors—governors, county commissioners, mayors—have had of the political presence and policy needs of older Americans. While the original OAA was as much about recognizing a legitimate and growing population as it was about service delivery, subsequent years found both the OAA and the network moving much more in a problem-resolution direction. This critical shift was a result of a variety of factors, most notably the growing numbers of the oldest segment of the older population and the enormous pressures building on state Medicaid programs to cover care costs associated with this very old population. Over a period of some four decades, the network experience captures a shifting perception of elders from a group be recognized, honored, and made comfortable in the community to one where the expenses of maintaining the safety, dignity, and autonomy of vulnerable elders must be weighed against the high budgetary costs of doing so. The network remains involved in both recognizing the contributions of the old and meeting their growing health-related needs, but, over time, the balance has shifted in the latter direction.

Early Developments

Important as the OAA has been in making social services available to older people, it was a relatively minor item among the myriad pieces of legislation enacted during the Great Society period of the 1960s. Without question, the major aging-related policy event of the time was the enactment of Medicare, the federal health insurance program for the elderly and for people with permanent disabilities. Yet had it not been for the struggle surrounding Medicare, the OAA probably would never have been passed. Many different individuals and organizations mobilized on behalf of Medicare's enactment, including quite a few whose interests extended beyond the world of acute health care. A variety of advocates wanted the federal government to recognize the presence and needs of older Americans in a broader and more symbolic way than Medicare alone could do.

Equally important, many professionals and providers of non-health-related services also wanted federal financial support for a range of interventions they were prepared to make on behalf of community-based elders. In a manner fully in keeping with Lowi's (1969) interest-group liberalism construct, many of those interests were ultimately recognized in specific provisions within the law. These included support for senior centers, transportation, nutrition, educational training, and research, among other endeavors. As is often the case with in-kind programs, it was advocates and services providers who were more active than seniors themselves in legislative testimony and lobbying (Binstock, 1972).

As a result of these twin pressures, the OAA was passed as a piece of legislation that served both to give formal recognition to the presence of older Americans in national life and to provide them with community-based services beyond those associated with health care alone. Title I of the OAA was clear on both of these points, stating that U.S. elders are entitled to the "full and free enjoyment" of an encompassing range of programmatic objectives, including an adequate income, the best possible physical and mental health, suitable housing, the opportunity for employment, retirement in health and honor, a full range of community services, and efficient community service, among several others (Section 3001).

Beyond the general language used in pursuit of these wider-ranging objectives, the principal operative language of the OAA centered principally on the organization and provision of social services for older people living in their homes in their communities. Title II established the Administration on Aging within the federal Department of Health, Education, and Welfare (which became the Department of Health and Human Services in 1977). The Title III community grant program was by far the most important of the original titles in the Act, providing federal matching funds to designated state units on aging (SUAs) to oversee the disbursement of funding to nonprofit social service providers. Title IV authorized a program of research, demonstration, and training grants, and the original Title V established an advisory committee on aging within the Department of Health, Education, and Welfare.

Although the scope of the legislation was broad, early funding under the OAA was extremely modest: $7.5 million in 1966 and $10.3 million in 1967. These dollars were barely sufficient to help the new state agencies get off the ground and to fund a few service efforts, many involving local senior centers. Indeed, there was talk in 1970 of eliminating the program because so little was being done (Sheppard, 1971).

Further difficulties arose in the early years because the mission of the OAA—and, in turn, of the network—was ambiguous as well as broad. The most obvious and straightforward charge was for the fledgling network agencies, using Title III funds, to contract with providers so that social, nutrition, transportation, legal, and other services could be provided to program clients. However, the volume of funding available in any given area was so modest that such services could barely begin to meet the levels of legitimate need. Thus amendments to the OAA in the late 1960s and early 1970s called for planning and advocacy activities wherein the network was charged with inducing major line departments—health, mental health, transportation, and criminal justice—to do more on behalf of older citizens, who were judged to be relatively under-served as well as in absolute need. These were very different mandates, and the former held distinct advantages for the nascent agencies, notably, that service outputs, however meager, could be easily measured and accounted for. That was certainly a more manageable task than that of asking these small agencies to go largely hat in hand to major state-level departments asking them to do more for their older citizens (Hudson, 1974). As a result, the network's early years were marked primarily by setting down roots and developing a constituency-oriented services network around older people.

However, events in 1971 led to a massive and unexpected increase in the size and scope of the OAA program. The precipitating event was a speech that President Richard Nixon gave to the White House Conference on Aging held that year (Pratt, 1976). The president was opposing a 20 percent increase in Social Security benefits being proposed by the Democrats, and to please his audience of 4,500 older Americans, he focused his attention on the small but appealingly named Older Americans Act. To everyone's surprise, he announced a fivefold increase in appropriations under the act, increasing the amount to $100 million. Thus, despite the president's opposing the much more expensive increase in Social Security benefits, the audience gave the president a standing ovation for these remarks, and the Older Americans Act—almost overnight—emerged as one of the nation's largest social services programs. A *Wall Street Journal* editorial at the time of the act's final passage captured the disdain critics attached to programs associated with the Great Society:

Santa Claus Lives on Capitol Hill

The Older Americans Act, pocket vetoed last fall, passed the Senate February 20 by a vote of 82 to 9 and passed the House this week by a vote of 329 to 69. The bill authorizes $1.55 billion over three years to do all kinds of wonderful things for Americans aged 45 and up, almost all of which involve employing social workers and such to provide "social services" and manpower training. A new bureaucratic empire would be spawned, along with a host of new boards, commissions, and advisory councils. Almost all the measures duplicate programs already being run by HEW, Labor, and other agencies. (*Wall Street Journal*, 1973)

The OAA programs continued to grow rapidly throughout the 1970s. The Area Agencies on Aging (AAAs) were established as a direct result of the president's decision and a broader new federalism agenda of the administration. In addition, a major new congregate nutrition program was enacted, a development that widened not only the network's programmatic mandate but also its political base—congregate nutrition sites became favorite campaign stops for candidates interested in wooing the senior vote. This combined programmatic and political momentum generated ever-increasing appropriations under the OAA during the 1970s, escalating to $919 million by 1980.

Consolidation Phase

Beyond making it possible to begin constructing service systems, expanded funding under the OAA played an important political role for the network as the 1980s and the presidency of Ronald Reagan dawned. In a manner later recalled by Arthur Flemming (U.S. Office of the Assistant Secretary on Aging, 1996), commissioner on aging during the Nixon years, the growing institutional presence of more than 600 local agencies was to provide the aging services network at all levels of government with an important grassroots political presence enjoyed by few other social welfare constituencies. Largely because of this rising political presence, the OAA and the aging services network remained essentially level-funded during the early Reagan years while other health, human service, and labor programs experienced significant program consolidation and budget cuts. Thus the Omnibus Budget and Reconciliation Act of 1981 (OBRA'81) consolidated 55 categorical grant programs into nine block grants and cut funding roughly 25 percent across the board: the Comprehensive Employment and Training Act was eliminated, 400,000 individuals were removed from the Aid to Families with Dependent Children (AFDC) rolls, food stamp funding was cut 14.3 percent, and subsidies for low- and moderate-income housing were cut by more than half (Jansson, 2005). In contrast, funding for the OAA's Title III program was cut by only 2.8 percent between 1981 and 1982, and by 1990 it had increased to $719 million.

Despite this relative success in preserving the OAA's funding base, it nonetheless remained the case that appropriations under the act remained far short of what would be required to meet the needs of older Americans across a range of enumerated concerns. In the 1980s and 1990s, the principal tension in debates about the OAA centered on how to avoid formal means-testing of would-be beneficiaries while concentrating resources on those who might appropriately be deemed to be in greatest need. O'Shaughnessy (1991) reviewed the shifting language about eligibility that was seen in successive reauthorizations during those years. The 1978 amendments called on state and area agencies to give preference to elders with "the greatest economic and social needs." The 1984 amendments further refined that phrase by requiring states to give special attention to low-income minority individuals and by defining low-income to mean below the official federal poverty line. In 1984 and 1987, emphasis was also placed on servicing "geographically isolated" individuals and rural residents.

The uncertainty associated with these shifting definitions was further exacerbated by basic questions of interpretation: how to determine economic need without means-testing; how to determine how many minority group members received services when various sources reported different percentages; and how to determine what being socially disadvantaged meant when that term might refer to older women, people over, say, age 70, or those who had trouble with daily activities. Beginning in the late 1980s, two mechanisms were introduced that were at least partially aimed at remedying these concerns (Justice, 1997). Program participants were encouraged to make voluntary contributions for services received so that more people might be served, and, after much debate, cost-sharing strategies were introduced for selected services (including homemaker, personal care, and adult day care services), based on self-declared income. However—again in keeping with the symbolic spirit of universality—services under the OAA would not be denied to individuals who refused to contribute or to cost-share (O'Shaughnessy, 2008).

These uneven steps toward focusing services on vulnerable members of the older population were accompanied by parallel efforts to narrow the breadth of the services which might be offered to them. No fewer than 18 supportive or direct services were enumerated in the original OAA legislation (Section 321a), and, in fact, the section concluded with a nineteenth item permitting "any other services" in keeping with the purposes of the program (Hudson, 1994). This listing was gradually narrowed over time, and in 1987 states were required to designate as priority service areas those addressing the access, in-home, and legal services needs of older people.

In yet another important development that extends very much up to the present day, there was a gradual shift in emphasis from the delivery of purely social services to those emphasizing health-related concerns. A number of factors have contributed to this shift. The aging of the population in general and, equally importantly, the aging of the older population itself made the health needs of older Americans ever more manifest. At the same time, both older people and their advocates were pressing for more community-based alternatives to institutional care for frail and disabled elders. Increasingly, state officials came to support these efforts, both for reasons of consumer preference and in the hope that community alternatives might rein in escalating Medicaid costs tied to long-term care for the elderly (Weissert, Cready, and Pawelak, 1989).

These three interrelated trends—targeting particular populations, narrowing the scope of services delivered, and addressing health-related concerns—represented both the emerging programmatic and the political realities associated with an aging United States (Hudson, 1994). The programmatic reality was that since limited OAA dollars could go only so far, concentrating those dollars on the most pressing needs of the most vulnerable elders was emerging as a nearly unavoidable imperative. By the end of the 1990s, this emerging emphasis for OAA and network activity was becoming increasingly more entrenched. In related veins, disease prevention programs were undertaken, nursing home ombudsman programs were expanded, and funding for the nutrition program continued to shift away from congregate sites to in-home meal delivery.

The political reappraisal of the OAA and the aging services network was equally profound and not unrelated. The dueling "constructions" in the OAA between elders as a population to be recognized and celebrated, and as a population whose growing needs must be concretely addressed, shifted in the latter direction. This was especially true at the state level, where Medicaid expenditures were rising, budgets had to be balanced, and competing interests—education, transportation, public safety, and economic development—were always in play. In contrasting federal and state perspectives on needs-based programs such as the OAA, Justice (1997, p. 175) observes: "At the state level, outcomes are more visible. Here, refusing to acknowledge the limits of available funding is less feasible, because the inability of one program to adequately serve its intended recipients places more demand on other related programs . . . Some argue that the real reason that states are more willing to set program eligibility criteria based on functional or financial need is that they are stingy—refusing to fund programs as generously as the federal government."

Contemporary Developments

The consolidation phase of the 1980s and 1990s has yielded to what might be termed a concentration phase over the past decade or so. State-level developments and amendments to the OAA have both pointed in the direction of heightened attention to the needs of chronically ill elders (and, in several states, to younger adults with disabilities) and to the development of coordinated funding and administrative structures designed to meet those growing needs. Yet this undeniable trend is juxtaposed against high levels of variability in both the capacities and the agendas of the multiple state and substate network agencies concerned about aging. The vagaries of federalism and funding have meant that the development of coordinated community-based service systems for the frail elderly remains highly uneven across the country.

Some states and regions have succeeded in building truly cohesive systems while, at the other extreme, there are agencies (often small and/or rural ones) where efforts remain reminiscent of the early years of the OAA and the network.

The Home and Community Based Care (HCBC) Drumbeat

A number of factors have continued to hasten the network's move into community-based long-term care. Simple demography is, of course, the underlying cause, with one in eight Americans now being aged 65 or older, and with individuals aged 85 or older being the fastest-growing age category in the population. Against this backdrop is the historical and more recent policy reality (Brody, 1987; Hudson, 1996) that long-term care provision has been a public policy orphan when contrasted with major achievements in the areas of income maintenance (through Social Security) and acute health care (through Medicare). That has left most publicly supported long-term care funding to the means-tested Medicaid program. Medicaid funds 49 percent of all long-term care services in the United States, with private sources (including out-of-pocket expenses paid by recipients) constituting 28 percent (Komisar and Thompson, 2007). It is against this background that a number of modest federal initiatives, as well as pressures from state-level actors, have found the aging services network agencies to be in a position to fill at least some of the policy void.

Since the early 1990s, a mix of legislative, judicial, and administrative actions have come from the federal level. In 1990, the Americans with Disabilities Act (ADA) was passed, prohibiting discrimination based on disability. An important Supreme Court decision in 1999—*Olmstead v. L.C.*—determined that, based on the ADA, the unnecessary segregation of individuals with disabilities into institutions may constitute discrimination based on disability and, in turn, may require states to provide community-based services rather than institutional placement. Where an individual preferred to live in a community setting and was judged to be qualified for community living, the state was to work toward moving that person into such a less-restrictive alternative. The Deficit Reduction Act of 2005 also furthered the development and consolidation of HCBC efforts in the states by allowing them to make such services part of their Medicaid state plans rather than having to continue pursuing the waiver process.

Amendments to the OAA further heightened concern with home and community-based services (HCBS) issues. In 2000, the Family Caregiver Support Act was added to Title III of the OAA, providing formal recognition (and limited funding) in support of the role that the informal care system plays in promoting community-based long-term care alternatives. The 2006 amendments to the OAA represent the Act's strongest recognition yet of the role that the network it spawned should play in long-term care. Provisions in this legislation addressed health promotion and disease prevention, support for streamlined access to long-term care services, and enhanced options for elders to remain in their communities. The term "modernization" was invoked for a number of interrelated initiatives in the 2006 amendments. One component, the Choices for Independence Initiative, consisted of activities to inform consumers about existing community care options, to support the "nursing home diversion modernization program," and to fund evidence-based disease prevention programs (O'Shaughnessy, 2008).

The network's emerging place in long-term care has also been promoted by administrative activity that has taken place within the Department of Health and Human Services involving the Administration on Aging (AoA), the Centers for Medicare and Medicaid Services (CMS), and the Office of the Assistant Secretary for Evaluation and Planning. CMS launched the Real Choice Systems Change Grants to support community-based services and help retain the direct care workforce (Browdie and Castora, 2008). In addition, the Bush administration's New Freedom Initiative, as it pertained to aging and disability services, allowed Medicaid funding to cover one-time costs (e.g., security deposits) to support community living. This effort was later formalized into the Money Follows the Person demonstration program, which joined yet another CMS initiative, the Cash and Counseling program, not only to promote community-based living for vulnerable adults but also to provide them with a central role in the design and implementation of their own individual care plans (Browdie, 2008). Finally, AoA and CMS have awarded funds to the states, based on a successful model from Wisconsin, to establish Aging and Disability Resource Centers (ADRC) to help adults of all ages make informed choices about their options. As of 2008, 143 ADRC pilot programs had been established in 43 states (O'Shaughnessy, 2008).

State-initiated actions involving SUAs and AAAs in the administration and funding of community-based services have perhaps been even more notable than the wave of federal-level initiatives. These efforts involved both *state-only money* as well as funding that has been available through the Medicaid program since OBRA'81. By the late 1980s, state-only appropriations totaled $586 million, with Pennsylvania ($154 million), Massachusetts ($105 million), and Illinois ($70 million) being the leaders (U.S. General Accounting Office, 1991). By 2002, these state-level appropriations had grown considerably (Summer and Ihara, 2004), amounting to $1.4 billion nationwide and involving 45 states, with California contributing the highest amount ($324 million), followed by Pennsylvania ($218 million), Illinois ($213 million), and Massachusetts ($150 million). Today, most states have state-only funding for HCBC services and, according to a 2004 survey conducted by the SUAs' trade association, the National Association of State Units on Aging (NASUA), the SUAs also administer these programs in 32 states for individuals under 60 years of age.

Nonetheless, Medicaid has emerged as a deeper source of funding support, both because of its size (Medicaid long-term care spending totaled $95 billion in 2005) and open-ended funding (the federal government is obligated to reimburse the states for between 50% and 78% of their Medicaid expenditures). Dating to its passage in 1965, Medicaid's long-term care expenditures had been overwhelmingly directed toward nursing home care; as recently as 1994, such institutional care still comprised 81 percent of Medicaid's long-term care funding. For at least 30 years, however, there have been persistent efforts on the part of aging and disability advocates (in the name of supporting community residency) and budget officials (in the name of cost savings) to shift expenditures in the direction of community placement. These rebalancing efforts have met with considerable success, despite resistance from institutional providers and their legislative allies; allocations for HCBC had risen to comprise 41 percent of Medicaid long-term care expenditures by 2006 (Kaiser Commission on Medicaid and the Uninsured, 2009).

Importantly, the network has found itself well-placed to administer these community-based initiatives in a growing number of states. The 2004 NASUA survey found that 33 states were designated as the operating agencies for the Medicaid HCBC waiver programs. Moreover, in 21 of these states the SUAs administered the programs for both the elderly and younger individuals with disabilities (NASUA, 2004, cited in O'Shaughnessy, 2008). This is due in part to there literally being such a network, and in part to Medicaid being a quasi-insurance financing mechanism that is primarily in the business of paying providers for services rendered to Medicaid-eligible clients—therefore, it possesses no natural administrative arm. Medicaid has traditionally been in the business of reimbursing mainstream providers—hospitals, clinics, nursing homes, and medical suppliers—but it is not designed to shape the delivery of health care services. In the case of community-based care, where recipients are scattered and numerous localized direct-care providers—nurse, home health, and personal care aides—are involved, some administrative oversight arrangement is very much in need. In theory, and increasingly in practice, the aging services network is well positioned to take on that role.

The Network's Ongoing Variability

Despite the network's move into the world of HCBC, there continues to be remarkable differences in the capacities and orientations of network agencies nationwide. In part, some degree of variation is to be expected from 56 state and territorial agencies, 655 area agencies, and 233 tribal and Native American organizations, to say nothing of some 30,000 service contractors. Yet research reported by Kunkel and Lackmeyer (2008) makes clear just how enormous these variations are among just the Area Agencies on Aging. The average AAA budget is $8.9 million but the median is only $3.8 million, with the range being between $150,000 and $250 million. Similarly, the average number of client served is 8,607, but the median is only 3,020 and the range falls between 91 and 128,945. Finally, the average number of full-time AAA employees is 20, but the median number is only 6, and, again, the range is enormous, being between 1 and 650. Kunkel and Lackmeyer (speak indirectly to how misleading it may be to have reified these hundreds of agencies into one "network" when they refer to an adage among directors that "if you've seen one area agency, you've seen one area agency" [p. 20]).

There also continues to be a major tripartite division in the network agencies' organizational structures. Roughly one-half of the SUAs are located in state health or human services agencies, with the remainder being independent departments or commissions within state government (O'Shaughnessy, 2008). Of the area agencies, 41 percent are private nonprofit agencies, 32 percent are part of county government, another 25 percent were units with Councils of Government, and 2 percent were Indian tribes or other entities (Burns et al., 2006). Ironically, organizational variability even pertains to the U.S. Administration on Aging, which has moved in and out of several units within the Department of Health and Human Services (DHHS) over the years and whose head, after years of pressure from advocates, was elevated to the rank of Assistant Secretary from Commissioner in the early 1990s.

Beyond structural variations, network agencies are invariably pulled in multiple directions, depending on political vagaries that are to be found in their catchment areas. In the early years, the SUAs (and later the AAAs) were heavily dependent on OAA funding, it being the largest source of SUA funding in 28 states in 1986 (U.S. General Accounting Office, 1991). Moreover, the prevailing model of federal grants-in-aid (GIAs) to the states was highly categorical (i.e., federal law and regulations were directive and state programs operating under those GIAs had relatively little latitude). As the network agencies matured, they found increasing levels of political and monetary support in their respective environments, as shown by increases in state-only appropriations and by their growing role in Medicaid-funded HCBC programs. At the same time, various incarnations of new federalism loosened the federal reins, with planning and decision-making models becoming more decentralized. Always subject to at least three masters—AoA officials in Washington, D.C., state or area officials, and citizen input through formal public hearing processes—network agencies found themselves increasingly under the sway of state and local imperatives.

In locales where state leadership in both the executive office and within the SUAs has moved network agencies into the long-term care and Medicaid arenas, the state-level "aging network" has emerged as an influential force. Yet in other jurisdictions, the HCBC emphasis has been less notable. OAA funding represents 42 percent of the funding for AAAs nationwide, yet there remain some AAAs that get 90 percent or even 100 percent of their funding from that one source. Because OAA dollars available to any given SUA or AAA are relatively modest, and because there are numerous programmatic mandates for the use of those scarce dollars, network agencies that have not chosen or not been able to avail themselves of state-only or Medicaid dollars have remained as marginal players in HCBC. Richard Browdie, a long-time participant in and analyst of network developments, notes the need to "lift the floor" of network agencies. He observes that those network agencies which have done well in the past are those that continue to do so today, but those that have lagged are also those who tend to remain behind.

Conclusion

Both the Older Americans Act and the aging services network have expanded and matured in ways that would have been hard to imagine in the 1960s. Originally largely political symbols and programmatic afterthoughts, together this law and many of these agencies have emerged as significant players in the policy world of aging in the United States. Yet for all this growth and maturation, the demographic and budgetary environments in which they are operating have, if anything, expanded more rapidly than they have. The principal challenge now, as it has been for at least the past quarter-century, is to what degree efforts will be concentrated in the world of home and community-based care (where the OAA and many network agencies remain relatively minor players) and to what degree agencies will work to assure themselves a place in the wider community for older people (defined in terms more holistic than what their chronic care needs may be).

On balance, the principal successes of the aging services network appear to lie in its having committed itself to serving the most vulnerable clients among the old (and, more recently, many younger adults with disabilities). In the present period, this might appear to be little more than manifest destiny for agencies dedicated to the well-being of older Americans. As indicated, however, this was far from always being the case, with pressures and preferences in many areas pointing toward celebrating the accomplishments of relatively healthy elders and creating interesting opportunities for those individuals in the community. It was not until well into the 1980s that the network balance clearly tipped in favor of keeping fragile elders in the community and out of institutions, as well as away from activities associated with senior centers, recreation, and community-involvement. An ongoing tension between congregate and in-home meal providers around the allocation of the $350 million in Title III nutrition money—the largest budget item in Title III—serves as a reminder that this debate is not completely resolved. A more recent contribution to this dilemma has been the growing level of interest in involving seniors in civic engagement, educational, and volunteer activities, demonstrating once again that these individuals should be understood as contributing members to society, not just as the recipients of expensive care services in their later years (Wilson and Simson, 2006; Kahana and Force, 2008).

It nonetheless remains the case that both many in the aging services network and officials in the Department of Health and Human Services and the Administration on Aging in Washington are committed to the OAA and the network having a central place in community-based long-term care. Here, the challenge is one of magnitude and leverage. Where state and area agencies have been able to play a key role, it is not because of the availability of OAA dollars, which, being allocated on a population basis, remain modest and relatively constant. Rather, it is because there is no other obvious administrative apparatus to deliver this set of services and because governors, commissioners, and mayors have needed to get a handle on the issue. Older people and their families are demanding community-based alternatives, and the costs associated with institutional placements are high and growing. Aggressive leadership within the network has worked to turn this challenge into an opportunity for many agencies, and there is evidence that a large number of them have undertaken this role with a high degree of success (O'Shaughnessy, 2008)

The variations in organizational capacity among network agencies will not, however, go away, at least in the near term. Over time, OAA dollars have become an increasingly minor item in the coffers of network agencies, and the language in state and area plans required under the OAA remains broad and permissive. The signals from Washington point in the right direction for home and community-based care (HCBC), but it is the state and area-level commitment of authority and of Medicaid and state-only resources that will allow the aging services network to have a meaningful role. This, however, is happening, and it is not unreasonable to hope that in the future a combination of increasing service demand and determined leadership will leave fewer and fewer agencies behind.

Notes

1. This chapter does not address Title V of the Older Americans Act, the Community Service Employment for Older Americans program, which is administered through the Department of Labor and for which appropriations in FY 2008 were $522 million.

References

Binstock, R. H. 1972. Interest group liberalism and the politics of aging. *Gerontologist* 12 (3, part 1): 265–80.

Brody, S. 1987. Strategic planning: The catastrophic approach. *Gerontologist* 27 (1): 13–38.

Browdie, R., and M. Castora. 2008. The aging network: State of the states. *Public Policy and Aging Report* 18 (3): 26–29.

Burns, F., et al. 2006. Survey of Area Agencies on Aging: Preliminary Results. Presented at the Annual Conference of the National Association of Area Agencies on Aging, August 6–10, Chicago, Ill.

Hudson, R. B. 1974. Rational planning and organizational imperatives: Prospects for area planning in aging. *Annals of the American Academy of Political and Social Science* 415 (1): 41–54.

———. 1994. The Older Americans Act and the defederalization of community-based care. Pp. 45–75 in P. Kim (ed.), *Services to the Aging and Aged*. New York: Garland.

———. 1996. Social protection and services. Pp. 446–66 in R. H. Binstock and L. K. George (eds.), *Handbook of Aging and the Social Sciences*, 4th ed. New York: Academic Press.

Jansson, B. 2005. *The Reluctant Welfare State*, 5th ed. Belmont, Calif.: Thomson Brooks/Cole.

Justice, D. 1997. The aging network: A balancing act between universal coverage and defined eligibility. Pp. 168–77 in R. B. Hudson (ed.), *The Future of Age-Based Public Policy*. Baltimore: Johns Hopkins University Press.

Kahana, J., and L. T. Force. 2008. Toward inclusion: A public-centered approach to promote civic engagement by the elderly. *Public Policy and Aging Report* 18 (3): 30–35.

Kaiser Commission on Medicaid and the Uninsured. 2009. *Medicaid and Long-Term Care Services and Supports*. Washington, D.C.: Henry J. Kaiser Family Foundation.

Komisar, H. L., and L. S. Thompson, 2007. *National Spending for Long-Term Care*. Washington, D.C.: Health Policy Institute, Georgetown University.

Kunkel, S. R., and A. Lackmeyer. 2008. Evolution of the aging network: Modernization and long-term care initiatives. *Public Policy and Aging Report* 18 (3): 19–25.

Lowi, T. J. 1969. *The End of Liberalism*. Chicago: Norton.

O'Shaughnessy, C. 1991. *Targeting Services to Older Persons under Title III of the Older Americans Act*. Washington, D.C.: Congressional Research Service, Library of Congress.

————. 2008. The aging services network: Broad mandate and increasing responsibilities. *Public Policy and Aging Report* 18 (3): 1–18.

Pratt, H. J. 1976. *The Gray Lobby*. Chicago: University of Chicago Press.

Sheppard, H. 1971. *The Administration on Aging—or a Successor*. Report to the Special Committee on Aging, U.S. Senate, 92nd Cong., 1st sess. Washington, D.C.: U.S. Government Printing Office.

Summer, L. L., and E. Ihara. 2004. *State-Funded Home and Community-Based Service Programs for Older People*. Washington, D.C.: AARP Public Policy Institute.

U.S. General Accounting Office. 1991. *Administration on Aging: More Federal Action Needed to Promote Service Coordination for the Elderly*. Report No. GAO/HRD-91-45 (Apr.). Washington, D.C.: U.S. General Accounting Office.

U.S. Office of the Assistant Secretary on Aging. 1996. Arthur Flemming, videotape interview with the author, Washington, D.C., October 4.

Wall Street Journal. 1973. Santa Claus lives on Capitol Hill. (Mar. 15).

Weissert, W. G., C. M. Cready, and J. E. Pawelak. 1989. The past and future of home and community-based long-term care. *Milbank Quarterly* 66 (2): 493–507.

Wilson, L., and S. Simson (eds.). 2006. *Civic Engagement and the Baby Boomer Generation*. Binghamton, N.Y.: Haworth Press.

15. New Challenges and Growing Trends in Senior Housing

Jon Pynoos, Ph.D., Caroline Cicero, M.P.L., and Christy M. Nishita, Ph.D.

Federal housing programs created in the 1960s and 1970s face undeniable new challenges, such as the aging of baby boomers and the increasing number of very old persons. With the increasing size and needs of the aging population, there is still a demand and purpose for senior housing. Policy now provides for supportive housing that meets the requirements of frail older adults, and the growing policy trend is toward moving long-term care out of nursing homes and assisted living facilities and into aging people's homes. Increasing long-term care and health care costs, as well as innovative design trends, broaden the previous senior housing criterion of "age plus need" beyond supportive housing to address how aging-friendly communities can accommodate their residents' health care, transportation, service, social, and self-care needs as their abilities change.

New trends in living arrangements, life expectancies, and the definition of special-needs groups require flexibility in thinking about senior housing models, funding sources, and eligibility requirements. Future housing policy will, of necessity, emphasize aging in place. Toward that end, it will decrease the separation between housing and long-term care / health care, accentuate public/private partnership models, and require the implementation of new design guidelines that meet the needs of people of all ages and abilities.

The History of Senior Housing

In the first half of the twentieth century, older people were seen both as financially needy and as desirable tenants, and therefore in need of housing assistance. When older people became eligible for public housing in the late 1950s, projects were oriented to active, healthy elderly people. At that time, the federal government had a bricks-and-mortar approach to housing policy: housing and services were treated as separate domains, each with its own set of policies, programs, regulations, and funding sources (Pynoos, 1992). While housing projects included some special features for older people, such as emergency call buttons, few services were tied to the complexes. The services that were provided had to be paid for through nonhousing sources. The primary roles of the manager were caring for the property and collecting rent.

In 1959, Section 202, a special housing program for elderly and disabled persons, was created as part of the National Housing Act, further indicating that there was a need for elderly-specific housing. Now, fifty years later, the program provides capital advances and project-based rental assistance to nonprofit sponsors for the development of supportive housing projects. The original designers of the program did not want Section 202 housing to function as nursing homes or even as homes for the aged. Consequently, buildings were developed for ambulatory, independent older persons, although several features to prevent accidents, such as grab bars and emergency call buttons, were included. In addition, space for services and common activities was allowed. Typically, 5 to 10 percent of the units were made accessible for persons with disabilities. Services such as meals, however, were not standard. When they were offered, residents or project sponsors were responsible for paying for the meals. In the case of services such as home care, they must be provided by outside agencies. This arrangement distinguishes senior housing from most assisted living.

Critics raised serious concerns about the impact of senior housing; they contended that segregated living arrangements would isolate the old from the rest of society. Social contacts and the formation of friendships would be restricted to those in the housing complex. Older persons would be unable to share their experiences with younger persons, ultimately resulting in low morale and feelings of uselessness (Golant, 1987). Critics predicted that seniors with severe physical and mental impairments would not be able to leave their residential units. Even proponents were concerned that senior housing would lead to isolation, depression, and ghettoization. There was tremendous relief when early studies indicated that, in fact, the opposite was true (Carp, 1987). The majority of older persons had numerous links to social networks outside their buildings through clubs and organizations, visits from families and friends, and communication by phone and mail. For the most part, older residents were highly satisfied with their new housing. The new communities promoted friendship, activities, and support. Living among same-aged peers offered opportunities for understanding and support with common age-related issues such as poor health or retirement (Golant, 1987). Age-segregated housing also provided higher levels of security against crime than had many of the residents' former homes and apartments.

Residents in Section 202 housing pay no more than 30 percent of their income in rent and have their own private apartments. The U.S. Department of Housing and Urban Development's (HUD) Section 202 program has built approximately 270,000 units available for older persons, with another 60,000—built between 1965 and 1992— that were designated for younger disabled residents (Government Accountability Office, 2005). After 1992, HUD's Section 811 program funded disabled units. The 202 program is an undeniable benefit to those seniors who secure units. Fifteen percent of older renters nationwide pay less than 20 percent of their income in rent. However, the fact that there are ten people on the waiting list for every one Section 202 unit is reflected in the fact that there are still 53 percent of older renters who pay 30 percent or more of their income for housing (American Community Survey, Table B25072, 2007). Moreover, Section 202 housing sponsors are challenged to meet the changing needs of an increasing number of frail older residents who have aged in place. HUD has funded service coordinators to help such residents in many buildings obtain supportive services from outside community agencies, but a gap exists between what is needed and adequate funding for services.

Legislation Sanctioning Senior Housing

Some citizen groups have lobbied against housing for older people because it has kept out younger families with children, who also have a great need for affordable rental housing that does not exceed 30 percent of their income. This issue came to a head with the contentious passage of the Fair Housing Amendments Act (FHAA) of 1988. The FHAA prohibits discrimination in housing but makes an exception for senior housing, with certain stipulations. It precludes discrimination in the sale or rental of housing based on familial status; property owners cannot prevent occupancy by families with children. The FHAA also follows Title VIII of the Civil Rights Act of 1968, which prohibits discrimination in the sale, rental, or financing of dwellings based on color, religion, sex, or national origin. The FHAA expands this law to prohibit discrimination based on disability. The term it uses, *handicap*, is defined as "a physical or mental impairment which substantially limits one or more such person's major life activities; a record of having such an impairment; or being regarded as having such an impairment" (*Federal Register*, 54 (13): 3245). This rule applies to all types of dwellings, including apartments, condominiums, cooperatives, and mobile homes.

At the same time, the FHAA grants a nondiscriminatory exemption if senior housing meets certain requirements. It allows for elderly-only housing, owing to the special health and social needs of older adults. This exemption in the FHAA was the result of long and laborious negotiations in Congress. Advocates for older adults insisted that some housing should be reserved to accommodate many older adults' preferences for an age-homogenous environment, as well as for their special needs (Morales, 1990). The result was that landlords may qualify for senior housing if one of three conditions are met: (1) the housing is subsidized and is specifically designed and operated for older people; (2) all residents are 63 years of age or older; or (3) 80 percent of the households have at least one person who is 55 years of age or older. Along with the third condition, the housing must also provide "significant facilities and services specifically designed to meet the physical or social needs of older persons" (42 U.S.C. § 3607 (b)(2)(C)(i)). The third circumstance is used most often by landlords because of its lower age limitation and greater flexibility in requiring that only 80 percent of the households meet this requirement.

Nevertheless, there has been much confusion because neither the statute nor the regulations define what constitutes "significant facilities and services." The statute merely states that these amenities must be "specifically designed to meet the physical or social needs of older persons." Such amenities include social and recreational programs, continuing education, information and counseling, homemaker services, an accessible physical environment, emergency and preventative health care programs, congregate dining facilities, and transportation. However, the regulations then state that the "housing facility need not have all those features to qualify for the exemption" (24 C.F.R. §11.304 (b)(1)). Overall, the housing provider must demonstrate that the structure and its amenities have been designed, constructed, or adapted to meet the particular needs of older persons. The "significant facilities and services requirement" is based on the premise that older persons tend to have health problems to a greater degree than younger persons and that older persons have more leisure time than younger persons. Disability advocates disputed the broad and vague regulations surrounding the "significant facilities and services" requirement, as managers could claim to operate "senior housing" without providing the needed supportive services to older residents.

A similar contentious battle occurred around housing younger persons with disabilities in Section 202 federally subsidized housing complexes for older Americans. In the late 1980s and early 1990s, an expansion of the definition of "handicapped" led to an increasing number of younger persons with mental disabilities and substance abuse problems moving into these housing projects, partly because of limited housing options. By 1993, approximately 50 percent of the public housing projects for older Americans contained younger persons with disabilities. The *mixed housing* issue rose to prominence on the federal government's agenda due to three factors: media accounts of disturbances in public housing; public housing managers' reports of problems; and government studies suggesting difficulties integrating these two populations (Pynoos and Parrott, 1996). Advocates representing elderly persons fought to preserve age-specific housing, while persons who have disabilities fought to maintain entry into these housing projects. Ultimately, it was a victory for elderly Americans, because the Housing and Community Development Act of 1992 permitted Public Housing Authorities the option of designating public housing sites as elderly-only, disabled-only, or mixed housing.

Despite the successes of the federal Section 202 program in providing affordable shelter for hundreds of thousands of low-income seniors, most older people do not live in elderly rental housing, whether subsidized or market rate. Approximately 4 million out of 112.5 million total U.S. households are headed by renters aged 65+, and 18 million households are owned by older adults. Of the oldest old, aged 85+, there are more than twice as many homeowners as renters (American Community Survey, Table B25007, 2007).

In addition, more than 10 million older adults live alone—27 percent of all older Americans. Thirty-four percent of all older females live alone, as do 17 percent of all older men. One-fifth of all older adults are females living alone. For those older people who do not live alone, 65 percent live in family households, 30 percent live in nonfamily households, and 5 percent live in group quarters (American Community Survey, Table B09017, 2007).

The Section 202 program is a project-based model, whereby the housing subsidy is attached to the unit. Low-income older renters have another option, however, that can allow them to age in place in approved market-rate rental units. With HUD Section 8 Tenant-Based Housing Choice Vouchers, the housing subsidy follows the resident, so that older residents have the potential to use their vouchers to rent an apartment of their own choosing. Approximately 340,000 older renters use Section 8 vouchers, which are dispensed to Public Housing Authorities by region (McCarty, 2008).

A Shift in Senior Housing Policy: Is Aging in Place the Right Policy?

Undoubtedly, supplying affordable rental housing is an important federal and local policy for that segment of the elderly population who live in substandard housing units, including very low-income owners (Golant, 2008). However, the majority of older residents are homeowners. For older persons whose housing is not deficient and who desire to age in place, federal policy toward housing for elderly people must continue to shift its focus and direct its resources toward long-term residents and the homes in which they have aged in place (Pynoos et al., 2008).

Eight percent of U.S. homeowners, in 6 million housing units, have lived in their houses for 40+ years, and another 9 percent have lived in their homes for 30–39 years. In contrast, just 2.5 percent of renters have lived in their same units for at least 30 years (American Community Survey, Table B25038, 2007). Older people form attachments over the years in which they live in their homes that contribute to their desire to stay in them until they die (Saegart, 1985; Brown and Perkins, 1992; Bayer and Harper, 2000; Wilhelmson et al., 2005). Aging in place is thus the appropriate policy, because it is the lived experience of most older persons.

How Will Older People's Health Care Needs Be Met if They Age in Place?

Current approaches to meeting older people's health care needs if they age in place emphasize elasticity in the conventional housing stock, particularly in terms of its ability to accommodate a wide spectrum of frail older persons and younger persons with disabilities. This trend has shifted long-term care policy toward community-based care. For example, early in the 1980s, Section 2176 of the Omnibus Budget Reconciliation Act allowed states to apply for Medicaid waivers that paid for nonmedical services for older adults who would otherwise face institutionalization (Pynoos and Redfoot, 1995). Maintaining older adults in the community is also well aligned with the *Olmstead* decision, issued by the Supreme Court in 1999, that requires states to administer programs and services to persons with disabilities in the "most integrated setting appropriate" to their needs. Because the states have borne the brunt of financial responsibility for long-term care through Medicaid, they have been more innovative than the federal government in their policies that bridge housing, aging in place, and the need for long-term care. In addition to their assisted-living Medicaid waiver programs, several states operate service-enriched supportive housing programs that also aim to rein in long-term Medicaid funding by limiting nursing home stays.

Federal housing policy necessitates coordination between the Administration on Aging and the Centers for Medicare and Medicaid Services (CMS) to meet the needs of U.S. elderly people who are aging in place in their own homes. Designating HUD funds for home repair or home maintenance programs is a step in the right direction, but it is inadequate to meet service and health care needs of older residents. With the Obama administration, congressional members who understand the needs of an aging society have been reconstructing previously dormant legislation that could fill the gaps in the continuum of care between independent living and skilled nursing. These bills, some of which would fund environmental assessments of elders' homes, aim to decrease Medicare expenditures and increase the home safety of older adults by targeting high-cost beneficiaries whose multiple chronic conditions put them at risk of institutionalization.

Aging in place takes place in a community context as well. Naturally Occurring Retirement Communities (NORCs) exist primarily because older persons' community ties to their neighborhoods motivate them to age in place alongside others in the same stage of life and/or because there are few other options they find appealing or affordable. The federal government has played a role in supporting these housing communities through the Older Americans Act's demonstration project funding, which has provided supportive services and case management. However, the vast majority of older people live in suburban homes that they own (American Community Survey, Tables B01003 and B25007, 2007). Suburban areas where large numbers of baby boomers are aging in residential communities of single-family homes have the potential to become NORCs. While 20 million older adults live in the suburbs of major U.S. metropolitan areas, twice as many baby boomers (40 million), soon to move into the category of retirees, live in the suburbs.

Long-term care that is person-centered rather than institution-centered will focus on modifying the environments where older persons live and on coordinating long-term care services. The Money Follows the Person (MFP) rebalancing demonstration project is CMS's strategy to assist states in transitioning older persons out of institutional care and back into their communities. HUD is encouraging local housing authorities and state housing agencies to house these residents (Centers for Medicare and Medicaid Services, 2009). Innovative localities could look beyond transition housing for such persons in designated senior apartments and also initiate MFP programs in single-family homes.

Several strategies are promising in terms of making the single-family housing stock better fit the needs of an aging population. For example, home modifications to existing residential environments can make it safer and easier to carry out daily activities such as bathing, cooking, and climbing stairs. Modifications include grab bars, roll-in showers, handrails, ramps, and wheelchair-accessible kitchens. Increasing evidence suggests that home modifications have an important impact on the ability of chronically ill or disabled persons to live independently. Home modifications are also an important part of multifactorial interventions to prevent falls, including medical and environmental risk assessments, exercise, educational programming, and follow-ups (Gitlin et al., 2006).

Future Directions: Achieving Aging in Place

In the future, housing policy will need to emphasize aging in place. However, achieving this goal requires new approaches to providing suitable housing, financing long-term care, and blurring the lines between different levels on the continuum of care. In light of the aging of baby boomers, a recent emphasis has focused on the creation of more aging-friendly communities and environments that emphasize person-centered care. Ultimately, the goal of aging in place will require innovative new approaches and broader conceptualizations of supportive environments.

Visitability and Universal Design

To avoid the necessity of home modification and retrofitting, there is a movement to build elder-friendly, newly constructed homes with accessibility features already in place. Visitability and universal design provide housing that is beneficial not only to older persons, but also to persons of all ages, including those with disabilities. These design movements are part of the growing trend that recognizes the elasticity of the housing stock to support increasingly disabled residents.

Visitability is a small set of basic accessibility features that enable older adults and persons with disabilities to access the main level of single-family homes. The concept of visitability does not require a completely accessible house. This is important in the United States, because single-family housing and complexes with less than four units do not fall under the requirements of the 1988 Fair Housing Amendments Act (FHAA), which requires such features as accessible entrances, corridors wide enough for wheelchairs, and raised electrical outlets. The FHAA is intended to assist residents, friends, and relatives who are functionally impaired (as well as future residents) to get around the home, and it therefore represents a civil rights approach to housing usability. The four main features of visitability include a zero-step entrance, interior doors with a minimum width of 32 inches, an accessible route inside the house, and a half bathroom on the first floor (Nishita et al., 2007).

The visitability movement has been gaining momentum, as some local jurisdictions have been willing to speed up permit processing or even waive some of the building fees for developers adopting visitability in constructing new homes (Pynoos et al., 2008). By 2008, visitability codes had been adopted in nearly 60 cities and states. The great majority of the approximately 30,000 visitable homes built in conjunction with these codes resulted from mandatory rather than voluntary programs, and half of all visitable homes have been built in Pima County, Arizona—which includes Tucson, the second-largest city in the state (Maisel, Smith, and Steinfeld, 2008). Yet on the federal level, the Inclusive Home Design Act—legislating visitability—has not been passed. Consequently, there is a long way to go in increasing wide-spread access to and federal support of visitable single-family homes.

Universal design promotes homes that are accessible, adaptable, and usable by persons of all ages and abilities. It differs from visitability by applying to the entire home and including features such as counters of variable heights, lever door handles and faucets, easy-to-use switches, supportive bars in the bathroom and shower, features that accommodate different levels of sight, and bathrooms and kitchens designed to accommodate wheelchairs and walkers. Features of universal design, which, from a lifespan perspective, are more conducive to all users than standard design, apply not only to housing but also to public spaces and commercial properties.

Various barriers limit the spread of design features that expand a home's usability. Developing uniform standards for consumers with diverse health conditions and disabilities is challenging. Advocacy groups face opposition from builders who oppose legal directives out of (1) concern that the increased cost of accessibility features negatively affects the affordability of housing, (2) a reluctance to offering more features to homebuyers who do not request them, and (3) a general resistance to regulations. Developers prefer voluntary programs or incentives that waive building permit fees. Progress in this area therefore requires both an educated group of consumer advocates who are convinced enough about the benefits of universal design to take on the building industry and consumers themselves who request special design features (Pynoos et al., 2008).

Greater Attention to the Broader Environmental Context

In the future, meeting the needs of seniors will require reaching beyond the confines of individual houses or residential complexes and into the larger community. The Americans with Disabilities Act of 1990 brought attention to accessibility needs in the broader community. While age-specific housing has many benefits, including those associated with security and mutual support among residents, it may not be the setting of choice for most older people. New models of housing, such as Village Networks, senior cohousing, and intergenerational intentional communities, have been developed in recent years and promote elders' self-determination and empowerment in selecting their optimal living arrangements. These models for retirement comprise the new Aging in Community movement, whereas the European village model builds on older people's efforts to age in place in connection with neighbors (Cohen, 2009; Durrett, 2009).

The *village model* for senior housing is part of the recent Aging-Friendly Communities movement (Scharlach, 2008). These neighborhoods (which require mixed-use zoning designations from the local jurisdiction) co-locate housing, restaurants, retail shops, medical care, and community services, and they offer access to public transportation and walkable streets. Such neighborhoods are based on a traditional village design but are innovative in their technology and approach. The field of urban planning regards this same concept as Smart Growth (Cicero and Pynoos, 2008), and recent efforts to implement its features stem from environmental concerns over sprawl and transportation-induced air pollution. Environmentalists support the same tenets in their advocacy for greener and more sustainable cities and neighborhoods. Like universal design on a smaller scale, a policy that promotes elder-friendly communities is desirable for persons across all stages of the lifespan. Several design movements and planning trends are working toward the same goals on behalf of different constituents. If the makers of aging policy, city planners, housing developers, and environmental advocates work together across disciplines and agencies, their mutual goals can be realized for the benefit of current elders and future generations (Cicero and Pynoos, 2008).

Conclusion

Senior housing is no longer defined solely by age, but instead is increasingly focused on the special medical and social needs of frail elders. These needs include a preference for avoiding institutionalization and for bringing long-term care into the home, so their lifelong communities can be maintained. With the aging of baby boomers, and increased life expectancies in general, the impetus of senior housing is now on maintaining older adults in their homes despite physical limitations and environmental barriers. Home modifications and innovative original design features can mitigate the impact that the built environment has on elders. A shift in housing policy will require innovation on the part of the federal government, which funds seniors' medical care and social service programming. Continued and increased commitment will be required as well from state agencies that fund long-term care and simultaneously seek ways to minimize costs. Finally, this shift must be implemented by visionary local jurisdictions that oversee housing construction and rehabilitation, in addition to overall city and neighborhood design.

References

American Community Survey. 2007. Tables B01003, B09017, B25007, B25038, and B25072. www.factfinder.census.gov.

Bayer, A. H., and L. Harper. 2000. *Fixing to Stay: A National Survey on Housing and Home Modification Issues.* Washington, D.C.: AARP.

Brown, B. B., and D. D. Perkins. 1992. Disruptions in place attachment. Pp. 279–304 in I. Altman and S. M. Low (eds.), *Place Attachment.* New York: Plenum Press.

Carp, F. 1987. The impact of planned housing. Pp. 43–79 in V. Regnier and J. Pynoos (eds.), *Housing the Aged.* New York: Elsevier Science.

Centers for Medicare and Medicaid Services. 2009. Money Follows the Person grants. www.cms.hhs.gov/DeficitReductionAct/20_MFP.asp [retrieved April 8, 2009].

Cicero, C., and J. Pynoos. 2008. In the aging zone: How cities can be more elder friendly. *Aging Today* 29 (1): 7, 10.

Cohen, R. 2009. Aging in community. Pp. 75–82 in S. Marohn (ed.), *Audacious Aging.* Santa Rosa, Calif.: Elite Books.

Durrett, C. 2009. *The Senior Cohousing Handbook.* Gabriola Island, BC: New Society.

Gitlin, L. N., W. W. Hauck, L. Winter, M. P. Dennis, and R. Schulz. 2006. Effect of an in-home occupational and physical therapy intervention on reducing mortality in functionally vulnerable older people: Preliminary findings. *Journal of the American Geriatrics Society* 54 (6): 950–55.

Golant, S. M. 1987. In defense of age-segregated housing. Pp. 49–56 in J. A. Hancock (ed.), *Housing the Elderly.* New Brunswick, N.J.: Center for Urban Policy Research.

———. 2008. Low-income elderly homeowners in very old dwellings: The need for public policy debate. *Journal of Aging and Social Policy* 20 (1): 1–28.

Government Accountability Office. 2005. *Federal Housing Programs that Offer Assistance for the Elderly.* Report No. GAO-05-174 (February). Washington, D.C.: U.S. Government Accountability Office.

Maisel, J., E. Smith, and E. Steinfeld. 2008. *Increasing Home Access: Designing for Visitability.* Washington, D.C.: AARP Public Policy Institute.

McCarty, M. 2008. *An Overview of the Section 8 Housing Programs.* Congressional Research Service Report to Congress RL32284. Washington, D.C.: Congressional Research Service, Library of Congress.

Morales, J. 1990. Senior housing as a children's issue: New cases implement Fair Housing Amendments. *Youth Law News* 5 (Sept./Oct.): 1–9.

Newman, S. J., R. Struyk, P. Wright, and M. Rice. 1990. Overwhelming odds: Caregiving and the risk of institutionalization. *Journal of Gerontology* 45 (5): S173–83.

Nishita, C. M., P. S. Liebig, J. Pynoos, L. Perelman, and K. Spegal. 2007. Promoting basic accessibility in the home: Analyzing patterns of diffusion of visitability legislation. *Journal of Disability Policy Studies* 18 (1): 2–13.

Pynoos, J. 1992. Linking federally assisted housing with services for frail older people. *Journal of Aging and Social Policy* 4 (3–4): 157–77.

Pynoos, J., C. Nishita, C. Cicero, and R. Caraviello. 2008. Aging in place, housing, and the law. *University of Illinois Elder Law Journal* 16 (1): 77–107.

Pynoos, J., and T. Parrott. 1996. The politics of mixing older persons and younger persons with disabilities in federally assisted housing. *Gerontologist* 36 (4): 518–29.

Pynoos, J., and D. L. Redfoot. 1995. Housing frail elders in the United States. Pp. 187–210 in J. Pynoos and P. S. Liebig (eds.), *Housing Frail Elders: International Policies, Perspectives, and Prospects.* Baltimore: Johns Hopkins University Press.

Saegart, S. 1985. The role of housing in the experience of dwelling. Pp. 287–309 in I. Altman and C. M. Werner (eds.), *Home Environments.* New York: Plenum Press.

Scharlach, A. 2008. Good places to grow old: New realities for an older America. *Aging Today* 29 (1): 6, 8.

Wilhelmson, K., C. Andersson, M. Waern, and P. Allebeck. 2005. Elderly people's perspectives on quality of life. *Ageing and Society* 25: 585–600.

16. Taxation and the Elderly

Christopher Howard, Ph.D.

As a general rule, governments rely on two methods to promote the well-being of elderly citizens: transfers and taxes. Transfers usually attract more attention from scholars and policy makers, and understandably so. Income transfers, notably Social Security, are crucial to millions of senior citizens. In-kind transfers such as Medicare and Medicaid are equally important. The growth of these transfers is the main reason why poverty among elderly people dropped dramatically during the latter half of the twentieth century. These transfers also help reduce income inequality.

This chapter will examine the role that the second method, taxation, plays in the lives of elderly people. The focus will be on the national level, which means that income taxes and payroll taxes will take center stage.[1] As we shall see, U.S. tax policy has a significant impact on elderly people, but the exact nature of that impact varies. Some tax policies reduce poverty, or inequality, or both. The progressive rate structure of the individual income tax is a good example. Other tax policies have little effect on poverty and actually aggravate inequality among elderly people. Foremost among these are tax expenditures for retirement pensions, housing, capital gains, and dividends.

Income and Payroll Taxes

During their 60s, most Americans experience a remarkable transformation. Their ratio of taxes paid to benefits received changes, sometimes dramatically. Instead of paying taxes to support other people (e.g., the elderly, the disabled, or poor people), they start getting back more each year than they pay. Younger workers are now helping to subsidize their income and their medical care. Individuals can claim Social Security retirement benefits as early as age 62, and they are eligible for Medicare when they turn 65. On average, Americans retire from work at about age 63. This does not necessarily mean they stop working altogether or start receiving Social Security, but it does mean that their income and their taxes will usually fall. Other chapters in this volume analyze the benefit side of this transition; this chapter examines the tax side.

Tax burdens rise and fall with income. Over the course of a lifetime, taxes should therefore peak when individuals are in their 40s and 50s and decrease as they reach their 60s and 70s. According to the 2007 Current Population Survey, the median household income that year was approximately $50,000 for the entire nation. The highest earners were between the ages of 50 and 54 ($64,802). Median income declined to about $54,000 for people in their early 60s, and then dropped significantly for people between the ages of 65 and 69 ($40,296). The typical household over the age of 75 had an annual income of $23,230—less than half the national average.[2]

As incomes decline, so too do marginal tax rates, making the individual income tax one of the most progressive sources of revenue in the United States. The top bracket in 2008 was 35 percent, applied to taxable incomes greater than $357,700. The next two brackets were 33 and 28 percent, respectively. Incomes between $32,550 and $78,850 were taxed at a 25 percent rate. Given that the average income was roughly $50,000, we might think of this as the middle-class tax bracket. There is a 15 percent tax bracket for the poor, near-poor, and lower-middle class, and then a 10 percent bracket for the seriously poor (incomes under $8,000). Most Americans drop down at least one tax bracket as they transition from their peak earning years into retirement. The combination of less income and progressive tax rates usually means they pay less income tax as they grow older.

Income taxes are used to finance a wide range of government functions, from national defense to agricultural research. A significant fraction of this tax revenue is spent on antipoverty programs such as Medicaid, food stamps, public housing, and Supplemental Security Income (SSI). Thus income taxes help low-income Americans, including those who are elderly, pay for health care, food, and shelter. And, because most income taxes are paid by the affluent (Joint Committee on Taxation, 2007), these programs help reduce inequality as well.

Payroll taxes are deducted from workers' paychecks and are used to finance social insurance programs such as Social Security, Medicare, and disability insurance. The tax rate for Medicare is the same across all incomes. The financing of Social Security, the largest payroll tax, is regressive because income above a certain threshold ($102,000 in 2008) is not subject to taxation.[3] The effective payroll tax rate is therefore lower for more-affluent workers. For many Americans, especially those with below-average incomes, payroll taxes take a larger bite out of their paycheck than do income taxes. Of course, some people continue working past the formal age of retirement (i.e., when they become eligible for Social Security or private pension benefits). They may shift from full-time to part-time work with their current employer, or they may change jobs entirely. In 2007, one-fifth of all elderly individuals and one-third of elderly households earned income from employment (Purcell, 2008). Thus most older Americans pay less in payroll taxes than they did before they retired.

One tax that becomes more important as people age is the corporate income tax. Over half of all elderly Americans receive some income from assets. They draw down on their bank accounts, cash in various bonds, collect dividends from stocks and, in some cases, receive income from trusts or rental property (U.S. Social Security Administration, 2006; T. Fisher, 2007). Because certain types of asset income are subject to corporate income tax, holders of those assets are effectively taxed as well, albeit indirectly. The Congressional Budget Office estimated that the effective corporate income tax rate for elderly households was 6.4 percent in 2005, while the average rate for all U.S. households was 3.1 percent. Nevertheless, this difference wasn't enough to outweigh the decrease in individual income and payroll taxes to which elders are subject. The total effective federal tax rate on the elderly was 17.2 percent in 2005, compared with 20.5 percent for the entire population (Congressional Budget Office, 2007a).

Tax Expenditures

Tax policy does more than identify what can be taxed and at what rate. It also defines which individuals or activities are eligible for preferential treatment. The U.S. tax code is riddled with tax credits, tax deductions, special tax rates, deferrals of tax liabilities, and exemptions from taxation. These are the main reason why the effective tax rates paid by taxpayers are so much lower than the marginal rates.[4] All of these tax breaks are counted as *tax expenditures*. Tax expenditures are considered to be equivalent to direct expenditures because the government is deliberately distributing money to certain individuals or corporations. For example, as a matter of policy, the U.S. government supports charitable organizations. It accomplishes this goal directly by contracting with charities to provide important goods and services to needy citizens. But the government also offers indirect support by allowing taxpayers to deduct their charitable contributions from their taxable income. Government support is recorded as a *budget outlay* in the first instance and a *revenue loss* in the second. In theory, if the government eliminated the charitable tax deduction, it would then collect more tax revenue and could use that additional money to support charities directly (Joint Committee on Taxation, 2007).

Although many tax expenditures do benefit specific industries (hence the term *corporate welfare*), the biggest items and most of the money promote social policy objectives. As described below, various tax breaks for retirement pensions, medical care, housing, and income support cost the U.S. Treasury hundreds of billions of dollars each year in forgone revenues.[5] The United States spends as much on tax expenditures with social welfare objectives as it does on all traditional means-tested programs, such as Medicaid and food stamps. Compared to other wealthy democracies, the United States relies heavily on tax policy to make social policy (Howard, 2007). While few of these tax expenditures are aimed explicitly at elderly people, several of them do provide substantial help to older Americans.

Retirement Pensions

Tax expenditures for retirement pensions offer the most obvious support to elderly people, and the U.S. tax code extends favorable treatment to both public and private pensions. Most retirees, for example, do not pay income tax on their Social Security benefits. Most European countries, in contrast, do subject public benefits to taxation (Adema and Ladaique, 2005). The congressional Joint Committee on Taxation (2007) estimates that this tax expenditure cost the national government more than $20 billion in 2007.[6] Admittedly, this sum was small relative to the cost of Social Security. But that $20 billion was more than the government spent on Head Start and subsidized school lunches combined.

The larger tax subsidies are directed at employer pensions. Companies are allowed to deduct their contributions to pension plans when calculating their taxable corporate income. Workers defer paying taxes on the investment income until they retire, when most of them will be in a lower tax bracket. In 2007, the cost of this tax expenditure surpassed $100 billion, with this figure covering traditional defined-benefit pensions as well as newer 401(k) plans. There are additional tax breaks for individual retirement accounts ($15.5 billion) and for Keogh plans covering the self-employed ($8.8 billion). Altogether, the United States is not collecting more than $130 billion in tax revenues each year to support these pensions. Anyone who refers to them as "private" pensions is overlooking the extent to which they are underwritten with public monies. The impact of these tax expenditures is broad, considering that one-half of all workers currently participate in some type of tax-favored retirement plan, and one-third of all people aged 65 or older receive income from employer pensions (Congressional Budget Office, 2007b; Purcell, 2008).

Medical Care

The story for medical care is similar to retirement pensions. The smaller tax expenditures are linked to public programs. The U.S. government does not tax the cash value of Medicare benefits, generating tax expenditures of $40 billion in 2007. Given that most Medicare recipients are elderly, this provision is aimed squarely at them. There are also smaller (less than $5 billion) tax expenditures for medical care given to members of the military, their dependents, and veterans.

The larger tax expenditures underwrite benefits in the private sector. Companies can deduct their health insurance premiums from their taxable income, and that provision costs the government more than $100 billion a year in forgone revenue. This is projected to be one of the fastest-growing tax expenditures, increasing from $106 billion in 2007 to $145 billion in 2011. At that point, it will cost more than the tax expenditure for company pensions and more than anything related to housing (Joint Committee on Taxation, 2007). The government also offers tax breaks for the self-employed who buy health insurance ($4 billion) and for Health Savings Accounts ($0.3 billion).

These various tax breaks help elderly people to the extent that they carry private health insurance after they retire. Of those workers who had health insurance before they retired, and who retired at age 65 or later, only about one-third continued to be insured through their former employer during their first year of retirement (Johnson, 2007).[7] That insurance supplements their Medicare coverage. Because of their greater numbers and greater likelihood of having employer coverage, current workers are therefore the primary beneficiaries of this tax expenditure. Finally, individuals who incur significant out-of-pocket medical expenses may qualify for a separate tax expenditure ($8 billion). Elderly people are more likely to have such expenses than the nonelderly.

Housing

Anyone looking at the federal budget would conclude that housing is a low priority. Budget outlays for housing assistance totaled $40 billion in 2007, which was less than 2 percent of the entire budget (U.S. Office of Management and Budget, 2008). Most of this money went to rental housing for poor and near-poor people, such as Section 8 vouchers and public housing. But that is not the main way the U.S. government makes housing policy. The tax code is far more important. The home mortgage interest deduction, for example, cost the government almost $75 billion in 2007. It provided, on average, almost $2,000 in tax relief to more than 35 million homeowners. The tax deduction for property taxes paid on owner-occupied residences cost another $17 billion. People often sell their homes for more than they originally paid, producing a capital gain. The tax code allows them to exclude much of this gain from their taxable income, to the tune of $29 billion a year. Other, smaller tax breaks for those who build or finance rental housing and owner-occupied housing added another $6 billion (Joint Committee on Taxation, 2007). The sum of these tax expenditures was more than $125 billion, or three times what the government spent on housing through traditional outlays.

Such subsidies are important to elderly people. Homeownership varies directly with age. People over the age of 65 are almost twice as likely to be homeowners as those under 35.[8] Although we tend to think that elderly homeowners have paid off their mortgages, one-quarter of them have not, and that figure has been growing (Peterson, 2006; J. Fisher et al., 2007). These individuals may still benefit from the mortgage interest deduction, and all elderly homeowners may take advantage of the tax break for property taxes paid on their homes.

More importantly, homes are the single largest asset for most older Americans. Checking and savings accounts are the most commonly held financial assets, while vehicles and homes are the most common nonfinancial assets for Americans aged 65 or older. However, the value of the typical home is much greater than these other assets. More than 80 percent of elderly people owned their homes in 2004, and the median value of their residences was between $125,000 and $150,000. The median value of all their assets, financial and nonfinancial, was about $200,000 (Bucks, Kennickell, and Moore, 2006). Years and years of mortgage interest deductions, taken during their working years, thus helped elderly people build up substantial equity in their homes.

Once retired, "they see their homes—rather than savings accounts—as piggy banks that can be tapped through home equity loans or refinancing to provide ready cash" (Peterson, 2006). Reverse mortgages, available to people aged 62 or older, have also become popular in the United States. In effect, reverse mortgages allow senior citizens to stay in their homes and convert their home equity into an annuity. Alternatively, some elderly people may sell their homes, move into less-expensive quarters, and pocket the difference. However it is derived from their homes, this extra income can be used to supplement Social Security and cover everyday living expenses. It can also help elderly people meet more difficult challenges. The odds that older Americans will convert their homes into income are greater for those over the age of 75, for widows and widowers, and for people who have chronic illness or an acute health shock such as a stroke (Coile and Milligan, 2006). All of these situations can make it harder for elderly people to live independently, leading them to seek in-home assistance or nursing home care. Neither option is cheap, and nursing homes can be expensive. That is why home equity can be so important. In effect, tax expenditures for homeowners lie at the intersection of housing, health, and income support policies.

Income Support

Besides pensions, the government has other ways of enhancing the income of older Americans via the tax code. The most targeted measure is a tax credit for elderly or disabled people. It is relatively small, costing less than $2 billion annually (Joint Committee on Taxation,

2007). This provision is designed to benefit people of modest means. In 2007, the tax credit was available to individual taxpayers whose incomes were below $17,500, and to married couples filing jointly whose incomes were under $25,000, as long as they could prove they were over 65 or permanently and totally disabled.[9] This provision helps fight poverty among elderly people, albeit on a modest scale.

The Earned Income Tax Credit (EITC) is a much larger provision, designed to boost the incomes of poor and near-poor people. It costs the government $45 billion in forgone taxes and tax refunds (Joint Committee on Taxation, 2007), making it much larger than the classic welfare program, Temporary Assistance for Needy Families. Nevertheless, elderly people do not benefit much from the EITC. First, eligibility is tied to employment, and the majority of older Americans do not work. Second, the EITC is designed to channel most of the aid to families with dependent children. Along with the Child Tax Credit, the EITC serves as the U.S. equivalent of family allowances found in many European nations.

The biggest tax expenditures in this category, however, benefit those who receive stock dividends and realize capital gains. In 2007, reduced rates of tax on dividends and long-term capital gains cost the U.S. treasury $127 billion. The Joint Committee on Taxation (2007) estimates the cost of more than 170 tax expenditures, and this one was the single most expensive. Moreover, favorable tax treatment for dividends and capital gains has grown considerably in recent years (Joint Committee on Taxation, 1999, 2007), a direct result of the Bush administration's tax policies. For a minority of elderly people, this tax expenditure is important. Around one-quarter of elderly families own stock, with smaller fractions owning shares in mutual funds or trusts. The average cash value of each type of asset was close to $50,000 in 2004. Elderly people were somewhat more likely than the nonelderly to own such assets, and the average size of these assets for elderly people was also above the national average (Bucks, Kennickell, and Moore, 2006). Some of this wealth will later be distributed to heirs, and once again the tax code plays favorites. The exclusion of capital gains at death cost the U.S. Treasury an additional $52 billion.

Distribution of Burdens and Benefits

The distribution of tax burdens and tax breaks is, of course, every bit as important as their absolute size. One useful way of capturing these patterns is to examine effective tax rates—that is, how much people actually pay. Table 16.1 compares effective tax rates among various income groups, both for elderly people and for the nation as a whole. We begin with elderly people. In 2005, the total effective federal tax rate for the average elderly household (with no dependent children) was 17.2 percent. That figure included all individual income taxes, corporate income taxes, payroll taxes, and excise taxes. Yet that average concealed wide disparities. The lowest quintile of older Americans paid a tax rate of 3.0 percent and the middle quintile a rate of 6.5 percent, while the highest quintile paid 24.1 percent. The richest 1 percent of elderly people paid at a rate of 30.8 percent. Overall, the U.S. tax system is progressive from the perspective of older Americans (Congressional Budget Office, 2007a).

Certain taxes are more progressive than others. Individual and corporate income taxes rank at the top. The poorest one-fifth of elderly people essentially pay no income taxes. At the other end of the spectrum, the richest fifth of elderly people pay more than 20 percent of their income in taxes. Because income taxes are the main federal taxes paid by elderly people, progressivity here is enough to ensure progressivity overall. Payroll tax rates, in contrast, gradually rise with income and then decline as one moves from the fourth to the fifth income quintiles. The payroll tax rate for those in the upper 5 percent of elderly people is the same as for those in the second quintile. Excise taxes on items such as alcohol and tobacco are the least significant source of revenue. The average elderly household pays only 0.8 percent of their income for these taxes. Excise taxes are clearly regressive, with the largest bite taken out of the poorest elderly people (Congressional Budget Office, 2007a).

For all households, federal taxes are also progressive, though not quite to the same degree as for elderly people. To illustrate disparities in incomes, economists often report the ratio of high to low incomes, and we can do the same with effective tax rates. With incomes, higher ratios mean greater inequality; with tax rates, higher ratios mean more progressivity. The ratio of effective tax rates between the top and bottom quintiles was 8.03 for elderly people and 5.93 for the entire nation

Table 16.1 Effective Federal Tax Rates (in Percentages), 2005

Tax	Lowest quintile	Second quintile	Third quintile	Fourth quintile	Highest quintile	Top 5 percent	All quintiles
Elderly households							
Individual income	0.0	0.2	1.5	4.5	12.0	14.3	7.9
Corporate income	0.7	1.3	1.9	2.9	9.5	12.2	6.4
Payroll	0.5	1.4	2.0	2.5	2.1	1.4	2.1
Excise	1.8	1.3	1.1	1.0	0.5	0.4	0.8
Total	3.0	4.1	6.5	10.8	24.1	28.4	17.2
All households							
Individual income	−6.5	−1.0	3.0	6.0	14.1	17.6	9.0
Corporate income	0.4	0.5	0.7	1.0	4.9	7.4	3.1
Payroll	8.3	9.2	9.5	9.7	6.0	3.5	7.6
Excise	2.1	1.3	1.0	0.8	0.5	0.3	0.8
Total	4.3	9.9	14.2	17.4	25.5	28.9	20.5

Source: Data from the Congressional Budget Office, 2007a.
Note: Numbers may not add up to the totals, due to rounding.

in 2005 (table 16.1). Individual income taxes are more progressive for the nonelderly than for elderly people, largely because the Earned Income Tax Credit and the Child Tax Credit help eliminate income taxes and generate tax refunds for many working families with children. These gains are offset by payroll taxes, which are not progressive and are naturally larger for workers than retirees. Another way to measure the progressivity of the tax code is to ask what share of the total tax burden is borne by different income groups. In 2005, the richest one-fifth of all taxpayers paid more than two-thirds (68.7%) of all federal taxes, while the richest one-fifth of elderly people accounted for four-fifths (80.4%) of all federal taxes paid by elderly people (Congressional Budget Office, 2007a).[10] However, as we shall see, these individuals also receive a large share of tax expenditures.

For all incomes, the effective tax rates are lower than the marginal rates, and the difference between them is due mostly to tax expenditures. The poorest elderly people, for instance, pay no individual income taxes. The main reason is that their Social Security benefits are not taxed, and Social Security constitutes almost all of their income. These older Americans also benefit from the special tax credit for elderly people, discussed earlier.

As the income of elderly people rises, their sources of income change. Employer pensions, asset income, and earnings grow in importance, while Social Security diminishes. For the top quintile, Social Security represents less than a fifth of their income. Their combination of employer pensions and asset income is twice as large as Social Security benefits (U.S. Social Security Administration, 2006). Consequently, the more affluent elderly people rely on different tax expenditures from the less affluent. For one thing, their Social Security benefits probably will be subject to income taxation. But these individuals will reap significant savings from other, larger tax expenditures.

Half of all U.S. workers participate in some sort of tax-favored retirement plan. That could be a traditional defined-benefit pension, in which workers are guaranteed a certain amount each month when they retire. It could be a 401(k) plan or individual retirement account (IRA), in both of which the benefits are less certain. Yet no matter what form a pension takes, the beneficiaries are likely to be more affluent. Only 20 percent of workers earning less than $20,000 participate in these kinds of pension plans, compared with 80 percent of workers earning more than $80,000. Less-affluent workers are less likely to be employed by companies that offer pensions; and these workers have enough trouble making ends meet that they cannot afford to open an IRA. The skew is even worse for 401(k) plans, which have gradually been supplanting defined-benefit pensions across the corporate United States. Only 6 percent of workers earning less than $20,000 contribute money to a 401(k) account. In contrast, more than half of workers earning above $80,000 have this type of pension plan. Moreover, affluent workers are able to put more money into their pension accounts each year (Congressional Budget Office, 2007b). Through tax expenditures, the United States spends well over $100 billion each year to promote all these pensions. Most of that money helps individuals who lived comfortably during their working years and will continue to do so in retirement.

The sizable tax breaks for financial assets, such as dividends and capital gains, work in much the same way. According to the 2004 Survey of Consumer Finances, about one out of every five U.S. families owned stock independent of any retirement account. In the bottom quintile, the rate was one out of twenty families; in the top quintile, it was more than two out of five. Members of the top quintile were ten times more likely to have pooled investment funds (e.g., mutual funds) than were members of the lowest quintile (Bucks, Kennickell, and Moore, 2006). Older Americans who own such assets are unlikely to live anywhere near the poverty line. Once again, the biggest tax expenditures favor the well-to-do.

Tax breaks for housing would appear to be widely available, given that four-fifths of elderly people own a home. Not all of these homeowners, however, take advantage of the home mortgage interest deduction. If that amount of interest is not large enough to push the value of their itemized deductions beyond the value of the standard deduction, the mortgage interest deduction is irrelevant. The bigger one's mortgage, the more likely the interest deduction. So who has large mortgages? The more affluent Americans who live in more expensive homes. Almost three-fourths of the money spent on the home mortgage interest deduction went to taxpayers with at least $100,000 in income in 2006. Property taxes on homes can also be deducted, and these same people are the most likely to benefit. At the other end of the spectrum, individuals earning less than $50,000—who accounted for 60 percent of all tax returns—claimed less than 5 percent of the total home mortgage interest deduction (Joint Committee on Taxation, 2007).

U.S. housing policy, rooted in the tax code, is aimed at the privileged few. For example, if you are fortunate enough to qualify for the top quintile of income, earning more than $100,000, the government could help you buy a $500,000 home that carries a $400,000 mortgage. You will receive a hefty mortgage interest deduction for years. Over time, your house might appreciate in value until it reached $700,000 or more. Even if the home did nothing more than hold its value, the lucky owner will build up substantial equity by the time he or she retires. Moving into a smaller but still nice $300,000 condominium will be a possibility. As needed, these homeowners could convert that equity into cash for living expenses and medical bills. They could use that money to join exclusive golf clubs or travel abroad. Less-affluent retirees may also own their own homes, but they won't have as much equity, and they probably won't be able to downsize as easily. In short, U.S. housing policy means that the privileged few will have more options than most retirees, and their standard of living will be higher.

Students are often surprised to learn that inequality among elderly people is greater than inequality among the rest of the population. After all, they know that Social Security fights poverty and inequality, and that many elderly people rely heavily on Social Security. They know that practically all elderly people are covered by Medicare. How could inequality be worse? Well, over time, some older Americans have been able to accumulate substantial wealth through their homes or other assets, and they later converted that wealth into income. Those assets have been crucial in making a minority of retirees much better off than the typical senior citizen (Wolff, Zacharias, and Kum, 2007). Even though the tax code overall is progressive, both before and after retirement, certain tax expenditures foster inequalities that cumulate over decades and are evident among elderly people.

Politics

Taxation is often a site of partisan conflict in the United States (Witte, 1985; Bartels, 2008). The 2008 presidential campaign offered a vivid example, as Senators McCain and Obama clashed frequently over the size and distribution of the tax burden. McCain, the Republican nominee, wanted to cut taxes for everyone, with the largest benefits going to the more affluent. Obama, the Democrat, supported tax increases on the wealthiest 5 percent of Americans to provide tax cuts for the rest of the country. In effect, McCain wanted to continue the tax policies of the George W. Bush administration, which had long been opposed by many Democrats, while Obama proposed returning the tax code to its former shape under President Clinton. Compared with Democrats, Republicans believe that the overall tax burden should be smaller and the tax code less progressive.

With respect to the broad contours of tax policy, elderly people tend to be closer to the Democrats. Pollsters often ask whether people feel their income taxes are too high, too low, or about right. In 2006, 58 percent of all respondents to the General Social Survey said their taxes were too high, compared with 41 percent who said they were about right (almost no one said their taxes were too low).[11] Older Americans were not as troubled by income taxes; less than half of people aged

65 or older considered their taxes to be too high. Most of the elderly felt their taxes were about right. In contrast, 65 percent of Americans between the ages of 40 and 64 said their income taxes were too high, and only a third felt their taxes were about right. The difference in attitudes between these groups thus mirrors the differences in their tax burdens. It also makes sense, considering that individual income and payroll taxes, two of the most visible taxes, are much lower for retirees than for workers. Older Americans don't feel as taxed as they used to be. In addition, elderly people tend to support the principle of progressive taxation more than the nonelderly. Nonetheless, this finding does not mean that elderly people will usually vote Democratic, for many issues besides taxation matter to them.

Partisanship, however, does not pervade all aspects of tax policy. Democratic and Republican officials have been creating, expanding, and protecting tax expenditures for years. President Clinton worked hard to create tax breaks for education and expand the existing Earned Income Tax Credit. He teamed up with congressional Republicans to pass the Child Tax Credit. Clinton tried and failed to create a new tax credit for long-term care. President Obama continues to call for expanding the EITC and the child care tax credit and making tax breaks for homeowners more widely available. Tax expenditures have been particularly attractive to the New Democrats, who tried to move their party away from more direct forms of governmental intervention such as social insurance, grants, and regulation. On the Republican side, President Nixon pushed for a new tax expenditure for IRAs, and President Reagan spoke glowingly about the EITC as he expanded it. The 2008 Republican Party platform promised to protect tax breaks for homeowners and to expand health insurance coverage by modifying the tax code. Republicans have embraced tax expenditures in part because they create a bulwark against more direct forms of government involvement. If tax breaks help many companies offer health insurance to their workers, then the demand for national health insurance will be diminished. If the tax code encourages individuals and companies to contribute to retirement pensions, then calls to expand Social Security will be muted. Republicans have sought to help low-income Americans by expanding the EITC rather than welfare or the minimum wage (Howard, 1997, 2007).

Public opinion helps explain why tax expenditures have bipartisan appeal. On the one hand, most Americans want government to spend more on Social Security, health care, education, and aid to poor people. This generalization is certainly true of ordinary Democrats, and it even fits most Republicans (Page and Shapiro, 1992; Gilens, 1999; Howard, 2007). On the other hand, most Americans do not trust government very much (Hetherington, 2005). What are elected officials supposed to do when their constituents want key problems addressed but lack confidence in government's ability to act? They use tax expenditures. The government's main role is therefore limited to financing; the task of providing goods and services falls to individuals and corporations. Instead of building homes, the government helps people buy homes from private builders and lenders. Instead of providing health insurance directly, the government gives companies incentives to buy private insurance for their workers. Moreover, tax expenditures do not require a new government bureaucracy. These programs can be grafted onto the existing tax system through additional lines or schedules on tax forms. And for those constituents (mostly conservative) who didn't want government to address social problems in the first place, officials can always refer to tax expenditures as tax cuts (Howard, 1997, 2007).

Finally, by working with and through the private sector, tax expenditures pick up significant support from interest groups. Organizations representing home builders, realtors, lenders, and construction unions rally around various tax breaks for housing. That money helps keep them in business. Banks, mutual funds, and other financial institutions want to keep tax incentives for retirement pensions because those pension funds, representing hundreds of billions of dollars, can be invested with their firms. Associations of hotel and restaurant owners testify before Congress in favor of the Earned Income Tax Credit; the bigger the EITC, the less pressure those employers feel to boost the pay of their low-wage workers. While business interests are often opposed to a larger welfare state, they make an exception when that growth works to their benefit. By and large, the individuals who ultimately benefit from tax expenditures do not organize on behalf of these programs (Howard, 1997, 2007). This is quite different from the politics of Social Security and Medicare, in which AARP plays a central role (Campbell, 2003).

Conclusion

Tax policy does more than raise the revenues needed to finance spending programs. The distribution of tax burdens influences how much income inequality exists in society. And through tax expenditures, governments can indirectly spend money on a host of social problems by reducing taxes for those who help to solve these problems. In a sense, the Internal Revenue Service (IRS) is the most comprehensive welfare agency in Washington. IRS officials make housing policy, health policy, retirement policy, education policy, and family policy, in addition to their usual job of collecting taxes.[12]

Despite their diversity, older Americans can always find something to like in the tax code. The less-affluent members among them will appreciate the progressive rate structure of the individual income tax. They will be glad that their main source of income, Social Security, is tax free. More-affluent seniors will benefit from major tax expenditures affecting their homes, their pensions, and other financial assets. Those in the middle will pay little to no tax on their Social Security benefits, will receive some benefit from other tax expenditures, and will likely move into a lower tax bracket after they retire. Considering that older Americans are unusually active in politics, and are growing in numbers, we should not be surprised that elected officials have found ways to tailor the tax code that help as many of them as possible. Yet normatively, we still might ask why the government spends tens of billions of dollars each year to help affluent people, while many Americans continue to live below or near the poverty line.

Notes

1. To learn more about taxes at the state and local levels, see Applebaum et al. (2005); McNichol (2006); and Martin (2008). For example, local property taxes become relatively more important to elderly people as their incomes decline and the value of their property (e.g., their home) increases.

2. These figures come from the Current Population Survey's (CPS) *2007 Annual Social and Economic Supplement*, Table HINC-02, at http://pubdb3.census.gov/macro/032008/hhinc/new02_000.htm.

3. The threshold for income subject to Social Security taxes is adjusted each year for inflation.

4. For example, while the top individual income tax rates were 33 and 35 percent in 2005, the effective tax rate on the wealthiest fifth of the popu-

lation was less than 16 percent. The effective rate on the richest 5 percent of taxpayers was less than 20 percent that year (Congressional Budget Office, 2007a).

5. Altogether, "the total estimated revenue loss from individual tax expenditures was more than 7 percent of GDP in 2006, and more than three times the federal budget deficit" (Gist, 2007, p. 9).

6. The Joint Committee on Taxation reports untaxed Social Security and railroad retirement benefits as a single item. Together, they cost $22.4 billion. Because Social Security benefits are so much larger, the vast majority of this tax expenditure goes to Social Security recipients.

7. The trend, however, has been for fewer employers to offer health insurance coverage to their retired workers and to charge those retirees a larger monthly premium to retain coverage (Johnson, 2007).

8. The homeownership rate for age 65+ was 80.2 percent, compared with 41.2 percent for adults under the age of 35. These figures come from the U.S. Census Bureau's study of housing vacancies and ownership for the second quarter of 2008, Table 7, at www.census.gov/hhes/www/housing/hvs/qtr208/q208tab7.html.

9. For more information, see Internal Revenue Service Publication 524, *Credit for the Elderly or the Disabled*, at www.irs.gov/pub/irs-pdf/p524 .pdf.

10. Table 16.1 offers a snapshot, and we may also want to know about change over time. Since the late 1970s, the overall effective tax rate has fluctuated between 15 and 20 percent for senior citizens. There was no clear trend up or down. The overall tax rate in 2005 (17.2%) was about average for this period. The same variations can be observed in income, payroll, and excise taxes (Congressional Budget Office, 2007).

11. Author's calculations based on the General Social Survey at http://sda.berkeley.edu/.

12. Whether the IRS is well suited to make these policies and whether tax expenditures are effective in achieving their objectives are important topics that will have to be analyzed elsewhere. Suffice it to say that many analysts have serious reservations about these practices.

References

Adema, W., and M. Ladaique. 2005. *Net Social Expenditure, 2005 Edition: More Comprehensive Measures of Social Support*. Paris: Organisation for Economic Cooperation and Development.

Applebaum, R., S. P. Roman, M. Molea, and A. Burnett. 2005. Using local tax levies to fund programs for older people. Pp. 294–304 in R. B. Hudson (ed.), *The New Politics of Old Age Policy*. Baltimore: Johns Hopkins University Press.

Bartels, L. 2008. *Unequal Democracy: The Political Economy of the New Gilded Age*. Princeton, N.J.: Princeton University Press.

Bucks, B. K., A. B. Kennickell, and K. B. Moore. 2006. Recent changes in U.S. family finances: Evidence from the 2001 and 2004 Survey of Consumer Finances. *Federal Reserve Bulletin* 92 (Feb.): A1–38.

Campbell, A. L. 2003. *How Policies Make Citizens: Senior Political Activism and the American Welfare State*. Princeton, N.J.: Princeton University Press.

Coile, C. and K. Milligan. 2006. *What Happens to Household Portfolios after Retirement?* Issue Brief No. 56 (Nov.). Chestnut Hill, Mass.: Center for Retirement Research at Boston College. http://crr.bc.edu/briefs/ what_happens_to_household_portfolios_after_retirement_.html.

Congressional Budget Office. 2007a. *Historical Effective Federal Tax Rates, 1979 to 2005*. www.cbo.gov/ftpdocs/88xx/doc8885/12-11-His toricalTaxRates.pdf.

———. 2007b. *Utilization of Tax Incentives for Retirement Saving: Update to 2003*. Congressional Budget Office Background Paper. www.cbo .gov/ftpdocs/79xx/doc7980/03-30-TaxIncentives.pdf.

Fisher, J. D., D. S. Johnson, J. T. Marchand, T. M. Smeeding, and B. B. Torrey. 2007. No place like home: Older adults and their housing. *Journals of Gerontology, Series B: Social Sciences* 62 (2): S120–28.

Fisher, T. L. 2007. Estimates of unreported asset income in the Survey of Consumer Finances and the relative importance of Social Security benefits to the elderly. *Social Security Bulletin* 67 (2): 47–53.

Gilens, M. 1999. *Why Americans Hate Welfare*. Chicago: University of Chicago Press.

Gist, J. R. 2007. *Spending Entitlements and Tax Entitlements*. Washington, D.C.: AARP Public Policy Institute. http://assets.aarp.org/rgcenter/ econ/2007_10_benefits.pdf.

Hetherington, M. J. 2005. *Why Trust Matters: Declining Political Trust and the Demise of American Liberalism*. Princeton, N.J.: Princeton University Press.

Howard, C. 1997. *The Hidden Welfare State: Tax Expenditures and Social Policy in the United States*. Princeton, N.J.: Princeton University Press.

———. 2007. *The Welfare State Nobody Knows: Debunking Myths about U.S. Social Policy*. Princeton, N.J.: Princeton University Press.

Johnson, R. W. 2007. *What Happens to Health Benefits after Retirement?* Issue in Brief, Work Opportunities for Older Americans, Series 7 (Feb.). Chestnut Hill, Mass.: Center for Retirement Research at Boston College. http://crr.bc.edu/briefs/what_happens_to_health_benefits_after_retire ment__5.html.

Joint Committee on Taxation [of the U.S. Congress]. 1999. *Estimates of*

Federal Tax Expenditures for Fiscal Years 2000–2004. Washington, D.C.: U.S. Government Printing Office.

————. 2007. *Estimates of Federal Tax Expenditures for Fiscal Years 2007–2111.* Washington, D.C.: U.S. Government Printing Office.

Martin, I. W. 2008. *The Permanent Tax Revolt: How the Property Tax Transformed American Politics.* Stanford, Calif.: Stanford University Press.

McNichol, E. C. 2006. *Revisiting State Tax Preferences for Seniors.* Washington, D.C.: Center on Budget and Policy Priorities.

Page, B. I., and R. Y. Shapiro. 1992. *The Rational Voter: Fifty Years of Trends in Americans' Policy Preferences.* Chicago: University of Chicago Press.

Peterson, J. 2006. Fewer elderly paying off mortgages. *Los Angeles Times* (July 22), A1.

Purcell, P. 2008. *Income and Poverty among Older Americans in 2007.* Washington, D.C.: Congressional Research Service, Library of Congress.

U.S. Office of Management and Budget. 2008. *Historical Tables, Budget of the United States Government, Fiscal Year 2009.* Washington, D.C.: U.S. Government Printing Office. www.whitehouse.gov/omb/budget/fy2009/pdf/hist.pdf.

U.S. Social Security Administration. 2006. *Income of the Aged Chartbook, 2004.* www.ssa.gov/policy/docs/chartbooks/income_aged/.

Witte, J. E. 1985. *The Politics and Development of the Federal Income Tax.* Madison: University of Wisconsin Press.

Wolff, E. N., A. Zacharias, and H. Kim. 2007. *How Well Off Are America's Elderly? A New Perspective.* Levy Institute Measure of Economic Well-Being. Annandale-on-Hudson, N.Y.: Levy Economics Institute of Bard College. www.levy.org/pubs/lmw_apr_07.pdf.

17. Age Discrimination in Employment

Laurie A. McCann, J.D., and
Cathy Ventrell-Monsees, J.D.

Employment discrimination laws are premised on the concept that each individual has the right to be judged based on one's abilities, not on one's membership in a protected class. The Age Discrimination in Employment Act (ADEA), enacted in 1967, embodies not only this premise, but also the same purposes and prohibitions of Title VII of the Civil Rights Act of 1964.[1] However, more than 40 years after the ADEA's enactment, age discrimination continues to impede the achievement of equal treatment for older persons in the workplace.[2]

One possible explanation for ageism's perseverance may be that historically, society has perceived age discrimination as more of an economics issue than a question of fundamental civil rights. Beginning with the government report that first documented the problem of age discrimination in the United States, ageism has been viewed as different from and less serious than racism or sexism in the workplace. This perception has relegated the ADEA to second-class status among the country's civil rights statutes. In light of the aging of the workforce and the pervasiveness of age discrimination in the workplace in the twenty-first century, the question arises whether the ADEA can adequately address these challenges.

The Age Discrimination in Employment Act (ADEA): Legal and Legislative History

The ADEA was enacted during this country's civil rights movement in the 1960s. As part of the Civil Rights Act of 1964, Congress directed the Secretary of Labor to "make a full and complete study of the factors which might tend to result in discrimination in employment because of age and of the consequences of such discrimination on the economy and the individuals affected."[3] Secretary W. Willard Wirtz's report[4] confirmed that age discrimination in employment was a pervasive and debilitating problem and advised Congress that legislation was needed to deal with the problem.

Although the report eliminated any doubts for Congress concerning the gravity and magnitude of the age discrimination problem, Secretary Wirtz made another and more critical conclusion: age discrimination was fundamentally different from other forms of discrimination. Wirtz concluded: " 'Discrimination' means something very different, so far as employment practices involving age are concerned, from what it means in connection with discrimination involving—for example—race."[5]

According to Secretary Wirtz, in contrast to discrimination based on race, religion, color or national origin, age discrimination does not result from "dislike or intolerance" or from "feelings about people entirely unrelated to their ability to do the job."[6] He continued: "There are no such prejudices in American life which apply to older persons and which would carry over so strongly into the sphere of employment."[7] Wirtz went so far as to conclude that it was inconceivable that society would hold malice for a "minority group in which we all seek . . . eventual membership."[8] In sum, although older workers needed protection from discrimination, such discrimination originated from progress, not malice.[9] Consequently, Wirtz advised Congress that although it would be easy to extend the legislative solutions crafted for other forms of discrimination to age discrimination, it would also be wrong.[10] In a decision that would have lasting implications for the effectiveness of the ADEA in eliminating age discrimination, Congress enacted separate legislation instead of simply adding "age" to the protected categories under Title VII. Yet, at the same time, Congress copied Title VII's prohibitions verbatim[11] and inserted them into the ADEA.

From the ADEA's inception, Congress chose not to fully condemn ageism. The statute's reach was initially limited to employees aged 40 to 65, thereby continuing to permit mandatory retirement at arbitrary ages. In 1978, Congress raised the upper age limit to 70.[12] It was not until 1986 that Congress eliminated the ADEA's upper age limit to protect employees age 70 or older.[13] However, even after Congress eliminated mandatory retirement for most employees, it continued to allow mandatory retirement for large groups of employees, including

tenured faculty,[14] company executives, and public safety and law enforcement personnel. In short, the first twenty years of congressional
action against ageism, as reflected in the ADEA, demonstrate a reluctance to commit to the complete abolition of age discrimination in
employment.

Age Discrimination: Civil Rights or an Economic Issue?

Congress's lack of zeal for eliminating age discrimination altogether
was also evident during the passage of the Older Workers Benefit
Protection Act (OWBPA)[15] in 1990. The compromise and debate surrounding the OWBPA poignantly manifested recalcitrance to treat
freedom from age discrimination as a civil rights issue.

As originally drafted, the OWBPA was simple; it would have overturned the U.S. Supreme Court's decision in *Public Employees Retirement System of Ohio v. Betts*, 492 U.S. 158 (1989), which held that
the ADEA did not forbid an employer from discriminating based on
age when providing employee benefits, unless it was doing so to try to
force the older workers to retire. As Justice Thurgood Marshall noted
in his dissenting opinion, the *Betts* decision meant that older workers could be legally denied benefits based on only an employer's "ab-
ject hostility to, or his unfounded stereotypes" about older workers.[16]
However, after sixteen months of intense debate and compromise, a
number of exceptions had been carved out of the ADEA's prohibition
of age discrimination in employee benefits. The OWBPA's exceptions
legitimize age discrimination in the provision of certain common employee benefits, which the courts had uniformly condemned before the
Betts decision.

The debate surrounding the passage of the OWBPA made it obvious that the right of older employees' to receive benefits was viewed
not as a question of discrimination, civil rights, or equality, but as an
economic issue to be resolved by the minimal standards of the tax
code or employee benefits statutes. Indeed, one of the arguments pro-
pounded by the employer lobby in opposition to the OWBPA was that
the ADEA should permit employers to deny benefits based on age if
the practice was legal under the Employee Retirement Income Security
Act (ERISA). ERISA generally sets minimum standards for the provision of employee benefits. ERISA, however, was never designed to
prohibit age discrimination in employee benefits. The injustice of us-

ing ERISA's minimum standards as the benchmark for determining a violation of the ADEA was articulated by then-counsel for pensions of the U.S. House of Representatives Committee on Education of Labor, Phyllis Borzi. At the annual Certified Employee Benefits Specialists' symposium, she highlighted how absurd it would be to suggest that a pension plan could lawfully exclude all African Americans from a pension plan so long as it did not discriminate in favor of the highly paid—the ERISA standard—and yet that was precisely what was being suggested as the standard for age discrimination.

Unfortunately, older employees continue to be denied benefits that are an accepted part of overall compensation. For example, on July 14, 2003, the Equal Employment Opportunity Commission (EEOC) issued a proposed regulation that allows employers to reduce or terminate retiree health benefits to individuals aged 65 or older (eligibility for Medicare) without incurring liability under the ADEA.[17] A legal challenge to the regulation was unsuccessful,[18] and the regulation took effect on December 26, 2007.[19] In 2008, the U.S. Supreme Court ruled that a Kentucky state pension plan that provides more generous benefits to workers who become disabled before reaching the plan's normal retirement age than workers who become disabled after reaching normal retirement age does not discriminate on the basis of age.[20] This decision opens the door for employers not only to deny benefits to older workers on the grounds of their age-based eligibility for retirement benefits, but also to justify all kinds of policies that discriminate based on age. As the dissent explained, "if the ADEA allows an employer to tie disability benefits to an age-based pension status designation, that same designation can be used to determine wages, hours, health care benefits, reimbursements, job assignments, promotions, office space, transportation vouchers, parking privileges, and any other conceivable benefit or condition of employment."[21] Most recently, in *Gross v. FBL Financial Services, Inc.*, 129 S. Ct. 2343 (2009), the Supreme Court expressly widened the gulf between Title VII and the ADEA by imposing a significantly more onerous burden of proof on age discrimination victims than on other discrimination victims.

The Civil Rights Act of 1991

The Civil Rights Act of 1991 (CRA) significantly widened the gap between the treatment of age discrimination and other forms of discrimination. Of the seven U.S. Supreme Court decisions issued from 1989 to 1991 that the CRA overturned,[22] four affected the interpretation of the ADEA,[23] because traditionally courts have used Title VII case law to guide their analysis of the ADEA when the provision of the two statutes are similar. Congress overturned the Title VII decisions because they severely weakened the protection of fundamental civil rights. Yet those Supreme Court decisions live on for age discrimination victims because Congress failed to amend the ADEA to prevent the application of the decisions to cases under the ADEA. As a result, scores of ADEA cases have been lost, based on Title VII decisions that were overturned for race and gender discrimination victims.[24]

The CRA also neglected age discrimination victims by providing for compensatory and punitive damages awards under Title VII and the Americans with Disabilities Act, but not under the ADEA.[25] The emotional trauma and injury inflicted by discrimination can be as significant in a case of age harassment as it is in a sexual harassment case. Yet Congress's failure to provide for such damages in an age case implies that the older victim does not deserve a remedy. Most recently, however, the Lilly Ledbetter Fair Pay Act, which was enacted on January 29, 2009, to overturn a 2007 Title VII decision,[26] also amended the ADEA to ensure that age discrimination victims would not continue to face the unreasonable time limitations for filing a charge of pay discrimination that were established in the 2007 *Ledbetter* decision.

In sum, the assessment of age discrimination as less wrong or malevolent than other forms of discrimination influenced Congress to devise a separate statutory solution rather than include ageism as part of the civil rights legislation. And until the recent passage of the Lilly Ledbetter Fair Pay Act, other legislative efforts have exacerbated the segregation of age discrimination law by strengthening Title VII and ignoring the ADEA.

Congress's acceptance in the 1960s of the belief that age related to one's ability to work may be understood in the context of other age-based legislation such as Social Security and Medicare, which are premised on economic need and an inability to work after a certain age. But these premises clash with the central tenet of discrimination laws that requires a focus on an individual's unique talents, qualifications, and abilities, regardless of one's membership in a designated class. Congressional action in age discrimination legislation has failed to reconcile this clash, as Congress continues to permit certain types of age discrimination in employment and thus acknowledges that age may be relevant to performance at certain times in certain jobs.

Age as Not a "Suspect Classification"

The assessment of age bias as less serious or wrong than other forms of discrimination has also been embraced by federal and state courts from the trial court level to the U. S. Supreme Court. This judicial philosophy has been most evident in equal protection challenges to age-based employment provisions, where the Supreme Court has repeatedly held that age is not a "suspect classification" and thus unworthy of the highest level of protection under the Equal Protection Clause of the Fourteenth Amendment.[27] "A *suspect class* is one "saddled with such disabilities or subjected to such a history of purposeful unequal treatment, or relegated to such a position of political powerlessness as to command extraordinary protection from the majoritarian political process" (*Massachusetts Bd. of Retirement v. Murgia*, 427 U.S. 307, 312 (1976)). Classes recognized as suspect include race, nationality, and alienage. Gender classifications also are examined under a higher, intermediate level of scrutiny than are age classifications. The designation of a classification as suspect imposes a stringent burden on the entity to prove that the challenged classification serves a "compelling state interest" to survive an equal protection challenge. Because this burden is so difficult to meet, the use of suspect classifications are consistently struck down as violations of the Equal Protection Clause.

In stark contrast, the Supreme Court views age classifications under the least stringent test—the rational basis standard. Age classifications need only be rationally related to the furtherance of a legitimate state interest. As a result of this more lenient standard, arbitrary age discriminatory polices have received rubber-stamp approval. In *Massachusetts Bd. of Retirement v. Murgia*, 427 U.S. 307 (1976), a unanimous Supreme Court upheld a Massachusetts law that required all state police officers to retire at age 50, regardless of physical fitness. In *Vance v. Bradley*, 440 U.S. 93 (1979), the Supreme Court upheld a federal statute requiring federal foreign service officers to retire at age 60; and in *Gregory v. Ashcroft*, 501 U.S. 452 (1991), a state law calling for the mandatory retirement of state court judges at age 70 had no problem surviving rational basis review.

The Supreme Court's rationale for concluding that age classifications do not warrant the strict scrutiny standard of review is essentially the same logic that precluded age from being added to Title VII's protected classes. The Court stated: "While the treatment of the aged in this Nation has not been wholly free of discrimination, such persons, unlike, say, those who have been discriminated against on the basis of race or national origin, have not experienced a 'history of purposeful unequal treatment,' or been subjected to unique disabilities on the basis of stereotyped characteristics not truly indicative of their abilities . . . old age does not define a 'discrete and insular' group . . . in need of 'extraordinary protection from the majoritarian political process.'"[28] In sum, the courts have been consistently unsympathetic to constitutionally based claims of age discrimination, which may reflect their conviction that "ageism is not a vice, or at least not enough of an evil to warrant judicial intervention."[29]

The Place of Ageist Comments

Similarly, courts tend to easily reject ageist comments as evidence of age discrimination, instead characterizing the comments as stray remarks or colloquialisms. For example, in *Reeves v. Sanderson Plumbing Products, Inc.*,[30] several months before Mr. Reeves was fired, his supervisor told him he was so old that he "must have come over on the *Mayflower.*" Two months before firing Mr. Reeves, the same supervisor told him that he was "too damn old to do the job" when Reeves was having difficulty starting a machine. The U.S. Court of Appeals for the Fifth Circuit discounted these statements as not relevant evidence of discrimination because they "were not made in the direct context of Reeves' termination."[31]

Surprisingly, the U.S. Supreme Court has repeatedly and clearly rejected this extremely restrictive view of ageist comments as not being relevant evidence.[32] Yet courts continue to discount or ignore blatantly ageist comments. One of the most disturbing examples of this trend is a case challenging a reduction-in-force where the vice president in charge of layoff decisions had commented that "there comes a time when we have to make way for younger people." In debating the relevance of the statement to the age discrimination claim, the court began by noting that because the comment had been made a couple of years before the reduction-in-force, it could not be used as evidence.

But then the court went on to say that the statement "reflects no more than a fact of life and as such is merely a 'truism' that carries with it no disparaging undertones. Moreover, statements about age may well not carry the same animus as those about race or gender. Unlike race or gender differences, age does not create a true we/they situation—barring unfortunate events, everyone will enter the protected age group at some point in their lives . . . [The vice president's] remark should be seen for the non-actionable reflection on generational passage that it was."[33]

Numerous courts have favorably cited this decision and agreed with its premise. Yet the ADEA was enacted because Congress determined that there is *no time* when an older person must make way for a younger person in the workplace because of age. The premise of the ADEA is that each individual has the right to remain a productive member of society and to be judged based on his or her individual abilities and contributions to their profession and community, not on his or her age. Less-capable and less-productive workers may need to make way for more-capable and more-productive workers. But the ADEA makes it clear that older workers need not make way for younger workers simply because they are older.

The Legacy of the Wirtz Report

It has become accepted theory, relying on the 1965 Wirtz Report, that age discrimination is different from other forms of discrimination. The questions to ask more than 40 years later are whether Secretary Wirtz's conclusions were correct, or complete at the time, or stand true today. Wirtz concluded that race discrimination originated from prejudice, while age discrimination did not. That may be true, but the analysis and conclusions are incomplete. It is generally recognized that race discrimination derives from stereotypes as well as from malice and prejudice.[34] While there is no doubt that racism derived in part from malice, dislike, and intolerance in the 1960s, the Wirtz Report ignores the impact of racial stereotyping as one of the causes of race discrimination in employment. Yet there can be no question that whites in the 1960s viewed blacks as inferior and that racial stereotyping played an important role in discriminatory employment practices.

The Wirtz Report further disregards the inclusion of sex discrimination in Title VII, a form of discrimination that did not derive from malice or animus. Rather, sex discrimination in employment was premised in large part on the view that women were not physically, mentally, or emotionally able to do the job. Yet Congress enacted the same prohibitions and protections for women as they did for blacks in Title VII. The Wirtz report makes no mention of this disparity in reasoning. Both racism and sexism at that time were premised in part on stereotypes—an inability to work at the same standards as the favored group, just as ageism was premised on stereotypes.

The term *ageism* was coined by Robert N. Butler, M.D., to describe the "deep and profound prejudice against the elderly which is found to some degree in all of us."[35] Butler describes ageism as "a process of systematic stereotyping of and discrimination against people because they are old, just as racism and sexism accomplish this with skin color and gender . . . Ageism allows the younger generations to see older people as different from themselves; thus they subtly cease to identify with their elders as human beings."[36]

Ageism is an attitude—a negative evaluation—that serves to prejudicially orient individuals toward older persons as a group.[37] The consequence of this attitude is discrimination; people avoid interacting with older people, and they victimize older people or otherwise do injury to them based on their age alone.[38]

In the words of U.S. Congressman Claude Pepper, "ageism is as odious as racism or sexism."[39] Ageism, like racism, sexism, or ethnicity, segregates on the basis of a characteristic that the individual neither has chosen nor has the power to change.[40] Like African Americans and women, older Americans face discrimination because of inaccurate stereotypes that are ingrained in society as well as in the workplace.[41] Consequently, the theory that age discrimination should be treated differently from other forms of discrimination is fundamentally flawed.

Why Age Discrimination's Secondary Legal Status?

In light of the above, why is age discrimination more acceptable to our society than other forms of discrimination? Why does discrimination based on age not elicit the same level of outrage as discrimination based on gender?

One rationale is that because older persons encounter age discrimination for only part of their lives, age discrimination is not as wrong or injurious as race or sex discrimination. This argument, however, is logically flawed. After all, although a Hispanic individual does not become a member of a minority group until he immigrates to the United States, the discrimination directed against him in this country is no less wrong or debilitating. For the same reason, simply because individuals are old for only a portion of their lives does not mitigate the discrimination they do encounter in their later years.

Similarly, the inequity of age discrimination has been downplayed because—unlike race or gender—age is viewed as not immutable. This excuse for relegating the seriousness of age discrimination was summarized by age-discrimination scholar Howard Eglit: "A law which discriminates against blacks can never be eluded by its targets, nor will it ever harm whites. A law which makes an age distinction, however, need not victimize forever. It can be outgrown."[42]

The flaw in this argument is obvious. Benjamin Button aside, individuals can age in only one direction.[43] Consequently, although one can always surpass the *minimum* age at which one can drive a car or vote, one can never overcome a *maximum* age limitation. Specifically, "while aging is a process of change which is experienced by everyone, the attainment of 'old age'—the condition on which age discrimination is based—places an individual in a class to which he will always belong."[44] It has also been suggested that because certain benefits, such as Social Security and Medicare, accompany aging, age discrimination is not invidious. The availability of benefits intended to serve very different purposes cannot, however, compensate for the injury of discrimination.

Another purported justification for not treating the right to be free from age discrimination as a fundamental civil right is the perceived absence of a history of unequal treatment of older persons. One commentator summarized this argument as follows: "If we consider the history of black militancy, which is centuries old, or the struggle for women's rights which goes back to Seneca Falls (1848) and beyond—and if we consider what kinds of discrimination blacks and women have complained of, how pervasive they were or are, it is obvious that age discrimination is a social problem of a different order entirely."[45]

While the nature and history of ageism may not be identical to those of racism and sexism, they are more alike than different. First, Congress did acknowledge a historical basis for enacting protections against age discrimination in the 1965 Wirtz Report. Second, rather than looking backward for guidance in addressing the inequitable treatment of ageism in the workplace compared with the treatment of racism or sexism, a current look is in order, as the histories of race or sex discrimination provide inadequate guidance in dealing with the racism or sexism of this new century.

The United States has made tremendous strides in the treatment of minorities and women. Americans elected their first African American president, and women now increasingly hold positions of power in the corporate sector and in government. In contrast, Americans' negative attitude toward aging and older workers has not evolved in such a positive direction. In the 2008 presidential election, John McCain's age called into question his competence to be president. The United States is still a society in which young is good and old is bad.[46]

Finally, the distinction between age discrimination and other forms of discrimination continues to be rationalized on the basis that age discrimination is not the result of malice toward older persons. This argument falls flat when age and sex discrimination are compared. Sexism in the workplace is not the result of malice. Sexism is based on stereotypes concerning women's abilities and on assumptions about the appropriate role for women in our society.[47] While African Americans undoubtedly have been the victims of irrational malice, most experts agree that in the United States there has been a substantial reduction in racism based on such malice.[48] Race discrimination is increasingly based on unfounded stereotypes about minorities' abilities, as opposed to malice or dislike.[49]

The most common cause underlying ageism, sexism, and racism in the workplace is stereotyping. Research about age stereotypes demonstrates that most individuals harbor specific beliefs about older people, that most of those beliefs are inaccurate, and that the stereotypes have persisted in disadvantaging older persons for decades.[50] Numerous studies support the claim that ageism against older workers is common within society in general and particularly within the business community.[51]

The "Great Recession": A Perfect Storm for Age Discrimination?

Until the recent crisis in the U.S. economy, most of the discussion surrounding older workers had turned to how smart employers should take steps to hire and retain older workers to address looming labor and skills shortages. Circumstances, however, can and do change rather quickly. In the words of the Equal Employment Opportunity Commission's outgoing general counsel, Ronald Cooper, the aging demographics of the U.S. labor force, combined with the ever-worsening economic crisis, "create a perfect storm" for age discrimination to escalate.[52] Indeed, the excitement about the value of older workers is waning already. In a recent article about how, as a result of the market meltdowns, older workers would *need* to remain in the workforce, the author commented that "with pensions and retiree health benefits largely things of the past—and financial markets devastating 401(k)s —companies are at risk of losing their competitive edge if they become *storehouses of embittered older employees who put in only the minimum effort to keep their jobs*" (italics ours).[53] In the words of Dr. Robert Butler, "like racism and sexism, ageism remains recalcitrant, even if below the surface. But it can be—and has been—churned up from its latent position."[54]

Conclusion

Historically, Congress, the courts, and society have viewed age discrimination as less malevolent than race or sex discrimination and have treated freedom from ageism as something less than a civil right. In our society, "racism is taboo, and sexism may be following close behind. 'Ageism' still has a long way to go."[55] Stereotypes about age and ability persist, in part, because of society's failure to fully attack and condemn ageist policies and practices. Thus a comprehensive and concerted effort is needed to recognize that age discrimination is as debilitating to the individual and as harmful to society as other forms of discrimination. Most importantly, older workers, employers, and society must internalize and practice the premise of the ADEA—that individuals must be judged based on ability, not age.

The old explanations and rationalizations for the different views and treatment of ageism compared with other forms of discrimination are increasingly difficult to justify in this day and age. It is time for a twenty-first-century study of the causes and the victims of ageism in the workplace that reexamines the basic questions about age discrimination: Who is the older worker of the twenty-first century? Contrast her to the older worker studied by Secretary Wirtz in 1965, who was most likely a white male in his early 60s who spent his entire career at one company. That older worker is an anomaly today, if he even exists, in a workforce where most will work for many different employers in many different jobs and may change careers as well.

What does age discrimination in the workplace look like in the twenty-first century? In the 1960s, Congress was most concerned with employment policies and practices that explicitly denied workers jobs based on age. The greatest concern today is unconscious or implicit ageism in the workplace that has become so ingrained and automatic that supervisors are unaware it exists.[56]

Is ageism as prevalent a problem as racism or sexism in the workplace and in society? Studies show that unconscious ageism persists at much higher levels than unconscious racism or sexism.[57] Stereotyping based on age is more automatic, ingrained, and prevalent than racism or sexism. It is time for Congress and society to act with greater resolve to stop this tragic waste and loss of talent, energy, and wisdom.

Notes

1. 29 U.S.C. § 621(b) (1967). Congress enacted the ADEA "to promote the employment of older persons based on their ability rather than age; to prohibit arbitrary age discrimination in employment; to help employers and workers find ways of meeting problems arising from the impact of age on employment."

2. In fiscal year 2008, 24,582 charges of age discrimination were filed with the Equal Employment Opportunity Commission (EEOC), a sharp increase from the 19,103 charges that had been filed the year before and significantly higher than any figure for the previous 15 years. See www.eeoc.gov/stats/charges.html.

3. Section 715 of the Civil Rights Act of 1964, Pub. L. No. 88-352, 78 Stat. 241, 265 (1964).

4. Report of the Secretary of Labor, *The Older American Worker: Age Discrimination in Employment* (1965), reported in the EEOC's *Legislative History of the Age Discrimination in Employment Act of 1967* (1981) (hereinafter "Wirtz Report").

5. Wirtz Report at 2.

6. Id.

7. Id. at 6.

8. Id. at 3.

9. Id.

10. Id. at 1.

11. *Lorillard v. Pons*, 434 U.S. 575, 584 (1978).

12. The 1978 amendments also removed the age cap altogether for fed-

eral employees and established a right to jury trials. Age Discrimination in Employment Act Amendments of 1978, Pub. L. No. 95-256, 92 Stat. 189-93 (1978).

13. Age Discrimination in Employment Act Amendments of 1986, Pub. L. No. 99-592, § 2(c), 100 Stat. 3342 (1986).

14. The exemption that allowed for the mandatory retirement of tenured faculty at age 70 expired on December 31, 1993. Age Discrimination in Employment Act Amendments of 1986, Pub. L. No. 99-592, § 6(b), 100 Stat. 3342, 3344 (1986). It was subsequently replaced, however, in the 1998 reauthorization of the Higher Education Act by a safe harbor that allows institutions of higher education to offer age-based early retirement incentives to tenured faculty without violating the ADEA. 29 U.S.C. § 623(m) (1998).

15. Pub. L. No. 101-433, 104 Stat. 978 (1990).

16. *Public Employees Retirement System of Ohio v. Betts*, 492 U.S. at 182.

17. 68 Fed. Reg. 41542 (2003).

18. *AARP v. Equal Employment Opportunity Commission*, 489 F.3d 558 (3d Cir. 2007), *cert. denied*, 128 S. Ct. 1733 (2008).

19. 72 Fed. Reg. 72938 (2007).

20. *Kentucky Retirement Sys. v. Equal Employment Opportunity Commission*, 128 S. Ct. 2361 (2008).

21. Id. at 2376.

22. *Wards Cove Packing Co. v. Antonio*, 490 U.S. 642 (1989); *Patterson v. McLean Credit Union*, 491 U.S. 164 (1989); *Martin v. Wilks*, 490 U.S. 755 (1989); *Price Waterhouse v. Hopkins*, 490 U.S. 228 (1989); *Lorance v. AT&T Technologies, Inc.*, 490 U.S. 900 (1989); *West Virginia Univ. Hosp. v. Casey*, 499 U.S. 83 (1991); *EEOC v. Arabian American Oil Co.*, 499 U.S. 244 (1991).

23. *Wards Cove Packing Co. v. Antonio*, 490 U.S. 642 (1989) (disparate impact); *Price Waterhouse v. Hopkins*, 490 U.S. 228 (1989) (mixed-motive cases); *Lorance v. AT&T Technologies, Inc.*, 490 U.S. 900 (1989) (timeliness of claims); and *West Virginia Univ. Hosp. v. Casey*, 499 U.S. 83 (1991) (expert fees).

24. For example, in *EEOC v. City Colleges of Chicago*, 944 F.2d 339 (7th Cir. 1991), the holding in *Lorance v. AT&T Technologies, Inc.*, 490 U.S. 900 (1989), that a discriminatory plan or policy must be challenged within 300 days of its adoption regardless of when it actually applies to the victim, was applied to the ADEA to render a challenge to a discriminatory early retirement incentive plan untimely. For years, the fact that the CRA's clarification of the proper analysis of a disparate impact claim was not added to the text of the ADEA was viewed by courts as evidence that

Congress did not intend the theory to even apply to the ADEA. And, even after the Supreme Court declared in *Smith v. City of Jackson, Mississippi,* 544 U.S. 228 (2005) that age discrimination victims could use the theory, the employer-friendly analysis of the overturned *Wards Cove* Title VII decision was held to continue to apply to the ADEA. The Court's subsequent decision in *Meacham v. Knolls Atomic Power Laboratory,* 128 S. Ct. 2395 (2008), that employers bear the burden of proving that their actions were based on a "reasonable factor other than age," in disparate impact cases under the ADEA was an important victory. However, it is still significantly more difficult to prove disparate impact under the ADEA than under Title VII.

25. The ADEA's provision of double (liquidated) damages in cases of a willful violation of the law is no substitute, because it only doubles the amount of back pay and does not compensate for other types of injuries, such as the emotional toll and injury that age discrimination inflicts.

26. *Ledbetter v. Goodyear Tire & Rubber Co.,* 550 U.S. 618 (2007).

27. The Fourteenth Amendment to the U.S. Constitution commands that no state shall "deny to any person within its jurisdiction the equal protection of the laws." The issue in equal protection cases is whether a statute or practice that classifies groups differently violates this principle.

28. *Massachusetts v. Murgia,* 427 U.S. at 313, 314.

29. H. C. Eglit, *Age Discrimination,* 3 vols. (Colorado Springs, Colo.: Shepard's/McGraw-Hill, 1986), vol. 2, p. 40.

30. 530 U.S. 133, 151 (2000).

31. Id. at 152.

32. The Supreme Court in *Reeves* ruled that remarks are relevant evidence of age discrimination if their content indicates age animus and the speaker of the remarks was "primarily responsible" for the adverse action. Id. at 151.

33. *Birkbeck v. Marvel Lighting Corp.,* 30 F.3d 507, 512 (4th Cir. 1994).

34. J. Waller, *Face to Face: The Changing State of Racism across America* (Cambridge, Mass.: Da Capo Press, 2001), pp. 25, 33.

35. R. N. Butler, *Why Survive? Being Old in America* (Baltimore: Johns Hopkins University Press, 1975), p. 11. See also S. de Beauvoir, *Coming of Age* (New York: W.W. Norton, 1973).

36. Butler, p. 12.

37. J. Levin and W. C. Levin, *Ageism: Prejudice and Discrimination against the Elderly* (Belmont, Calif.: Wadsworth, 1980), p. 73.

38. Id. See also J. Levin, *The Functions of Prejudice* (New York: Harper & Row, 1975).

39. 123 Cong. Rec. 27, 121 (1977).

40. Eglit, vol. 3, pp. 1–4.

41. E. B. Palmore, *Ageism Negative and Positive*, 2nd ed. (New York: Springer, 1999), p. 98; C. R. Lawrence, III, "The Id, the Ego, and equal protection: Reckoning with unconscious racism," *Stanford Law Review* 39 (1987): 317, 330.

42. Eglit, vol. 2, p. 30.

43. Id.

44. Note, "Age discrimination in employment," *New York Law Review* 50 (1975): 930.

45. L. M. Friedman, *Your Time Will Come: The Law of Age Discrimination and Mandatory Retirement* (New York: Russell Sage Foundation, 1985), p. 12. This same reasoning was relied on by the Supreme Court in *Massachusetts v. Murgia*, 427 U.S. at 313, to uphold Massachusetts' mandatory retirement statute.

46. *General Dynamics Land Systems, Inc. v. Cline*, 540 U.S. 581, 591 (2004): "One commonplace conception of American society in recent decades is its character as a 'youth culture,' and in a world where younger is better."

47. See, for example, *Price Waterhouse v. Hopkins*, 490 U.S. 228, 250–52 (1989) (discussion concerning sex stereotyping). Sexist stereotyping continues to be severe, particularly for women managers and leaders. See Catalyst, Inc.'s research report, *Women "Take Care," Men "Take Charge": Stereotyping of U.S. Business Leaders Exposed* (Oct. 2005). www.catalyst .org.

48. E. B. Palmore, *Ageism: Negative and Positive*, 1st ed. (New York: Springer, 1990), p. 180.

49. L. Duke, "White's racial stereotypes persist: Most retain negative beliefs about minorities, survey finds," *Washington Post* (Jan. 9, 1991), p. A1.

50. Levin and Levin, pp. 70–96.

51. J. N. Lahey, *Do Older Workers Face Discrimination?* Issue in Brief No. 33 (Chestnut Hill, Mass.: Center for Retirement Research, Boston College, 2005); M. Bendick, Jr., L. E. Brown, and K. Wall, "No foot in the door: An experimental study of employment discrimination against older workers," *Journal of Aging and Social Policy* 10, no. 4 (1999): 5.

52. K. P. McGowan, "EEOC official sees age, disability bias as growth areas in Commission litigation," *Daily Labor Report* [Bureau of National Affairs] (Dec. 5, 2008), p. C-2.

53. J. Marquez, "Retirement out of reach," *Workforce Management* (Nov. 3, 2008): 1.

54. R. N. Butler, "Dispelling ageism: The cross-cutting intervention," *Annals* 503, No. 1 (1989): 138, 140.

55. Friedman, p. 64.

56. C. W. Perdue and M. B. Gurtman, "Evidence for the automaticity of ageism," *Journal of Experimental Social Psychology* 26, No. 3 (1990): 199, 200.

57. B. R. Levy, "Eradication of ageism requires addressing the enemy within," *Gerontologist* (Oct. 2001): 578. See also B. R. Levy and M. R. Banaji, "Implicit ageism," in T. D. Nelson (ed.), *Ageism: Stereotyping and Prejudice against Older Persons* (Cambridge, Mass.: MIT Press, 2004), pp. 54–55 (discussing research showing that antiage attitude is "among the largest negative implicit attitudes . . . observed").

Index